DI065157

GLOBAL PUBLIC HEALTH

Global Public Health

ECOLOGICAL FOUNDATIONS

Franklin White
Lorann Stallones
John Last

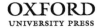

OXFORD
UNIVERSITY PRESS

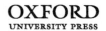

OXFORD
UNIVERSITY PRESS

Oxford University Press is a department of the University of Oxford.
It furthers the University's objective of excellence in research, scholarship,
and education by publishing worldwide.

Oxford   New York
Auckland   Cape Town   Dar es Salaam   Hong Kong   Karachi
Kuala Lumpur   Madrid   Melbourne   Mexico City   Nairobi
New Delhi   Shanghai   Taipei   Toronto

With offices in
Argentina   Austria   Brazil   Chile   Czech Republic   France   Greece
Guatemala   Hungary   Italy   Japan   Poland   Portugal   Singapore
South Korea   Switzerland   Thailand   Turkey   Ukraine   Vietnam

Oxford is a registered trade mark of Oxford University Press in the UK
and certain other countries.

Published in the United States of America by
Oxford University Press
198 Madison Avenue, New York, NY 10016

© Oxford University Press 2013

Library of Congress Cataloging-in-Publication Data
White, Franklin, 1946-
Global public health : ecological foundations / Franklin White, Lorann Stallones, John Last.
    p. ; cm.
Includes bibliographical references and index.
ISBN 978-0-19-975190-7 (hardback : alk. paper) — ISBN 978-0-19-987699-0 (ebook)
I. Stallones, Lorann.   II. Last, John M., 1926-   III. Title.
[DNLM: 1. World Health.   2. Ecological and Environmental Processes.   3. Public Health. WA 530.1]
362.1—dc23
2012032257

Contents

Preface

THE WORLD IS undergoing epic transformations and dramatic economic and political power shifts between and within countries. Some nations are experiencing exciting new stages of economic development, while others struggle to avert potential decline. People everywhere are striving to achieve social justice, improved living conditions, better health. Yet the prospects for future generations remain unclear and will depend on the actions of us now living. This is a critical time in the life of our planet. Will the economic systems fostered by today's decision makers prove sustainable? Will our planet be plundered or nurtured?

Will future generations inherit fair or unfair access to health and health care: health for all or only for a few? A key response to this is to ensure that we have well-grounded public health systems. An organized society seeks to promote, protect, improve, and restore the health of individuals, groups, and entire populations. Public health can be all of this: a vision, a discipline, an institution, and a practice. As a unifying enterprise, it offers many avenues through which practitioners may direct their energies. Combining social philosophy and values with scientific thought and advocacy, and working within the mandate received from society, practitioners formulate policies and actions and deliver these through programs, services, institutions, and related initiatives that emphasize health promotion and disease prevention.

A multidisciplinary field, public health encompasses diverse professional skill sets that range from epidemiology and the biomedical sciences to the social and behavioral sciences, nursing, medicine and animal health sciences, engineering, law, and much more, all engaged together in synergy to advance health from community to global levels. From this synergy, public health competencies emerge: the ability to apply those skills within specified roles for the benefit of its common vision of the highest attainable standard of health for everybody. Among its hallmarks is the mutual respect held among its practitioners: regardless of their diverse spheres of orientation, influence or application, public health is a team effort.

A process of renewal has been under way in recent decades, encouraging public health to focus more attention on the underlying determinants of health and to reengage the field in issues of social justice and environmental sustainability. Sometimes depicted as the "new public health," this stream of thought and activism runs prominently through the health promotion movement, suffusing public health as a whole. Another rallying call is "global health," which has captured many an imagination: on the heels of globalization in all forms from trade to culture, this emphasizes global cooperation for solutions. It differs from "international health," which takes its origins from the health situation of developing nations and the related need for development assistance. More often applied locally than globally, assistance flowed historically from developed nations (as it still does) but is now augmented by increasing south-south cooperation. These are among the many streams of thought and action in contemporary public health.

Why ecological foundations? Human interest in ecology originated in the dawn of prehistory in the struggles of our species coming to grips with its environment. This instinctive interest has undergone an ethical and scientific revolution as we discover ourselves and all other species to be threatened by the unsustainable practices of an increasingly man-made world, with its anthropogenic impacts ranging from local to global pollution and climate change. At its core, the environment is about the interplay of actions that promote or diminish the sustainability of life and health, and is best understood in how people live locally, in the control they have over their mode of living, and the quality of decision making, especially with regard to the prospects for future generations and for other species. When we examine our ecological foundations, we refer to both natural and man-made environments; and now increasingly, we must look to our planet. Public health is not only about human health, but also about the health of all living beings and of our planet.

By combining the terms "global public health" and "ecological foundations" we convey a perspective: that public health principles apply to all countries across the development spectrum, and that it is a global discipline. It is not sufficient, however, only to have global comprehension if this means a relatively narrow focus on policy actions taken only from that level. Health needs to be understood and approached from the community perspective, from the ground up. Global public health therefore encompasses local public health, especially when one considers the ecological basis for all health: in effect, there is but "one health."

With our best efforts at balance and objectivity, in this book we try to blend what is valuable from established wisdom with what is new. We attend to facts, giving credit where due, and refer to authentic experience from the real world. With this approach, we hope to stimulate a new dialogue about how the different streams of public health can work more synergistically, and we trust that the next generation of scholars and professionals will carry this spirit forward.

All future health professionals should find something useful in these pages: some will discover public health as their vocation; others will broaden to appreciate its importance, even as they enter other pathways. We do not attempt to be "all things to all readers"; for those who need more depth in any aspect of public health, there are more specialized texts. For many readers this book may be a point of departure from which they will search for more breadth, depth, and experience as they evolve their perspectives and skills. The ultimate beneficiaries are most people around the world; their future depends on whether their nations listen to their voices and respond with health initiatives that meet their needs and help them to find ways of making sound decisions about their own health. If this book makes a difference in how health professionals evolve their roles to shape a healthy future for generations, we will have achieved our purpose.

FW, LS, JL

Author Biographies

FRANKLIN WHITE IS a scholar-practitioner whose professional focus is on locally sustainable solutions for health and social development. He has held posts in Canada and abroad, notably with the Aga Khan University and the Pan American Health Organization (PAHO/WHO). Founder of the consulting firm Pacific Health and Development Sciences Inc., and adjunct professor at the School of Public Health and Social Policy, University of Victoria, and in Community Health and Epidemiology, Dalhousie University, he is a past president of the Canadian Public Health Association and a former chief examiner in Public Health and Preventive Medicine, Royal College of Physicians and Surgeons of Canada. He is a recipient of the Medal of Honor, the highest award conferred upon staff officers of PAHO/WHO.

Lorann Stallones is an internationally recognized occupational epidemiologist with extensive expertise in agricultural safety and health. Professor of epidemiology at Colorado State University, and director of the Colorado Injury Control Research Center and of the Institute of Applied Prevention Research, she directs the CSU Graduate Degree Program in Public Health, Colorado School of Public Health. She is deputy director, High Plains Intermountain Center for Agricultural Safety and Health and directs the Occupational Health Psychology training program, Mountain and Plains Education Research Center. Past president of the American College of Epidemiology, she is professor laureate in the College of Natural Sciences at CSU.

John Last is Emeritus Professor of epidemiology and community medicine at the University of Ottawa. He is the author of *Public Health and Human Ecology*, founding author of the *Dictionary of Public Health*, and former editor-in-chief of *Public*

Health and Preventive Medicine ("Maxcy-Rosenau-Last"), and he has written many book chapters, encyclopedia entries, original articles, and reviews on aspects of public health sciences. His honours and awards include MD honoris causa, Uppasala University; the Duncan Clarke Award (for contributions to preventive medicine); and the Abraham Lillienfeld Award for contributions to epidemiology. In 2012 John Last was admitted as an Officer of the Order of Canada in recognition of lifetime service in epidemiology and other public health sciences.

Acknowledgments

THE AUTHORS OWE gratitude to countless people with whom we have worked over the decades in several world regions and numerous countries at different stages of socioeconomic development.

This includes role models, mentors, colleagues, and students whose encouragement served as inspiration for this book, especially the many frontline practitioners who grapple daily with the realities of making public health work in diverse settings and whose on-ground experience is simultaneously the source and the proving ground for many of the ideas and observations presented within these pages.

We are grateful to all who helped in shaping the book itself, particularly those who advocated the need for a work that would be friendly to a wide range of students that would offer broad educational value and addresses not only the "how" but, more important, the "why."

A number of people provided specific input to this project by critiquing drafts, offering corrections and suggestions, advising on specialized content, drawing attention to important trends in the evidence base, facilitating permissions, and verifying sources. Others helped shape ideas and insights, supplied background for some of the case studies, or provided avenues to explore issues at various times leading up to and during the gestation of this work, sometimes in unrelated contexts. Some individuals provided several forms of inspiration, input and support.

In acknowledgment of these valuable direct and indirect contributions, we thank Saeed Akhtar, Nelson Ames, Mark Asbridge, Kate Browne, Geraldine Cooney, Graham Dickson, Brian Emerson, Trevor Hancock, James Hospedales, Anwar Islam, Syed Kadri, Perry Kendall, Jane Kneller, Joseph Konde-Lule, Karen Trollope

Kumar, Joseph Longenecker, Richard Mathias, Ian McDowell, Debra Nanan, Parvez Nayani, F Javier Nieto, Armando Peruga, Fauziah Rabbani, David Robinson, Ian Rockett, Bernie Rollin, M Abdus Salam, Nasra Shah, Michael Smalley, Leda Stott, Panduka Wijeyaratne, and Shehla Zaidi.

It has been a privilege to work with Oxford University Press under the guidance of Chad Zimmerman and his team, including the (unknown) external reviewers whose constructive reviews helped to bring our book to fruition.

We have undoubtedly omitted others who also deserve recognition (and to whom we apologize!). As authors, we take full responsibility for the final work, especially for any defects.

FW, LS, JL

GLOBAL PUBLIC HEALTH

Like education and justice, public health is one of the essential institutions of a well-organized society. It combines sciences, skills, and values that function through collective societal activities and involve programs, services, and institutions aimed at protecting, preserving, and improving the health of all the people. This chapter provides an overview of the aims and methods used in public health. But to understand where we are and what we have yet to do to improve the human condition requires that we review our past accomplishments and learn from past successes—and mistakes—that have punctuated human history, a task that this chapter takes up as well. It also offers a brief discussion of milestones in public health that have provided paradigm shifts in how we understand diseases, injuries, and health and how we protect and promote health.

1

HISTORY, AIMS, AND METHODS OF PUBLIC HEALTH

PUBLIC HEALTH IS the art and science of promoting and protecting good health; preventing disease, disability, and premature death; restoring good health when it is impaired by disease or injury; and maximizing the quality of life. Public health requires collective action by society; collaborative teamwork by nurses, physicians, engineers, environmental scientists, health educators, social workers, nutritionists, administrators, and other specialized professional and technical workers; and an effective partnership with all levels of government.[1]

The aims of public health are to promote and improve the people's health; protect good health; prevent disease, injury, and premature death; and ameliorate disability and suffering. There are many ways to achieve these aims and many overlaps and synergistic interactions among the methods we use to achieve them. Public health aims to provide benefit to the population as a whole, which requires defining the magnitude of a health problem; identifying the causes; understanding risk and protective factors for at-risk populations; developing, implementing, and evaluating prevention programs; and expanding the use of effective interventions to larger groups while monitoring impact and assessing their cost-effectiveness. Public health professionals are also involved in communicating the risks and benefits of actions, from individual to societal, so people can make informed decisions about lifestyle choices and policy makers can have impact on decisions that will improve health for all. By way of an introductory overview, the target areas for programs can be simplified by grouping them into the following five categories:

- Safe environments: control of physical, chemical, and biological hazards, including air, water, and food (see chapters 1, 2, and 7). This also includes the built environment and protecting against manmade and natural disasters; issues of sustainability and care for ecosystems also must be addressed from a public health perspective (chapter 9).
- Enhanced host resistance: fundamental to all host resistance is sound nutrition. This means well-balanced dietary intake of carbohydrate, protein, and fat containing all essential micronutrients (vitamins, minerals), and ensuring that this intake is neither too much nor too little (chapters 1, 6, and 7). Also key is immunization against vaccine-preventable diseases to protect the health of individuals and communities. Attention to other risks that reduce host resistance (e.g., smoking, inactivity) and good management of conditions that increase susceptibility (e.g., diabetes, tuberculosis, HIV/AIDS) is also critical (chapter 6).
- Health-promoting behaviors: public health aims to foster conditions and encourage habits that lead to health, such as good nutrition and regular exercise, and to discourage harmful, risk-taking behaviors such as drinking and driving and consumption of tobacco products (chapter 4). Advocacy (arguing, acting, or both in support of a cause, policy, or group of people) is often an essential activity in support of such aims.
- Protection of vulnerable groups: vigilance regarding inequitable distribution of health and social services and attention to the special needs of mothers, children, the disabled, the elderly, the poor, and the unemployed. This implies such provisions as effective reproductive care to ensure healthy mothers and infants and safeguarding children, disabled, and elderly, especially with regard to all forms of abuse, deprivation, and neglect (chapters 3, 4, 5, and 8).
- Prudent and accessible health care: all actions and interventions of the health care system should be evidence-based, or based on prudent action when evidence is not yet available, using the principle of do more good than harm (chapters 3 and 8). All services essential to health should be universal to an extent that is affordable and sustainable.

Definitions of Health

Health is described in the Preamble to the Constitution of the World Health Organization (1948) as, "A state of complete physical, mental and social well-being and not merely the absence of disease or infirmity."[2] This statement has been much criticized because of its vagueness, absence of measureable indicators, and the fact that it is almost entirely subjective.

Fortunately there are several acceptable alternative definitions, mostly varying with context. Discussions under the aegis of WHO and the Canadian Public Health Association in 1984 led to this one: "The extent to which an individual or a group is able to realize aspirations and satisfy needs, and to change or cope with the environment; health is a resource for everyday life, not the objective of living. It is a positive concept, emphasizing social and personal resources as well as physical capabilities."[3] This implies some control over many determinants of health by individuals, families, and social groups and connects well with a simplified yet salient definition of public health as "society's response to threats to the collective health of its citizens."[4]

A definition that accords with the status of humans as one among myriads of interdependent life forms is: "A sustainable state of equilibrium or harmony between humans and their physical, biological and social environments that enables them to coexist indefinitely."[5] This does not necessarily imply that the environment or life-supporting ecosystems must remain unchanged; however, it implies that the environmental capacity to adapt or adjust to change is not adversely affected by human activities and changes in aspects of the environment and the life-supporting ecosystem do not adversely affect human health. In the Preface we discussed the global context of this book. Simply defined, "global health" may be considered as the health of all people globally within sustainable and healthy living (local and global) conditions.[6]

A Brief History of Public Health

To understand where we are and what we have yet to do to improve the human condition requires that we review and learn from the past successes—and mistakes—that have punctuated human history. The history of public health is reflected in scientific advances that can be described through the accomplishments of individuals, but these accomplishments took place within the social context of the time and reflected more than individual successes. Further, some of the methods used to achieve this scientific knowledge would today be considered unethical, for example using children as subjects in experiments without parental consent or the children's assent. Such choices made in earlier times reflected a view of children as property, just as were women considered in many of the societies discussed in this chapter; orphans were given even less social recognition. Nonetheless, at various times in history there was considerable concern by some people about the role of social deprivation in contributing to early death. Therefore we need to consider the historical context in which physicians, nurses, and public health practitioners operate, as well as the social conditions that produce health and disease within the framework of the political and economic conditions of the day. The conditions of a given era, whether the present or the future (whatever it may bring), will always impact health and disease.

One way to consider the history of public health is as a series of paradigm shifts that accompany epochal insights and discoveries about ways to improve health or prevent debilitating and life-shortening disease. This approach works most of the time but lets us down when we recall that some of the most important discoveries occurred historically in haphazard sequence, only tenuously related, if related at all, to what was already known, and to prevailing beliefs and theories about what caused many of the most terrible diseases, as well as annoying but not lethal afflictions, of humankind. So for the most part, this account focuses on the great insights and discoveries, sometimes identified with names of those who made the discoveries, and illustrates the intermittent and accelerating pace of progress toward good health for all.

About a million years ago our hominid precursors discovered how to use fire to cook the meat they had hunted. They found that cooked meat tasted better, it didn't go bad so quickly, and eating it was less likely to make them ill. Our understanding of nutrition (an important public health science), food hygiene, and the art of cooking has been improving ever since. In those prehistoric times, judging from archeological evidence, there is little doubt that humans evolved as spiritual beings in search of meaning for their lives and relationships with their environment. This trait lies at the core of the gradual development of belief systems about health and disease.

As long as 9000 to 10,000 years ago, people discovered how to grow crops and tame animals. With the advent of agriculture came permanent settlements, and at about the same time people discovered that grain could be used to make flour and then high-density carbohydrate foods. The settlements led to efforts to control the flow of water for agricultural needs (irrigation) and were evident in Mesopotamia and Egypt during the Neolithic period (5700–2800 BCE).[7] Sophisticated urban water systems date from a later period, in the Bronze Age (2800–1100 BCE). Mohenjo-Daro, a major urban center of the Indus Civilization, developed one such system for water supply and sewage.[8] Water came from over 700 wells and supplied domestic needs, a system of private baths, and a Great Bath for public use. Rainwater collection in cisterns was practiced in an area north of Jordan around the same time, and groundwater collection systems were developed in Persia.[9] The system in Persia consisted of subterranean tunnels of connecting wells, using vertical shafts designed to collect and transport water from highland areas to low-lying farmland. This system is important because the technology was applied over extensive periods and the systems were so durable that some are still in use. About the same time advanced urban water technologies were developed in Greece and on the island of Crete. These included construction and use of aqueducts, cisterns, wells, fountains, bathrooms, and other sanitary facilities, which suggested lifestyle standards close to those of today. The Romans developed engineering skills and expanded these technologies for use on large-scale projects. But with the fall of the Roman Empire, water supply systems, sanitation, and public health declined in Europe. Europe reacquired high standards of water supply and sanitation only in the 19th century, largely as a result of efforts to improve human health and reduce the burden of disease resulting from unsanitary conditions and polluted drinking water.[7]

A secure food supply led to the first great population surge. Little settlements became villages, villages became towns, and towns grew into cities. Before long, civilizations with religions, laws, history, customs, traditions, and sciences arose in favorable settings: on lake shores, river estuaries, and fertile plains beside the great rivers in Egypt, the Middle East, India, and China. Our ancestors had begun their progress on the road to health, toward our present situation.

But it has been a long road, because as the human population increased, so did the variety and number of their diseases. Permanent human settlements transformed ecosystems, and the probability of respiratory and fecal-oral transmission of infection rose as population density increased.

Ecological and evolutionary changes in microorganisms and vectors account for the origins of measles, influenza, malaria, smallpox, plague, and many other diseases. Microorganisms evolve rapidly because of their brief generation time and prolific reproduction rates. Many microbes that previously had lived in symbiosis with animals began to invade humans, in which some of them became pathogenic. Some evolved complex life cycles that require more than one host species: humans and other mammals, humans and insects, humans and freshwater snails.

These evolutionary changes in host-parasite relationships occurred several millennia before we had written histories. Our oldest written records that have a bearing on health date back about 4000 years. The Code of Hammurabi (c. 2000 BCE) contains ideas that indicate insights into the effects on health of diet and behavior.[10] It also suggests rewards and punishments for physicians who did their jobs well or poorly.

Understanding that theories of disease have changed over time allows us to put into proper perspective historical approaches to disease prevention. Some cultures attribute diseases to malevolent supernatural forces, curses from enemies or sorcerers, or the anger of gods.[8] The Classical Greeks conceived a theory of imbalance among four "humors," loosely associated with personality types—choleric, phlegmatic, melancholic, and sanguine—and in the absence of contrary evidence, this theory persisted for centuries.[8] It led to empirical treatment regimens including poultices, blood-letting, and steam inhalations.[8] These same personality types are described in psychology today as descriptors of types of people, and research continues in relation to their contributions to mental and behavioral disorders.[11] Another theory held that diseases were caused by miasma, emanations of malign vapors or fumes from rotting vegetation in swamps and marshes.[8] This theory provided an explanation for some vector-borne diseases such as malaria and yellow fever but not other lethal epidemics, including typhus and plague.

Defining the Magnitude of the Problem

A *census* (discussed in chapter 5) is the single most important tool for the construction of a population profile, whether for health or other application (e.g., education, economic development). The earliest census was probably carried out about 1500 BCE in ancient Egypt. Censuses were used by the Romans to identify potential military recruits and eligibility for taxation, and they are conducted today at 10-year intervals in most countries for a much wider range of applications. Information provided by a census allows public health professionals to compute rates of diseases in order to assess the relative magnitude of risk for populations and to determine what types of health care services may be needed in a community.

Information about the impact of diseases, especially of epidemics, from those ancient times has come down to us in myths and religious accounts of pestilences and plagues, although we can't reliably identify the nature of any epidemics that afflicted ancient populations. The Greek historian Thucydides provided a meticulous description of the epidemic that struck the Athenians in the second year of the Peloponnesian War in 426 BCE, from which the Athenians never fully recovered; but modern epidemiologists cannot identify the disease. The causal organisms of other ancient epidemics is similarly a mystery: almost 1000 years ago "sweating sickness" recurred in epidemics many times in mediaeval Europe then vanished, never to be seen again; we have no idea what caused this lethal disease. Even the exact nature of the Black Death, the terrible pandemic that devastated Asia Minor and all of Europe in 1347–1350 is debated. It was almost certainly bubonic and pneumonic plague but some scholars argue that it may have been anthrax or fulminating streptococcal infection, or a combination of all these.

A systematic approach to defining disease problems emerged in the more recent past. The earliest attempt to systematically classify diseases was attributed to French physician and botanist Francois Bossier de Lacroix (1706-1777), better known as Sauvages.[12] Carl Linnaeus (1707-1778), the Swedish botanical taxonomist and a colleague of Sauvages, also wrote a treatise on disease classification: *Generus Morborum*.[13] At the beginning of the 19th century, the classification of disease in most general use was one by William Cullen (1710–1790) of Edinburgh, which was published under the title *Synopsis Nosologie Methodicae*.

The statistical study of diseases, however, began with John Graunt and his published work in *Natural and Political Observations...upon the Bills of Mortality* (London, 1662),[14] which was the foundation for the science of vital statistics. John Graunt demonstrated the importance of gathering facts in a systematic manner to identify, characterize, count, and classify health conditions of public health importance. The diagnostic categories in the *Bills of Mortality* tell us what was understood 400 years ago about the variety of human ailments and their causes. Progress in the use of medical statistics, as well as improved classifications and international uniformity, was made with the establishment of the General Registrar Office of England and Wales in 1837, under the direction of William Farr (1807–1883).[12]

The utility of a uniform classification of causes of death was recognized by the International Statistical Congress, and at the first meeting in Brussels in 1883, William Farr and Marc d'Espine of Geneva were asked to prepare an internationally applicable and uniform classification of causes of death. The resulting schemes were based on different principles. d'Espine classified diseases based on their nature (e.g., gouty, herpetic), whereas Farr classified diseases under five groups: epidemic, constitutional, local arranged according to anatomic site, developmental, and those resulting from violence.[12] The general arrangement proposed by Farr was used as the basis for the International List of Causes of Death. In 1891 at the International Statistical Institute meeting in Vienna, Jacques Bertillon (1851–1922) was asked to prepare a classification of causes of death, which he presented at the International Statistical Institute meeting held in Chicago in 1893.[12]

The Bertillon Classification of Causes of Death was adopted by several countries and first used in North America by Jesus Monjaras in San Luis Potosi, Mexico.[12, 15] In Ottawa, Canada in 1898, the American Public Health Association recommended adoption of the Bertillon Classification of Causes of Death by registrars in Canada, Mexico, and the United States and that the classification be revised every 10 years. The International List of Causes of Death, as Bertillon's Classification of Causes of Death came to be called, was revised in 1900, 1910, and 1920 under the direction of Bertillon. The Fourth and Fifth revisions of the International List of Causes of Death were carried out as a coordinated effort with the Health Organization of the League of Nations and the International Statistical Institute.

At the Fifth International Conference for the Revision of the International List of Causes of Death in Paris in 1938, the group recognized the need to have a corresponding list of diseases for morbidity statistics.[12] The group recommended that

TABLE 1-1

ICD revisions and years covered

Revision	Years Covered	Revision	Years Covered
1st	1900–09	6th	1949–57
2nd	1910–20	7th	1958–67
3rd	1921–29	8th	1968–78
4th	1930–38	9th	1979–89
5th	1939–48	10th	1990–present

the United States government continue to study the classification of causes of death when two or more causes were mentioned on the death certificate and to work with other countries to investigate this issue over the next ten years. In 1948 in Paris, the International Conference for the Sixth Revision of the International Lists of Diseases and Causes of Death adopted the classification system prepared by an expert committee appointed by the World Health Organization in 1946.[12] Table 1-1 illustrates the history of revisions, showing the years for which they were applied.

The 9th Revision of the International Classification of Diseases (ICD, launched 1979) developed supplementary classifications of Impairments and Handicaps and of Procedures in Medicine, amended coding rules for mortality and introduced rules for selection of a single cause for counting morbidity, changed definitions and recommendations for statistics in the field of perinatal mortality, and encouraged countries to work on multiple-condition coding.[12] Between the 9th and 10th Revision of the ICD, it became clear that the established ten-year interval between revisions was too short, resulting in delayed implementation of the 10th Revision (endorsed by the World Health Assembly in 1990) in 1994. The 11th revision is underway and this process will continue until 2015.

The 10th Revision of the ICD is currently in use. The ICD has been the international standard diagnostic classification for general epidemiological studies, health planning and management, and clinical use. These include the analysis of the general health situation of population groups and monitoring of the incidence and prevalence of diseases and other health problems in relation to other variables such as the characteristics and circumstances of the individuals affected, reimbursement, resource allocation, and quality and treatment guidelines.

Determining the Causes, Risks, Protective Factors, and Population Affected

Understanding the causes, risks, and protective factors for many diseases, and describing the populations at risk of them, has been accomplished throughout history by the astute observations of many people. There is no clear separation between understanding the causes of disease and implementing approaches to control or prevent them, since some of our understanding of causes comes from attempts to control disease, as does some of our understanding of health and what keeps people healthy. Therefore the next section deals with foundational work in understanding why disease occurs in specific locations among particular individuals.

SAFE ENVIRONMENTS

The role of the environment in health has been recognized since ancient times and in many cultures, as stated by the Greek physician Hippocrates (circa 400 BCE) in his treatise on *Airs, Waters, Places*. The Egyptian Ibn Ridwan wrote at the turn of the first millennium on the adverse effects of the urban environment in the city of Cairo.[16] European scholars followed, such as Agricola (1494–1555), whose treatise *De Re Metallica* documented the health hazards of mining and smelting,[17] and his contemporary Paracelsus (1493–1541), who became recognized as founder of the modern science of toxicology. His dictum, "everything is toxic, depending on the dose," is an important principle that underlies the concept of the now frequently used exposure-response curve.[18]

Of these contributions, we learned perhaps most from Paracelsus (his full name was Theophrastus Bombastus von Hohenheim), as we accept today that an association between an exposure and a biological outcome may be evidence for a causal relationship and for defining exposure levels that may be cause for concern. Although many pollutants of concern today also occur freely in nature (e.g., nitrogen and sulfur compounds, carbon monoxide and particulate matter), as their concentrations increase they become increasingly incompatible with physiological function and health (e.g., even oxygen is toxic at high concentrations). The study of such relationships (in animals and in humans) helps us prevent or alleviate such exposures and effects through the design of effective interventions.

OCCUPATION AND DISEASE

In Ancient Greece, a focus on aristocratic hygiene reflected, as well, the lack of concern about the health of workers (whether paid or slave) with little mention of occupational issues in historical medical literature. One reference to an illness of a miner can be found in Hippocratic writings.[8] In Roman writings there is evidence of recognition of hazards associated with work from Pliny mentioning diseases prevalent among slaves, references to dangers of certain occupations in poetry, and diseases specific to sulfur workers, blacksmiths, and gold miners.[8] Galen mentions that copper sulfate miners worked in a suffocating environment where the miners were naked during work because the fumes destroyed their clothing.[8] Accounts of diseases among workers continued to focus on miners and expanded in the 16th century to include the health of sailors, with concerns about scurvy and typhus fever as the sea routes expanded to the Far East and the New World.[8] Bernardino Ramazzini (1633–1714) was an Italian physician who published the first comprehensive treatise on occupation and diseases. He provided a foundation for occupational medicine when he reported his observations about the diseases for which workers in each occupation were vulnerable in *De morbis artificum diatribe* (Discourse on the Diseases of Workers, 1713).[19] But not until the middle of the 18th century were further significant contributions to occupational welfare made. A few are described next.

THEORIES ABOUT CAUSE

For over a thousand years after Hippocrates, people were afflicted with ever-present respiratory and gastrointestinal infections that cut deeply into the lives of everyone, especially children, who often died before adolescence, carried off by measles, scarlet fever, diphtheria, bronchitis, croup, pneumonia, or gastroenteritis. From time to time this steady drain on long life and good health was punctuated by terrifying epidemics—smallpox, typhus, influenza, and, most terrible, the plague—the black death. The causes of these periodic devastations, the reasons they happened, were a mystery. Many believed they were God's punishment for sin or the work of evil spirits. Ideas about contagion were rudimentary, even though it had been dimly understood since antiquity that leprosy, perhaps the least contagious of all the infectious diseases, was associated with overcrowding and uncleanliness.

Understanding the number of means by which diseases are spread has allowed for the development of public health approaches to control transmission of diseases. The Italian priest-physician, Girolamo Fracastoro (1478–1553) concluded that disease could pass by intimate direct contact from one person to others because he observed the dramatic epidemic of syphilis that was manifestly spread by sexual intercourse.[8] Fracastoro's other concepts, droplet spread and spread by way of contaminated articles such as clothing and kitchen utensils, were published in *De Contagione*, in 1546 and provided a systematic view of the role of contagion in the rise and fall of communicable diseases; as such it serves as a landmark in the evolution of scientific theory of communicable diseases.[20]

The nature of diseases caused by creatures not visible to the naked eye was a mystery that began to clarify when Antoni van Leeuwenhoek (1632–1723),[21] a Dutch linen draper and amateur lens grinder, perfected the first functioning microscopes. He gazed at and drew pictures of what he saw in drops of water, vaginal secretions, feces, his own semen, and the structures of plants and insects. He lacked formal scholarly training but in a series of 165 letters to the Royal Society of London, he described accurately and in detail the microscopic creatures that he saw. He did not suggest that these tiny creatures were capable of causing diseases, but he is celebrated as the first of the "microbe hunters" who sought and identified pathogenic microorganisms responsible for many diseases.

Recognition that insects can transmit diseases to humans was another major shift in identifying means to control diseases. In an attempt to reduce mortality among cattle from Texas cattle fever in 1889, Fred Kilbourne, Cooper Curtice, both veterinarians, and bacteriologist Theobold Smith discovered the role of ticks as vectors in the disease.[22] The discovery was the first time that insect vectors had been established in the transmission of disease and also established that adult ticks could infect nymphs. Understanding the life cycle of the tick provided a path to control by dipping the cattle to kill the ticks. Further, this discovery presaged the discoveries that led to understanding the role of insect transmission of trypanosomiasis of cattle by David Bruce (1895), malaria by Ronald Ross (1897), yellow fever by Walter Reed and his colleagues (1900), and typhus by Charles Nicolle (1909).[22]

Malaria was described by Hippocrates in the 4th century BC and is probably one of the most ancient diseases of humans.[23] Today (chapters 2, 5, and 6), at the dawn of the third millennium, it remains a public health priority. About 3.3 billion people (almost half the world's population) are at risk; endemic in 106 countries, in 2009 there were an estimated 225 million cases and some 800,000 people died, the vast majority of them children in sub-Saharan Africa and Asia.[22] The word itself comes from Latin roots (literally "bad air"), and in its prescientific history it was among a number of conditions known as "swamp fever." In those days people knew that swamps were not healthy places for human habitats, which in itself played a role in the location and sustainability of human settlements, and in efforts to reclaim such areas so as to make them more conducive for human habitation. However, the development of agriculture that resulted in clearing forests and vegetation, turning soil, and irrigating land created new collections of water and encouraged breeding of the anophopline mosquitoes in close proximity to human populations.[24] The extent of malaria in a community typically depended on the location of homes relative to the fields, housing conditions, the presence of livestock, and also the breeding and feeding habits of the mosquitoes.[22, 23] Only at the beginning of the 20th century, slightly more than 100 years ago, did people begin to systematically control the disease through attacking its insect propagators.[22] Over time agricultural communities experienced less malaria because of the development of resistance to the disease, improved approaches to agriculture that reduced habitat for mosquitoes, such as draining swamps, improved housing, including windows and screens, better nutrition and improved overall health, and moving of livestock away from homes.[23]

Economic and social forces, in addition to ecological conditions, also shape the distribution of malaria globally. In the United States, Europe, and Great Britain, declines in malaria coincided with increased political and economic power.[23] The growth of industrial capitalism and the spread of colonial rule, which incorporated local tropical economies into global markets and the concentration of land ownership at the expense of peasant farmers, also contributed to the persistence of malaria in areas where some of the population lived in inadequate housing and subsisted on poor diets.[22, 23] Social, economic, and political disruptions, including human conflicts that result in human migrations from malaria endemic regions, also have provided opportunities for malaria to return to areas where it had previously disappeared.[23]

The control of malaria at the end of the 19th century and in the early part of the 20th century focused on defending people against the disease by reducing exposure to mosquito populations. In 1900 Italian malariologist Angelo Celli published "Malaria According to the New Researches" describing the epidemiology and prevention of malaria based on the discovery of the malarial parasite and the role of anopheline mosquitoes.[23] He discussed the biological relationship between the parasites, the mosquitoes, and humans but added the influence of economic development, politics, and social conditions on the geographic distribution of the disease.[23]

Develop, Implement, and Evaluate Prevention Programs

One of the oldest techniques for control of disease is quarantine, which began during the 14th century to protect coastal cities from plague epidemics. Ships arriving in Venice were required to be anchored for 40 days before landing. The word quarantine is derived from this practice and the Italian words *quaranta giorni,* meaning "40 days."[25] Quarantine is still used today in various forms (chapter 6). However, as understanding of the causes of diseases progressed, other techniques for controlling diseases developed. Notable shifts in disease control based on evolving understanding of transmission and causes of disease are described next.

SANITATION, HYGIENE, AND HEALTH

As populations in cities grew there was increasing need to have systems to deal with the disposal of animal and human waste. The respect Romans had for public and personal hygiene was evident in the water supply and sewage systems they left behind and was also evident in the baths.[7] During the Middle Ages bathhouses served the dual purpose of hygiene and pleasure and were licensed by municipalities.[8] Ritual bathing was a part of ancient Hebrew culture, but routine bathing for hygienic purposes was practiced as well.[26] Washing was a major feature of Islamic countries through medieval and Renaissance periods, and frequent washing was a religious requirement. In Japan the tradition of public bathing dates back at least to 552 AD and was linked to Buddhism, which taught that such hygiene purified the body and brought good luck.[27]

During the 15th century, when syphilis became a public health problem, communal bathing fell into disfavor in Europe, much as it did in the United States at the height of the current AIDS epidemic. There was a resurgence of interest in public bathing in the mid-1800s when sanitary conditions were exceptionally bad.[8] Epidemics of cholera had plagued Great Britain, and the need for improved circumstances had been highlighted in 1842 by an *Inquiry into the Sanitary Conditions of the Labouring Classes*. In his report, Sir Edwin Chadwick (1800–1890) argued that disease was directly related to living conditions and that there was a need for public health reform. The Public Baths and Wash Houses Act of 1846 subsequently allowed local parishes in the United Kingdom to raise money to provide public baths and laundries.[8] The rapidly increasing urban population, often living in unsanitary conditions, resulted in viewing bathhouses as essential public services. This example serves to represent a number of shifts in health perspectives, from viewing bathing as a personal hygiene issue to recognizing it as a public health issue. It also illustrated the use of data to provide support for legislative action in the interest of people who do not have the economic resources to improve their living conditions.

Johann Peter Frank (1745–1821) studied medicine in Heidelberg and Strasburg, was a professor of medicine at Göttingen and Pavia, and taught in many other centers of learning, ending his career in Vienna where he was professor of medicine at the Allegemeines Krankenhaus, the Vienna General Hospital. Early in his career he began writing *System einer vollständigen medicinischen Polizey*, his great work on ways to improve population health. This appeared in a series of nine volumes from 1779 to 1827. His work dealt with every then-known way to protect and preserve good health, including communal hygiene, personal hygiene and cleanliness, and a suggested set of laws and regulations to govern the control of conditions in lodging houses and inns, medical inspection of prostitutes, brothels, communal kitchens, and bathhouses.[8]

John Snow (1813–1858) was a London physician and a founder of modern epidemiology. Snow's work on cholera demonstrated fundamental intellectual steps that must be part of every epidemiological investigation.[28, 29] He began with a logical analysis of the available facts, which established that cholera could not be caused by a "miasma" (emanations from rotting organic matter) as proposed in a theory popular at that time, but must be caused by a transmissible agent, most probably in drinking water. He confirmed this with two epidemiological investigations in the great cholera epidemic of 1854. He studied a severe localized epidemic in Soho, using analysis of descriptive epidemiological data and spot maps to demonstrate that the cause was polluted water from a pump in Broad Street. His investigation of the more widespread epidemic in South London involved an inquiry into the source of drinking water used in over 700 households. He compared the water source in houses where cholera had occurred with that in others where it had not. His analysis of information about cases and their sources of drinking water showed that the cause was water supplied by the Southwark and Vauxhall water company, which drew water from the Thames downriver, where many effluent discharges polluted the water (Table 1-2). Very few cases occurred in households supplied by the Lambeth company, which collected water upstream from London, where there was little or no pollution. John Snow reasoned that the cholera therefore must be caused by an agent in contaminated water. This was a remarkable feat, 30 years before Robert Koch identified the cholera bacillus. Snow's demonstration that polluted water can cause disease was another paradigm shift in understanding the ways in which diseases may be transmitted—and prevented.

ENHANCED IMMUNITY

Smallpox has been recognized as a disease for over 2000 years and was evident in Indian and Chinese writings around the 4th century AD.[30] The disease appears to have spread from Africa to India by way of early Arab merchants.[30] In the 9th century the Persian physician Al-Razi published an article on the epidemiology and clinical features of smallpox. From the time of the Crusades smallpox moved into Europe and then with the great European migrations that occurred from the 15th century onward, the disease was carried to Central, South, and North America,

TABLE 1-2

Cholera Mortality—London 4 week period July 9–August 5, 1854.[1]

Water Company	Houses Supplied	Deaths	Rate per 10,000 Houses
Southwark and Vauxhall	40,046	286	71.4
Lambeth	26,107	14	5.4
All Others	287,345	277	9.6

[1] Table 1-2 adapted from Snow J. On the Mode of Communication of Cholera, 2nd ed. London: Churchill 1855. Reprint with annotations by Wade Hampton Frost, New York: Commonwealth Fund, 1936: reprint New York: Hafner 1965.

South Africa, Australia, and some of the larger islands in the Pacific Ocean. The case fatality rate for smallpox ranged from 50% in the younger and older age groups to about 10% among those 5–14 years of age, but survivors were sometimes severely scarred and, if smallpox vesicles affected the eyes, blind. Recovery conferred lifelong immunity for most people with the secondary attack rate less than one in a thousand. Smallpox was not a highly infectious agent and usually spread only to close family contacts, but the virus was resistant to environmental conditions and could be spread through fomites, such as through the sharing or distribution of contaminated blankets. The occurrence was seasonal and spread favored low humidity and was inhibited by high humidity. No animal reservoir of the virus is known. The observation that infected people did not become infected again with smallpox led to experiments in China probably before the 10th century CE. Liquid obtained from a pustule was used to inoculate uninfected persons, who were in generally good health. Infection among these people was milder than natural smallpox and the practice of inoculation became widespread in parts of Asia. Lady Mary Wortley Montague, wife of the British ambassador to Constantinople, described this practice in a letter to a friend in 1717, and imported the idea to England on her return, following which the practice of inoculation became widespread there. The case fatality rate of inoculation was 2% or lower when the operator was skilled and lesions were less extensive than in natural smallpox. However, there was always illness and sometimes death involved, and the inoculation smallpox could cause outbreaks of severe natural smallpox in unprotected people, especially if more susceptible (e.g., underlying nutritional deficiencies and skin disorders). By the time Edward Jenner (1749–1823) was a child, this practice had become popular among educated English families as a way to provide some protection against smallpox.

Jenner knew the popular belief that people who had been infected with cowpox, a mild disease acquired from cattle, did not get smallpox. He reasoned that since smallpox in mild form was transmissible, it might be possible similarly to transmit cowpox. A smallpox outbreak in 1792 gave him an opportunity to confirm this notion. In 1796 he began a courageous and unprecedented experiment—one that would now be unethical, but that has had incalculable benefit for humankind.[30] He inoculated a 9-year old boy with secretions from a cowpox lesion. In the following months until summer 1798 he inoculated others, mostly children, to a total of 23. All survived unharmed and none got smallpox. Jenner published *An Inquiry into the Causes and Effects of the Variolae Vaccinae* (1798)[31]—perhaps the most influential public health treatise of all time. The importance of Jenner's work was immediately recognized, and although there were skeptics and hostile opponents, vaccination programs began at once. Jennerian vaccination was widely adopted all over Europe and in North America. By 1802 the vaccine had been successfully transported to India and by 1804 to Spanish colonies in South America, the Philippines, and China.

No account of smallpox history can be considered complete without noting that it is the first disease to be eradicated. The application of scientific principles, including (in addition to the vaccine) the critical roles of surveillance, operational leadership, and management, to the eradication of smallpox is an epic of modern public health history, presented in chapter 2.

NUTRITION

James Lind (1716–1794) was apprenticed to a surgeon when he was 15, and spent nine years as a naval surgeon, during which time he saw many cases of scurvy, a disease that disabled and often killed sailors on long ocean voyages.[8] Lind thought this disease might be caused by a diet lacking fresh fruit and vegetables. He conducted an experiment in which he gave different diets to each of several pairs of sailors. The sailors who received fresh oranges and lemons recovered rapidly from the scurvy, the others did not or got worse. Lind also initiated the first effective measures aimed at enhancing hygiene in the British navy, but he is best known for his work on scurvy, reported in *A Treatise of the Scurvy* (1753).[32] Not only was this a very early clinical trial, it also documented the role of diet in health. However, understanding the biochemistry lagged far behind the findings of this trial.

The foundation for increased understanding of the physiology and pathology of nutrition was created in the 18th century.[8] Justus von Liebig (1803–1873) formulated a unified concept of metabolic activity that influenced work on nutrition and nutrition chemistry. This was based on classifying nourishment requirements into proteins, carbohydrates, and fats according to the earlier work of Francois Magendie (1783–1855), who showed how proteins were used to build or repair and carbohydrates and fats were used for fuel.[8] Experimental evidence of the principle of conservation of energy for living organisms was provided by Max Rubner (1854–1932).[8]

In the United States, an American standard requirement of 3500 calories per man per day was set. Carroll D Wright (1840–1909) studied the protein, fat, carbohydrate, and fuel value of a variety of foods.[8] During the same period, William Atwater (1864–1907) observed that nutrition involved social and psychological considerations; in 1888 he called on social scientists to help explain why the poor considered foods with delicate appearance and of the highest price to be the most desirable. He and industrialist Edward Atkinson felt consumers should obtain dietary needs in the most economical manner; they advocated including food laboratories within the Agricultural Experiment Stations, which had been recently created by the US Congress. Appropriations were made to accomplish this in 1895.[8] These laboratories were to investigate and report on the nutritional value used in the human food supply and to suggest economical ways to obtain full, wholesome, and edible rations. Later in this chapter you will find a historical case study that illustrates the role of social and economic factors (Case Study—Joseph Goldberger and Pellagra).

Knowledge of history helps us appreciate how the adequacy of the science of the day, and misinterpretations of it, led to errors in thinking and decision making. This is a vital lesson for our own and future times. For example, the early scientific focus on fuel value of food and lack of understanding of vitamins and minerals resulted in condemning foods that are now considered essential. In particular, use of green vegetables, sweet corn, and canned tomatoes were considered poor food value due to small amounts of proteins, low energy value, or too expensive a source of protein. Oranges and green vegetables were viewed as appetizing but nonessential, ignoring the earlier work of Lind that established the fact that citrus fruits would prevent scurvy.[8]

While laboratory work supported the need for essential components in diet beyond proteins, fats, and carbohydrates, the work of naval surgeon T. K. Takaki (1858–1920) proved to be a breakthrough comparable to the earlier work of Lind. Takaki eradicated beriberi by adding fish, meat, and vegetables to the diet of the Japanese navy.[33] Experimental studies that isolated essential ingredients to prevent deficiency diseases such as rickets and beriberi were not accepted as evidence for preventive approaches to reduce disease in humans until 1912.[8]

Casimir Funk (1884–1967) announced the isolation of a chemical substance he believed to be an amine and therefore named it "vitamine."[8] Subsequently the "e" was dropped when it became clear that the substances were not amines, and the search began to identify chemicals that are known now as vitamins. Work quickly progressed in isolating vitamins associated with specific diseases, leading to the convention of using letters of the alphabet to name the vitamins. But further work revealed that vitamins alone may not prevent specific diseases. William Huntley, a medical missionary in India, concluded that while diet may play a role in rickets, lack of exercise outside and lack of exposure to sunshine seemed to be main factors in the disease.[8] T. A. Palm conducted a geographical survey of the distribution of rickets and found it was more prevalent where there was less sunshine.[8] Cod liver oil was known to cure rickets, but the link that explained why sunshine and cod liver oil could be associated with onset and cure of rickets was not made until the discovery of vitamin D. Sunshine acts on fats in the body to produce vitamin D. Cod liver oil contains vitamin D.

The ancient Greeks and others used iodine-rich seaweed to combat goiter (thyroid gland enlargement associated with metabolic dysfunction). In 1811, Bernard Courtois (1777–1838) noted a violet vapor arising from burning seaweed ash, subsequently identified by Joseph Louis Gay-Lussac (1778–1850) as iodine, a new element. Swiss physician Jean-Francois Coindet (1774–1834), in 1813, hypothesized that traditional treatment of goiter with seaweed was effective because of its iodine content and successfully treated goitrous patients with iodine.[34] Almost two decades later, in 1831, the French agricultural scientist Jean Baptiste Boussingault (1802–1887), then working in the Andes Mountains where goiter was endemic, was first to advocate prophylaxis with iodine-rich salt to prevent goiter and that iodine-rich salts could be used to treat it.[35] Sixty-five years were to pass, however, before Eugen Baumann (1846–1896) in 1896 was to discover the presence of iodine in the thyroid gland, thus affording a scientific basis for the importance of this element in human physiology. In the years 1907–1909, David Marine, a young physician in Cleveland, Ohio, began using iodine-fortified salt to prevent goiter.[36] His early effort to conduct a large-scale trial of iodized salt in Cleveland public schools was vetoed by another doctor who served as chairman of the school board. This delayed the determined Dr. Marine until 1916, when he teamed with O. P. Kimball to convince the Akron, Ohio school board to conduct the trial on elementary school girls (who had double the expected rate of goiter). The outcome was successful and the lead shifted to David Murray Cowie of the University of Michigan, who led a process resulting in collaboration with the salt producers association. By 1924 iodized salt was commonly available in the United States. Within a decade, over 90% of salt consumed in the US "goiter belt" was iodized. Goiter incidence plummeted (e.g., in Detroit from 9.7% to 1.4% within 6 years of using iodized salt).[37]

The rest of the iodine story is still a work in progress. Current efforts are focused on *global elimination of brain damage caused by iodine deficiency* (reviewed in chapter 6).

PRUDENT AND ACCESSIBLE HEALTH CARE

Provision of improved obstetric care to reduce maternal mortality began with the establishment of wards for obstetrical patients in the 1700s in London. Mortality rates for mothers and infants declined after the establishment of the special wards until around 1810–1820, when they began to rise again. To address the high maternal mortality that was becoming more common, the Hungarian physician Ignaz Semmelweiss (1818–1865) tried to transform traditional but ineffective treatment methods, using logic and statistical analysis to demonstrate efficacy, or lack of it, when he compared treatment regimens. He believed in the germ theory of disease and was convinced that the terrible death rates from puerperal sepsis (childbed fever) must be caused by pathogens introduced into the raw uterine tissues by birth attendants who did not disinfect their hands. He carried out a meticulous mortality study, comparing his own wards, where he insisted that all birth attendants must cleanse their hands in a disinfectant solution of bleach, with other wards run by senior obstetricians where hand-washing was not routine. His belatedly published comparative statistical analyses of the death rates from puerperal sepsis in his own and other wards of the *Allegemeines Krankenhaus* are a model of how to conduct such investigations, but unfortunately no one in Vienna heeded him and young women continued to die of childbed fever for another generation. In Boston, Oliver Wendell Holmes (1809–1865) made similar observations in 1847 and published them, but he, too, was ignored. Their observations and recommendations were applied in modified form later when Joseph Lister (1827–1912) began using carbolic acid to kill pathogens in obstetrical labor and surgical operating rooms.[8, 20]

Medical science advanced rapidly in the second half of the 19th century, with the application of the exciting discoveries of bacteriology, which transformed public health. The great bacteriologists of the late 19th century identified many pathogenic bacteria, classified them, developed ways to cultivate them, and, most important, worked out ways to control their harmful effects by using sera, vaccines, and "magic bullets" such as the arsenical preparations that Paul Ehrlich (1854–1915) developed to treat syphilis. In the interest of brevity only the work of the great Louis Pasteur (1822–1895) is described here. This French chemist evolved into a bacteriologist, and he was a towering figure of 19th century bacteriology and preventive medicine. In 1854, having just been appointed professor of chemistry in Lille, he was invited to solve the problem of aberrant fermentation of beer that made it undrinkable. He showed that the problem was caused by bacteria that were killed by heat. In this way he invented the process for heat treatment to kill harmful bacteria, first applied to fermentation of beer, then to milk—the process known ever since as *pasteurization*, that has saved innumerable people, especially children, from an untimely death. He went on to study and solve many other bacteriological problems in industry and animal husbandry. He developed attenuated vaccines, first to prevent chicken cholera, then in 1881 to control anthrax, which was a serious threat to livestock as well as an occasional human disease. Before this, in 1880, he began experiments on rabies, seeking a vaccine to control this disease, which without treatment is invariably fatal. Following the success of the anthrax vaccine he believed that an attenuated rabies vaccine could be made. This was almost 60 years before the virus was identified. He successfully tested his rabies vaccine in 1885 on a boy who had been bitten by a rabid dog. Pasteur became not just a national but an international celebrity.

Born in the same year as Louis Pasteur, the Austro-Hungarian monk Gregor Mendel (1822–1884) was another amateur scientist, a botanist. Experimenting with varieties of garden peas, he cross-pollinated them, observing and recording the results. Unfortunately he published his findings in an obscure journal, where they remained unnoticed for many years, but when they came to light 15 years after his death, Gregor Mendel was retroactively honored as the founder of the new science of genetics, which soon found many applications in clinical medicine with recognition of the fact that many inherited diseases were caused by genetic disorders. Almost 100 years after Mendel's death, other discoveries with great public health relevance, including development of genetically modified sterile insect vectors of disease, genetically resistant strains of food crops, and applications of genetic engineering to limit and even prevent some recessive inherited disorders. Genetics and genomic sciences (see chapters 6 and 9) may well transform public health during the 21st century.

CASE STUDY—JOSEPH GOLDBERGER AND PELLAGRA

The roles of social and economic factors that contribute to dietary deficiency diseases were studied intensively by Joseph Goldberger (1874–1929) and colleagues in their investigations of pellagra.[38] Pellagra was known in Spain and northern Italy,[39] first described by Don Gaspar Casal in 1735 among peasants in Spain, although he believed it to be a form of leprosy because of the nature of the skin rash.[40] Casal associated the disease with poverty and noted that the diet of pellagrins (that is, people with pellegra) consisted of cornmeal and little meat, thus suggesting that the cause was spoilage of corn. The introduction of American Indian corn into the Old World increased the food calorie yield per acre well beyond that of rye and wheat, and increased cultivation followed beginning in the second half of the 17th century. Cultivation of corn and its use as a staple crop moved from Spain to southern France, Italy, Romania, Russia, and Egypt, and pellagra moved as well. The theory that spoiled corn was the cause of pellagra persisted despite the lack of identification of an organism that could produce the symptoms in animals or in people.[39, 40]

The first cases of pellagra in the United States began to be reported in the early 1900s.[40] In 1906, eighty-eight cases were reported in a state hospital for the insane with a mortality rate of 64%. Reports of outbreaks rapidly increased first in other mental hospitals and moved to inmates of prisons, orphanages, and the general population. National data are incomplete, but by 1912, the state of South Carolina reported 30,000 cases with a mortality rate of 40%. By the 1920s there were 100,000 cases of pellagra per year with thirty-six states and the District of Columbia included in the reporting area, but nine southern states accounted for 90% of the cases. Overall the epidemic lasted from about 1906 to 1940 and resulted in 3 million cases with 100,000 deaths in the states involved in the reporting area.[40]

A commission convened to study the issue conducted a house-to-house survey in cotton mill districts and concluded there was no relationship between pellagra and diet, but rather that the disease was related to poor sanitation and that the disease occurred among people who lived with or next to homes where there was a case. No mention of poverty or the clustering of cases in the poorer areas of town where housing and sanitation facilities were worst was included in the report.[40] Laboratories were established in the affected areas and concerted attempts were made to find the causative infectious agent of the disease to no avail.

These failures and Goldberger's own observations when touring mental hospitals, orphanages, and cotton mill towns convinced him that germs did not cause the disease. In institutions, only the patients, inmates, and orphans contracted the disease, but staff never did. Goldberger knew from years of experience working on infectious diseases that germs did not distinguish between inmates and employees. He was also struck by the monotonous diet served at the institutions he visited: corn meal, molasses and meat, with the meat being mostly fatty pork.[39, 40]

Further, in the orphanages children between six and twelve years old were most affected, and he noted that infants were provided milk when it was available and older children worked and were fed a somewhat better diet. He experimented by providing a more varied diet with federal funds, including fresh meat once a week and sufficient quantities of milk for all the children. He began a similar study among patients in an asylum. Children and patients on the improved diets did not contract pellagra. When the money ran out, the diets reverted to the old one and pellagra returned to the institutions.[39, 40]

Critics who held to the theory of an infectious agent raised doubts about the results of his studies. Goldberger hoped to convince the opposition by studying healthy inmates on a prison farm that had never had a case of pellagra that he could induce the disease with an experimental dietary regime.[39, 40] With the cooperation of Mississippi's progressive governor, Earl Brewer, Goldberger experimented on eleven healthy volunteer prisoners at the Rankin State Prison Farm in 1915. Six of the eleven showed pellagra rashes after five months.[39, 40] However, the results were questioned because the governor had offered pardons to the participating inmates, and two were his friends. Several of the inmates were so ill they begged to be removed from the trial. Although the trial has been conducted in secrecy, the information began to appear in newspapers, and the governor was accused of having arranged the experiment to release his friends and was also convicted of embezzlement.[39, 40, 41]

Virtually complete elimination of pellagra did not occur until the 1940s with the identification of the specific micronutrient deficiency, nicotinic acid, and several other vitamins, including those in the B group including riboflavin.[40] Fortification of food resulted in the elimination of the disease. However, determining precisely why the epidemic occurred in the time and location that it did has never been thoroughly studied. It seems likely that this happened due to a change in processing of corn that resulted in de-germinating corn during the milling process which removes a layer of corn that contains lipid, enzymes, and cofactors including nicotinic acid.[40] The resulting corn meal is more stable and can be shipped without decay. Thus we are now aware that changes in food processing introduced for commercial benefit may result in disease outbreaks due to nutritional deficiencies that may occur as an unintended outcome.[40]

The Modern History of Public Health

It is common practice in writing histories to focus on what is already done, not what is still a work in progress. Hence, we have somewhat restricted the scope of the foregoing historical view to the work of early bacteriologists, nutritionists, pathologists, and public health interventionists. They represent an era that established the fact that microorganisms caused many diseases, that the germ theory was fact, not theory. But the same era ushered in awareness that it takes more than a "germ" to cause disease. For example, tuberculosis is caused by the tubercle bacillus acting in conjunction with poverty, ignorance, overcrowding, poor nutrition, adverse social and economic circumstances ,and other enabling and predisposing factors. Therefore prevention and control programs have to address much more than the direct agent involved in disease transmission to reduce the burden of disease (chapters 5 and 6).

Similarly, diarrheal diseases like cholera are caused by microorganisms, which get into the gut when ingested with contaminated water or food; in other words, they are more fundamentally caused by poor sanitary and hygienic practices. By late in the 19th century, many of these factors had been clarified. The stage was set for the health reforms of the "sanitary revolution," the beginnings of a social safety net, provision of immunizations, nutritional supplements for school children, prenatal care for pregnant women, and other essential public health functions that we address elsewhere in this book, some of which we may even take for granted.

Obviously more is needed than scientific discoveries. These must be applied, and this often requires changes in the established social and economic order. A different set of skills also is usually required to translate a scientific idea into an effective and efficient public health program. So other pioneers also appear on the road to health. They include journalists, creative writers, performing artists, cartoonists, administrators, professional leaders, and politicians.

Indeed, this has always been so, as shown by the role of activists throughout history, whether they be diarists such as John Evelyn (1620–1706), who alerted the English-speaking world with his 1661 submission to King Charles II and parliament: *Fumifugium: the Inconvenience of the Aer and Smoake of London Dissipated*, thereby bringing an important public issue to the attention of persons who set policy and wield power.[41] Consider also enlightened administrators such as Edwin Chadwick (1800–1890), whose *Inquiry into the Sanitary Conditions of the Labouring Classes* ushered in major reforms (discussed earlier) to improve the health prospects of people living in urban slums.[42] And do not put aside the likes of Florence Nightingale: best known for her work on sanitation and nursing conditions during the Crimean war, she was a pioneer in the graphical use of statistics to make a vivid case to authorities that dire health situations required attention.[43] A contemporary of William

Farr, at the Fourth International Statistical Congress (London, 1860), she urged adoption of Farr's classification of diseases for the tabulation of hospital morbidity in her paper *Proposals for a uniform plan of hospital statistics*.[12]

By now the reader will have observed that it is mostly men who are recognized in the history of public health, although this is rapidly changing as a result of positive shifts in the status of women, especially in western industrialized states during the 20th century. While it is beyond our scope to delve into the realm of women's rights as such, as an exemplar of this trend, and also as a lens through which we can appreciate the historical gender imbalance, we focus now on Alice Hamilton (1869–1970), a founder of occupational medicine in the United States.

Hamilton was the first woman academician at Harvard Medical School and first woman to receive the Lasker Award in Public Health (1947). She was appointed director of the Occupational Disease Commission of Illinois in 1910 when it was created by the state governor. First of its kind in the world, the commission was responsible for several worker's compensation laws in Illinois and introduced the novel notion that workers were entitled to compensation for health impairment and injuries sustained on the job. Hamilton was asked by the US Commissioner of Labor to replicate her research on a national level but was not offered a salary. She studied hazards posed by exposure to lead, arsenic, mercury, organic solvents, as well as radium (used in manufacturing watch dials). She remained in this unsalaried post from 1911 to 1921 when her program was cancelled after pro-business Republicans gained control of the White House. Hamilton was a supporter of peace and, along with Jane Addams and Emily Balch, traveled in Europe encouraging the end of World War I. The group became the Women's International League for Peace and Freedom. In 1919, she was offered and accepted the post of assistant professor of Industrial Medicine at Harvard Medical School. There were three restrictions on her appointment: she was not allowed to use the Faculty Club, she had no access to football tickets, and she could not march in commencement processions. Harvard did not admit women students until World War II, therefore all her students were males. After 1925, she was also appointed to the faculty of the Harvard School of Public Health. She published *Industrial Poisons in the United States* (1925) and *Industrial Toxicology* (1934) and following retirement in 1935, became a consultant to the Division of Labor Standards, US Labor Department. In 1943, she published an autobiography entitled *Exploring the Dangerous Trades*. Hamilton received many honorary degrees, distinctions, and awards, including a listing in Men of Science in 1944. It is noteworthy that her final academic rank was Assistant Professor Emeritus of Industrial Medicine, meaning despite her many accomplishments she was never promoted.[44]

This brings to a close our reconnaissance of public health history from prehistoric to modern times as a window on its aims and methods. In so doing, we have highlighted some of those who made observations and investigated them using the science of their times, and others who translated the resulting concepts of public health to the public at large and to enlightened politicians, who in turn are indispensable partners in a team that makes it possible for society to advance along the road to better health. The process continues in contemporary times with similarly dedicated individuals, whose work is now further enhanced by investigative journalism, TV documentaries, You-Tube videos, blogging, and other social media, all of which has a role.

Disciplines in Public Health

The field of public health comprises many disciplines. For example, for the purposes of accreditation of schools of public health in the United States five core knowledge categories are specified.[45] Accreditation requirements vary across countries (reflecting their priorities), but for illustrative purposes it is useful to review these five disciplinary categories briefly here:

- **Biostatistics**—collection, storage, retrieval, analysis, and interpretation of health data; design and analysis of health-related surveys and experiments; and concepts and practice of statistical data analysis
- **Epidemiology**—distributions and determinants of disease, disabilities, and death in human populations; the characteristics and dynamics of human populations; and the natural history of disease and the biologic basis of health
- **Environmental and occupational health sciences**—environmental and occupational factors including biological, physical, and chemical factors that affect the health of a community and workers
- **Health services administration**—planning, organization, administration, management, evaluation, and policy analysis of health and public health programs
- **Social and behavioral sciences**—concepts and methods of social and behavioral sciences relevant to the identification and solution of public health problems

Biostatistics is the application of statistics to biological and medical problems and is considered a basic science of public health. Epidemiology is a basic science of public health and is the study of the distribution and determinants of health-related states or events in specific populations and the application of derived knowledge from studies to the control of health problems. Social and behavioral sciences include the application of health promotion and health education to protect the health of the population. Environmental health sciences are concerned with the whole range of environmental determinants of health (physical, chemical, biological, social, and behavioral) and with diseases of environmental and occupational origins. Health services administration encompasses the role of public health practitioners in monitoring equitable distribution of services, ensuring policies are in place to support health and are working as intended, as well as evaluating costs related to public health programs and medical services.

For each of these disciplines there are a number of textbooks available. It is not our intention to replicate the detailed information already available in such texts, but rather to show the intersection of them in the context of general public health practice using an ecological perspective. Elsewhere in this book (chapters 2, 4, and 8) we explore the competencies required of public health practitioners and core public health functions at all levels from local to global.

Conclusion

Public health practice changes with new discoveries and the emergence of new diseases, as well as changes in social and economic circumstances and new ways of thinking. Understanding the fundamental principles that are used in developing public health programs can be enhanced by reviewing the history of public health as we have briefly done in this chapter. For those who wish to explore this further, there are a number of sources (Box 1-1) that discuss in more detail these and other historical accomplishments in public health. The future of public health belongs to those who continue to build upon this proud history through their vision, insights, efforts, and actions to promote and improve the health of present and future generations.

BOX 1-1
THE HISTORY OF PUBLIC HEALTH

Selected Sources

- McNeill WH. Plagues and People. Anchor Books. New York. 1998.
- Milestones in Public Health: Accomplishments in public health over the last 100 years. Pfizer Global Pharmaceuticals. New York, NY. 2006.
- Porter D. Health, Civilization and the State. Routledge Press. New York. 1999.
- Rosen G. A History of Public Health. Expanded Edition. Johns Hopkins University Press. 1993.
- Zinnser H. Rats, Lice and History. Transaction Publishers. New Jersey. 2008.

This chapter introduces the scientific and professional disciplines that form the foundation of an ecological approach to public health, especially regarding how health depends on the way in which people relate to their biological, physical, and social environments. The chapter will help public health professionals understand how this array of disciplines contributes to public health policies, programs, and approaches to foster health and well-being in communities and in the population as a whole. These are the same sciences that provide a basis for effective interventions that reduce risk from disease through developing and delivering effective methods of prevention and control. The chapter concludes with a selection of case studies to illustrate how public health sciences have proven critical in the search for effective interventions.

2

ECOLOGY AND PUBLIC HEALTH—THE SCIENCE BASE

PUBLIC HEALTH IS in essence ecological because health is determined in a multi-level environment that comprises all the physical, biological, social, cultural, behavioral, and spiritual forces that affect our development throughout our lives. All living organisms alter their environment to some extent by the mere fact of existing, but the interaction of humans and the environment is uniquely marked by the magnitude of the effect of the organism on the environment. The changes that people have produced are truly massive, with far reaching results on the nature of plant and animal life, the shape of physical features, and changes in climate.

In a broad sense, the structure of human society is determined by our biological characteristics and is modified by the immediate physical environment. However, the boundaries between the biological, social, and physical influences on human health and development are not clearly demarcated, and the three are in many ways overlapping and interdependent.

Biological Environment

Biological sciences include those disciplines involved in studying living organisms such as biology, botany, ecology, entomology, genetics, immunology, microbiology, nutrition, pathology, and zoology.

The biological environment consists of the plants and animals with which we share our world. It serves as a source of food, shelter, implements, fiber, drugs, disease agents, and nonhuman companionship. It is not quite right to say that we depend upon the biological world for our survival, with the implication that we stand apart from the biological environment and draw our sustenance from it. Rather our dependence is more like the dependence of a child on the family; but the child is also a part of the family, with innate capabilities that are the result of the endowment received from the family. From the moment of conception, the child's characteristics are modulated by the characteristics of the family. Likewise, human beings are a product of the biological environment; humans alter it, and are altered by it and remain a part of it.

Numerous noxious agents arise from the biological environment, including toxins and allergens from plant pollens, spores, organic house dust, feathers, moulds, and dander (dandruff) from the skin of animals, that can provoke severe allergic respiratory and dermatological disorders. Some of this is seasonal (e.g., hay fever), but other conditions can occur year-round. Plant juices from poison ivy and sumac can result in vesicular dermatitis while foods such as strawberries and seafood can cause allergic reactions ranging from mild urticaria to anaphylactic shock. Highly toxic substances can occur in potentially lethal amounts in nature: certain wild mushrooms are inedible, raw manioc root or cassava must be cooked to destroy the cyanide they contain, apricot kernels also contain cyanide and must be avoided as a food source, and bivalve mollusks can accumulate high levels of toxins produced by microscopic algae (dinoflagellates) when in bloom, which is why there is a regulated shellfish season in many parts of the world. Some plants may be therapeutic in certain dosages but toxic in overdoses such as cinchona tree bark (quinine) or foxglove leaves (digitalis). Others can be addictive, toxic, and therapeutic, such as the Oriental poppy (opium and its derivatives).

Reflecting their view of the biological world, ecologists have developed the concept of the ecological pyramid (Figure 2-1). This pyramid represents the flow of energy through the food chain, thus illustrating relationships between organisms in a particular ecosystem.

The base of the pyramid comprises organisms capable of synthesizing complex organic substances (e.g., carbohydrates) from simple inorganic materials by using light as an energy source (photosynthesis) or through chemical energy (chemosynthesis). These organisms are eaten by others, who are thus spared the necessity of starting at such an elemental level, and they in turn serve the nutritional needs of higher-order predators: this is also known as the "food chain." There is a rough correlation between increasing size, decreasing numbers, and higher-order predation. Also, as the food chain pyramid is ascended, there is a significant decrease in the efficiency of energy transfer.

Since the primary food synthesizers form the foundation of the pyramid, it follows that the nature of soil and vegetation in an area determines the nature of the

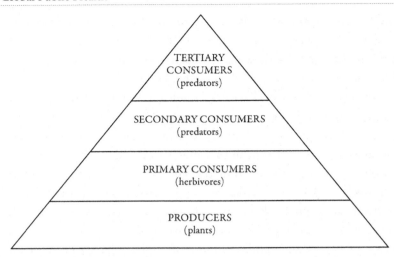

FIGURE 2-1 Ecological Pyramid.

animal life that depends on it for food. The nature of the vegetation depends substantially on three factors: the physical features of the area, humans inhabiting the area, and chance. Humans have exerted a profound influence on vegetation through agricultural activities and through the transport of plant species into areas where they previously did not exist.

Physical features such as topography, climate, rainfall, and the texture and chemical composition of the soil play a role in establishing terrestrial plant life. Similarly, the distribution and variety of marine vegetation are affected by analogous factors. Control is exercised by selection of species that are capable of existing best under a particular combination of these factors; the less fit are starved or crowded into a more specialized ecological niche or otherwise face extinction. The parallels between the influences exerted through these processes reveal that it is difficult to separate the physical and biological environment.

Human beings are an important contributor to the landscape. Our behavior operates through a number of ways, including use of fire and tools to clear land, selection of specific plants to nurture, importation of foreign species, breeding and cross-breeding livestock to develop more economically desirable forms, establishing water supplies independent of local climate, and changing soil characteristics in dramatic ways.

Ultimately, chance plays a role in many places, for instance, where certain types of plants are introduced inadvertently by animals, migratory birds, variations in currents of wind or water, or transported on people's clothing or shoes. Another manner by which chance changes are introduced is through mutation, which may be predictable in the aggregate, but specific mutations that allow one version to subsist a little more successfully and thus replace less adaptable forms cannot always be foreseen.

These, then, are the basic determinants of that part of the environment that is mostly green and waves in sea currents or in the breeze.

Animal life is influenced by the same set of factors, although the emphasis is placed a little differently. This is a very important additional factor of the nature of vegetation: vegetation affects plant eaters, and plant eaters in turn affect animal eaters, and so on through the entire ecological pyramid, thus reflecting a complex array of relationships from symbiosis to parasitism. The improved reproductive advantage of organisms with favorable traits is referred to generally as *natural selection,* the process that lies at the core of evolution.

Human beings emerged in an environment that was presumably optimal for our species, or at least highly satisfactory. There are fierce arguments about whether or not parallel evolution of different strains of hominids proceeded in different places. However this may be, as the number of people increased or people followed game for food, there was migration into many parts of the world, some of them clearly not optimal. Until quite recently, there was still ample room for expansion into areas where climate did not pose intolerable problems and where food, water, and shelter were available at reasonable expenditures of effort. Now such unoccupied territory is not easily found, and further increases in human population will cause greater population density, which will pose ever more severe demands on the readily available resources. An alternative to increasing the efficiency of utilization of present resources is the development of a means of living satisfactorily in areas where human habitation is now restricted by shortages of food or water or climate extremes of heat or cold. Thus, for example, much effort is currently devoted to making sea water potable and usable for irrigation, and to increasing the efficiency of harvesting food from the ocean, which itself is coming under increasing threat as a result of overfishing and unforeseen consequences of fish farming. As a result of such developments, there is a contentious debate about the Earth's carrying capacity. The limiting factor is fresh water. This issue will be addressed further in chapter 7.

Physical Environment

Physical sciences include disciplines that analyze the nature and properties of energy and nonliving matter, including chemistry, physics, earth sciences, engineering, and environmental sciences.

The physical environment has been traditionally viewed as the natural environment that includes geological structures, the topography, temperature, humidity, precipitation, solar radiation, air quality and composition, audible sound, and water availability, quality, and composition. However, in a more contemporary sense, our physical environment has also come to include built environments, such as buildings, industries, farming and mining communities, parks, playgrounds, and transportation modalities in which we live, work, and travel. Human settlements take many forms, some more conducive to good health, others less so. We examine the community foundations of public health in chapter 4, but within the domain of built environments it is also clear that we have created a wide range of micro-environments, which give rise to physical challenges to good health.

There are numerous examples of buildings and other enclosed spaces that have been constructed, ventilated, heated, or cooled in a manner that has contributed directly to outbreaks of diseases. Environmental health scientists in recent decades have focused on exposure to substances that cause chronic illnesses, such as pulmonary disease, cancers of various types, birth defects, and neurological disorders. The exposures have tended to be inanimate—chemicals, noise, and dusts—although organic exposures also play important roles, and all such influences may be confounded by factors that affect individual susceptibility. Examples of such work includes studies of air pollution associated with respiratory symptoms, impaired lung function, and aggravation of asthma; specific pesticide exposures associated with cancer, stillbirths, and birth defects; and lead exposures associated with declines in mental acuity among children.

Community studies of air pollution have documented that there are highly susceptible individuals within communities, such as older adults and individuals with pre-existing chronic conditions such as asthma and heart disease, who will be more likely to be hospitalized during periods of high levels of air pollution. Similarly, exposure to airborne hazards can be aggravated by ergonomic factors, such as level of exertion, rate and depth of breathing, and physical stature, while underlying immune conditions and personal habits such as smoking also can render some individuals more susceptible than others.

The physical environment also contributes greatly to the propagation and transmission of infectious agents and has long been studied from this perspective. As a result of such work, housing conditions are now widely used as a socioeconomic indicator of health: poor housing quality and overcrowding are associated with poverty and increased vulnerability to disease. For example, poor air quality within homes as a result of inadequate ventilation and presence of mold and smoke contribute to poor respiratory health in general and are implicated in the spread and/or outcome of tuberculosis.[1] The same principles of indoor air quality also apply to large buildings: Legionnaire's disease is a classic example of this, as is described in one of the case studies in this chapter.

Social Environment

Social sciences involve the study of human society and of individual relationships in and to society such as administration and management, anthropology, communication studies, criminology, economics, education, geography, history, leadership, political science, and sociology.

The social environment includes all things involved with the organization of people, for example, politics, economics, culture, religious faiths, philosophies of life, and occupations. A few thousand years ago, small bands of humans roamed forests and fields, subsisting on hunting and food gathering. Gradually this economic pattern was largely supplanted by planting and harvesting and the husbandry of

BOX 2-1
SOCIAL DETERMINANTS OF HEALTH

Individual
- Age
- Gender
- Ethnicity
- Migration status
- Occupation/employment status
- Socioeconomic status/poverty/educational attainment

Social
Family structure
- Separation, divorce
- Single-parent family
- Group marriage, commune
- Homosexual pair or group

Stage of family evolution
- Formation
- Child rearing
- Maturing family
- "Empty nest"
- Caring for older family members
- Bereaved survivor

(continued)

BOX 2-1 (Continued)

Social networks
- School based
- Neighborhood based
- Work based
- Church based
- Club/society based

Community
Culture
- Attitudes and beliefs

Political/social
- Access to credit
- Local policies

Society
Political
- State/provincial and national policies

domesticated animals. The development of these technologies greatly increased the carrying capacity of desirable acreage and, as land values came to reflect this and social systems appeared, human populations increased. Global population growth since the late 19th century (chapter 5) has been attributed mostly to improvements in nutrition, child survival, and sustained high birth rates.

Specialization of function within evolving economies was accompanied by development and growth of urban communities and the expansion of commerce. The process of urbanization was vastly accelerated by the industrial revolution and is continuing for reasons related to the complex nature of postindustrial societies. Human diseases evolved and changed as the pattern of life changed, as described in chapter 1.

Living in one place has the major disadvantages that things that were chasing you have a chance to catch up and things that you used to leave behind accumulate. Thus, in the history of diseases, early settlements provided an environment where disease agents formerly encountered occasionally and accidentally became adapted to the human condition and became common. Disease vectors and some animal reservoirs for microbial pathogens adjusted to life around human habitation. Certain animals that actually or potentially harbored disease agents pathogenic for man were domesticated, or otherwise became symbiotic with human settlement, thereby increasing the probability that those agents would be transmitted to and sometimes from people. Social factors that influence disease patterns include occupation, socioeconomic status, the cultural milieu (e.g. food preferences, religious practices, beliefs, and attitudes), and the network of family, friends, and working groups to which individuals belong. These factors influence disease patterns in populations through altering exposure to agents of disease and injury or by altering susceptibility when individuals are exposed to hazards.

Measuring Health

The definition and measurement of health has evolved not only with greater understanding of disease, the risk factors for disease, and their underlying determinants, but also with an increasing emphasis on well-being even when individuals are living with chronic and disabling conditions, by acknowledging the importance of mental and emotional health as well as physical diseases (chapter 1). This shift has allowed public health professionals to move beyond solely focusing on disease prevention to embrace the broader principles of health promotion. New concepts of health are emerging, and these, too, require measurement.

In order to appreciate disease prevention as an approach to health, one must develop an understanding of the natural history of disease (chapter 6). Central to this is a system of classification. *What is disease?* The word *disease* itself derives from "dis-ease" meaning the opposite of ease or comfort. It implies any departure from good health, or from normal physiological or psychological function, and therefore also encompasses "disorders." Operationally, disease is defined by clinical, pathological, and epidemiological criteria that enable systematic study and application. As discrete entities, diseases and disorders have been organized within classification systems into categories—infectious, chronic noninfectious, traumatic, psychological—then subclassified into specific conditions.

Measuring health in populations requires use of uniform indicators for the purpose of comparing health across different communities. The most basic indicators are based on births, deaths, illnesses, and injuries. As knowledge advances, classification revisions are updated; for example, the World Health Organization's International

BOX 2-2

See this website for more about evidence based public health:
   http://phpartners.org/tutorial/04-ebph/index.html
   Accessed January 2, 2012

Classification of Diseases (ICD) is in its 10th revision, with development of the 11th revision in process. Other bodies contribute, such as the International Health Terminology Standards Development Organization (IHTSDO), which focuses on clinical terminology for health records management, and the American Psychiatric Association, which provides the Diagnostic and Statistical Manual of Mental Disorders (DSM). Comparability of categorizing deaths by cause is accomplished through the International Classification of Disease (ICD) coding system (chapter 1). In recent decades new efforts have been made to define and measure health *per se*, not only inversely by measures of morbidity, mortality, and life expectancy, but also through means such as self-assessed health status, quality of life,[2] and happiness and indirect measures such as income inequality.[3]

HEALTH INFORMATION SYSTEMS

Many aspects of public health require analysis on an ongoing basis. Detailed descriptions of how to approach assessing the health of communities and of larger populations, including the topic of health indicators, are presented in chapters 4 and 5.

Evidence-Based Public Health

Evidence-based public health is defined as the development, implementation, and evaluation of effective public health programs and policies by applying principles of scientific reasoning, including systematic uses of data and information systems, and appropriate use of behavioral science theory and program planning models.[4,5,6]

STANDARDS OF EVIDENCE

The call for evidence-based[7] disease prevention and health promotion has triggered an international debate among researchers, practitioners, health promotion advocates, and policy makers on what should constitute standards of evidence for public health interventions. Such standards are needed to avoid invalid conclusions about the outcomes of intervention trials (internal validity) or about the expected outcomes of interventions when implemented in different sites, settings, and cultures (external validity or generalizability). In the interest of the targeted populations and cost-effectiveness of programs, evidence should meet the highest possible standards.

In evidence-based medicine, the randomized controlled trial (RCT) is widely accepted as the "gold standard" and the best strategy to reduce the risk of invalid conclusions from research. Nevertheless, in prevention, health promotion, and public health research, the RCT has limitations. The design is appropriate for studying causal influences at an individual level using interventions in a highly controlled context. However, many disease prevention, health promotion, and other public health interventions address people within group settings, such as schools, companies, communities, or larger population groups (states, countries). Some studies have used randomization of school classes and whole schools; however, such designs have their own methodological challenges, can be difficult to conduct, and often require long-standing relationships between researchers and the groups involved.

Therefore, other research designs, such as quasi-experimental studies and time-series designs, are also considered valuable strategies for developing the evidence base in public health. These research strategies have been used successfully to evaluate the impact of national legislation and policy measures to reduce the use of alcohol, tobacco, and illicit drugs. In certain situations, qualitative studies are also necessary to obtain insight into facilitating factors and barriers to developing and implementing effective programs and policies. For the sustainability of programs in communities, use of qualitative methods can increase the likelihood that proper commitment to program success is in place before implementing a program.

To increase the evidence base needed to ensure programs will be successful in new communities or among different populations, priority needs to be given to replication studies across communities and countries. Such studies are needed to understand what role variation in cultural and economic conditions plays when similar interventions are implemented in new settings. They also help identify which adaptations are needed in such settings to maintain outcomes found earlier. Most of the current public health and prevention research has been implemented in developed countries, especially in the United States. To a large extent the accessibility and use of evidence-based interventions and prevention knowledge worldwide may be hampered if such programs are not adapted to other situations. This said, it is important that public health researchers and practitioners also value the research that is increasingly carried out in developing countries, and the emergence of a literature that caters to this, especially because what is relevant varies with the health situation of particular countries. For example, the "10/90 gap" refers to the finding of the Global Forum for Health Research that only 10% of worldwide expenditure on health research and development is devoted to the problems that primarily affect the poorest 90% of the world's population.[8] Another underlying principle also applies: lessons learned from developing countries can be of value to developed ones as well (e.g., large-scale field trials of vaccines and micronutrients, related health systems research). Being able to locate and assess research from many parts of the world is an increasingly valuable asset for public health everywhere.

In the adoption of evidence-based prevention programs and the international trend to promote "best practices" across countries and communities, questions arise about the appropriate standard of evidence that needs to be available in order to decide about their adoption, reimplementation, or large-scale implementation.[9] It is difficult to provide general rules for such decisions that are valid across countries because of differences in cultural practices, health literacy, and economic circumstances. For further discussion of this and the challenges of "scaling up" interventions and sustainability see chapter 4.

AIM OF EVIDENCE-BASED PRACTICE

The aim of evidence-based practice is to improve preventive and health promotion practices, patient care, and health care delivery and to contain costs by demonstrating the links between interventions and health outcomes and by continuous monitoring of program outcomes. Evidence-based practice was originally developed in clinical medicine to provide clinicians with information about therapies that work and those that do not. Although the need for evidence-based practice is now widely accepted, it was not until 1952 when the randomized controlled trial appeared in a publication about the value of streptomycin in the treatment of pulmonary tuberculosis.[10] This approach provided the medical community with an experimental design that could be used in applied medical research, and it opened a new world of evaluation and control that has extended beyond application to selection of the most effective and efficient therapies to encompass evidence-based public health. British epidemiologist Archie Cochrane set out the principle that because resources would always be limited they should be used to provide equitable distribution of forms of health care shown to be effective using randomized controlled trials. He further suggested there be a critical summary of all relevant randomized controlled trials. This challenge led to the establishment of an international collaboration to develop a database on perinatal trials. Following his death in 1988 and named in his honor, this led to the opening of the first Cochrane Center in 1992 and the founding of The Cochrane Collaboration in 1993. The Cochrane Collaboration is an international network of people helping health providers, policy makers, patients, advocates, and caregivers make informed decisions about health care. The Cochrane Library provides over 4000 reviews that are updated and accessible (www.cochrane.org).

In 2010, the first joint Colloquium of the Cochrane and Campbell Collaborations was held in Keystone, Colorado. The Campbell Collaboration is a comparable international effort founded in 2000 to prepare, maintain, and disseminate systematic reviews of the effects of social interventions in education, crime, and justice and social welfare. Systematic reviews are designed to assess the best available evidence on a specific question through synthesis of the results of studies. Studies are screened for quality and include clear inclusion/exclusion criteria, a specific search strategy, systematic coding and analysis of included study, and a meta-analysis.

Shifting from evidence-based medicine to evidence-based public health requires recognizing different operational realities and therefore incorporating some different principles. Public health research involves more quasi-experimental studies and is less likely to have many randomized controlled trials to evaluate. The interventions involved tend to take longer than those in clinical medicine, and the training of those conducting them in local settings is often less formal than in clinical medicine, sometimes with no formal certification required, particularly when conducted by voluntary organizations and community advocates who have particular interest in a specific cause. To address some of these fundamental differences in the United States, the Guide to Community Preventive Services was developed under the leadership of the federally appointed Community Preventive Services Task Force. The Task Force oversees systematic reviews led by Centers for Disease Control and Prevention (CDC) scientists to consider and summarize results of systematic reviews, make recommendations for interventions that promote population health, and identify areas within the reviewed topics that need more research. The Task Force was established in 1996 by the US Department of Health and Human Services (DHHS) to develop guidance on which community-based health promotion and disease prevention interventions work and which do not. Systematic reviews involve identifying relevant intervention studies via a clearly defined search strategy, assessing the quality of the studies identified by using established criteria, and summarizing the overall evidence of effectiveness and applicability (which may vary enormously by setting) of the interventions being reviewed.

The potential benefits of evidence-based public health decisions include program planners having access to a wide range of interventions that are documented to be effective and, where possible to determine, were deemed cost-effective as well. Fewer resources will be wasted on programs that are not effective, and in the long term, community health outcomes will be improved. The implementation of fewer but more effective programs will also aid in institutionalization of public health practice on a national level and may serve to reduce the wide variation in public health delivery systems that currently exists. Topics reviewed to date include adolescent health, alcohol, asthma, birth defects, cancer, diabetes, HIV/AIDs, sexually transmitted infections and pregnancy, mental health, motor vehicle injuries, nutrition, obesity, oral health, physical activity, social environment, tobacco, vaccines, violence, and worksite health. Evaluation of the utility of this approach for community organizations and public health professionals is needed to determine whether there is increased use of the interventions that have been determined to be effective through the systematic review approach. Other countries also have comparable systems for assessing evidence as applicable in their contexts (e.g., in Canada the National Collaborating Centre for Methods and Tools, at McMaster University).[11]

COMMUNITY-BASED PARTICIPATORY RESEARCH

Traditional approaches that use outside experts and develop interventions that do not adequately address the context in which they are being delivered have led to disappointing results and probably have led to increased demands by community leaders and residents for more truly collaborative approaches (see Chapter 4 on community participation).[12] Community-based participatory research (CBPR) is a collaborative process of research involving researchers and community representatives; it engages community members, employs local knowledge in the understanding of health problems and the design of interventions, and commits community members to the processes and products of research. In addition, community members are invested in the dissemination and use of research findings and ultimately in the reduction of health disparities.[13] The approach has historical roots in development programs in emerging economies, where programs designed without input from those affected tended to be unsuccessful.

CBPR is a collaborative research process that recognizes the unique strengths of all participants and begins with a research topic of importance within a community. It aims to combine knowledge and action for social change to improve community health and to eliminate health disparities. Key elements of the approach are that it is participatory; it is cooperative, involving community members and researchers contributing equally; it invokes a colearning process; it involves systems development and local community capacity building; it is empowering for participants and leads to increased control for participants over their lives; and it achieves a balance between research and action. CBPR is an approach to social change, and while research is one part of the process, it is not the only one. For this reason it is sometimes referred to as "action research." There are three main goals in CBPR: learning knowledge and skills relevant for the program; developing relationships; and engaging in actions that are successful and that build self-sufficiency.

Competencies in Public Health

The preceding sections reveal that public health professionals need to acquire a range of knowledge, values, and skills so as to be capable of working with professionals from a wide range of disciplines. This multidisciplinary science base has also been organized by the profession into core competencies, so as to provide guidance for how it can be integrated within the design and assessment of training programs. It is for this reason that core competencies are now presented in this chapter. Contemporary education in public health is now substantially guided by core competencies; this integrates and expands on the traditional approach of addressing component disciplines separately.

In fact, this is becoming a global movement: public health professionals in many parts of the world are recognizing the need to specify the core competencies required for a trained public health workforce appropriate to their settings. In part this reflects the growing professionalism of the field in response to the increasing complexity of some public health issues. There is also recognition that many people enter this field from other areas of the health profession or even from outside the health professions, with clinical, management, or research backgrounds but without preparation in disciplines essential to competent public health practice. In some traditional settings it is common for individuals to be promoted based on seniority or even political consideration. A key need everywhere is to advance the public health human resource on the basis of professional competence.

This move to define public health core competencies is taking place in several parts of the world; it can be considered a work-in-progress everywhere it is taking place. In Canada, the competencies include public health sciences, assessment and analysis, policy and program planning, implementation and evaluation, partnership, collaboration and advocacy, diversity and inclusiveness, communication, and leadership.[14] Themes proposed for competencies in Europe are similar but worded differently. Grouped into themes, they include methods (epidemiology and biostatistics; qualitative); social environment and health; physical, chemical, and biological environment and health; health policy, organization, management and economics, health promotion and prevention, cross-disciplinary themes including strategy making; ethics and related themes.[15]

The purpose of this movement is to help guide the health human resource development efforts that are vital for public health organizations to achieve their aim to protect and promote the health of populations. For more detailed illustration, the approach being taken in the United States is relevant. The US approach recognizes three tiers of skill from entry level to senior managers across eight key domains, within which are defined specific professional and technical skills. The first tier applies to public health professionals who carry out day-to-day tasks of public health organizations and are not in management positions. Responsibilities of tier one professionals include basic data collection and analysis, fieldwork, program planning, outreach activities, programmatic support, and other organizational tasks.

Tier two competencies apply to individuals with program management and supervisory responsibilities and may include program development, program implementation, program evaluation, establishment and maintainence of community relations, management of timelines and work plans, and presentation of arguments, and recommendations on policy issues. Tier three competencies apply to senior management and leaders in public health organizations responsible for managing major programs or organizational functions, setting strategies and vision, and building the organizational culture, and they typically have staff reporting to them. The domains addressed are analytical assessment skills, policy development and program planning skills, communications skills, cultural competency skills, community dimensions of practice skills, public health science skills, financial planning and management skills, and leadership and systems thinking skills. Examples from each domain and the expected competency by tier are presented in Table 2-1.[16] These efforts to define core competencies are also supported by an evolving range of other documented guidelines and assessment toolkits that go beyond the scope of this limited introduction.

In the United States, the Association of Schools of Public Health includes five core disciplinary areas (discussed in chapter 1) which must be present for institutional accreditation purposes (biostatistics, environmental health sciences, epidemiology, health policy management, and social and behavioral sciences) and, in addition, an integrated interdisciplinary, cross-cutting set of overall competency domains (communication and informatics, diversity and culture, leadership, professionalism, program planning, public health biology, and systems thinking).[17] Although training requirements differ across countries, there is substantial similarity in the professional training needed for developing a competent public health workforce in all countries.

Conclusion

The knowledge base that contributes to development of successful public health programs is constantly undergoing change. Through critical review of the underlying science and the evolving knowledge base, public health professionals are able to develop more effective prevention programs. Using the evidence-based public health program approach coupled with a community participation, it is possible to modify programs as needed, ensure that successful programs continue, and eliminate unnecessary programs while ensuring sustainability of public health programs and policies within communities. Training of public health professionals needs to focus on core competencies so that professionals can apply their knowledge and skills to changing public health challenges.

TABLE 2-1

Core Competencies For Public Health Professionals[12]

Selected Examples

Analytical/Assessment Skills (selected from 13 specific competencies)

Tier 1	Tier 2	Tier 3
1A1. Identifies the health status of populations and their related determinants	1B1. Assesses the health status of populations and their related determinants of health and illness	1C1. Reviews the health status of populations and their related determinants of health and illness conducted by the organization

Policy Development/Program Planning Skills (selected from 10 specific competencies)

Tier 1	Tier 2	Tier 3
2A1. Gathers information relevant to specific public health policy issues.	2B1. Analyzes information relevant to specific public health policy issues.	2C1. Evaluates information relevant to specific public health policy issues.

Communication Skills (selected from 7 specific competencies)

Tier 1	Tier 2	Tier 3
3A1. Identifies the health literacy of populations served.	3B1. Assesses the health literacy of the populations served.	3C1. Ensures that the health literacy of the populations served is considered throughout all communication strategies.

Cultural Competency Skills (selected from 7 specific competencies)

Tier 1	Tier 2	Tier 3
4A1. Incorporates strategies for interacting with persons of diverse backgrounds.	4B1. Incorporates strategies for interacting with persons of diverse backgrounds.	4C1. Ensures that there are strategies for interacting with persons from diverse backgrounds.

Community Dimensions of Practice Skills (selected from 11 specific competencies)

Tier 1	Tier 2	Tier 3
5A1. Recognizes community linkages and relationships among multiple factors (or determinants) affecting health.	5B1. Assesses community linkages and relationships among multiple factors (or determinants) affecting health.	5C1. Evaluates the community linkages and relationships among multiple factors (or determinants) affecting health.

(continued)

TABLE 2-1 (Continued)

Public Health Sciences Skills (selected from 10 specific competencies)

Tier 1	Tier 2	Tier 3
6A1. Describes the scientific foundation of the field of public health.	6B1. Discusses the scientific foundation of the field of public health.	6C1. Critiques the scientific foundation of the field of public health.

Financial Planning and Management Skills (selected from 17 specific competencies)

Tier 1	Tier 2	Tier 3
7A1. Describes the local, states, and federal public health and health care systems.	7B1. Interprets the interrelationships of local, state, and federal public health and health care systems for public health program management.	7C1. Leverages the interrelationships of local, state, and federal public health and health care systems for public health program management.

Leadership and Systems Thinking Skills (selected from 9 specific competencies)

Tier 1	Tier 2	Tier 3
8A1. Incorporates ethical standards of practice as the basis of all interactions with organizations, communities, and individuals.	8B1. Incorporates ethical standards of practice as the basis of all interactions with organizations, communities, and individuals.	8C1. Incorporates ethical standards of practice as the basis of all interactions with organizations, communities, and individuals.

CASE STUDIES—SCIENCES IN SEARCH OF EFFECTIVE
PUBLIC HEALTH INTERVENTIONS

Case Study: Biological Sciences in Disease Control

Smallpox Eradication

One of the most frequently cited examples of the application of biological sciences to control human disease is the eradication of smallpox.[18, 19, 20]

The possibility of eradicating smallpox was first raised by Jenner himself in 1801 (see chapter 1) and in the same year Carl, in Prague, advocated smallpox eradication by a combination of surveillance and vaccination. Not until 1923, when an international register of infectious diseases was established as an agency of the League of Nations, was it possible to begin to understand the geographic extent of smallpox.[15] Many countries failed to report, so it was not until 1946 when the World Health Organization replaced the earlier organization that most countries of the world began providing regular reports of the occurrence of smallpox.[15] In Europe, countrywide elimination of endemic smallpox was achieved between 1930 and 1950 and by 1958 endemic disease was eliminated from that continent.[15]

Progressive increases in the number of smallpox-free countries were seen in the Americas and in Asia, but there was little change in Africa and the Indian subcontinent.[15, 17] In 1958 a Soviet delegation to the World Health Organization proposed worldwide eradication of smallpox; the proposal was approved by the World Health Assembly the following year.[15] Between 1959 and 1966, further gains in smallpox-free countries were made in South America and Asia, in particular the Peoples' Republic of China, but smallpox was rampant in the Indian subcontinent and in most of Africa.[15, 17] In 1967 the Intensified Smallpox Eradication Programme was established by WHO with the goal to eradicate smallpox in the next decade.[15] A Smallpox Eradication Unit was established at WHO in Geneva, funding was supplied by a regular budget, and a young American public health worker, D. A. Henderson, was appointed chief of the Unit.[15] The Unit first surveyed the incidence of endemic smallpox worldwide, assessed the quality and quantity of smallpox vaccine, especially in endemic countries that were mostly in the tropics, and assessed the effectiveness of national smallpox eradication programs in the endemic countries.[15]

Smallpox, at the time, was endemic in 33 countries, with imported cases reported in another 11 countries. The number of reported cases was 131,697, believed to be about 1% of the actual cases.[15, 17] Methods were available for large-scale production of a good freeze-dried vaccine, which provided transport and storage without requiring refrigeration. However, many endemic countries were using liquid vaccine whose stability under tropical conditions allowed perhaps 15–20% of the vaccine used in the field to be of acceptable potency.[15,17] Under the leadership of Dr. Isao Arita, from Japan, the WHO Smallpox Eradication Unit undertook a major campaign to upgrade the quality and increase the quantity of the vaccine.[15, 17] By 1970 a majority of the vaccine used in both developed and developing countries met WHO established standards for quality. Regional priorities were established by the Smallpox Eradication Unit.[15] West and Central Africa were targeted, and the program reached an effective conclusion by 1970.[15] Assistance was provided to Brazil and smallpox eradication was successful by 1971.[15] Indonesia also received assistance to repeat what had previously been accomplished in 1937. The major attention of the program then focused on the Indian subcontinent.[15, 17]

The approach taken to control importation of cases was intensive efforts to identify cases and to provide what is called "ring vaccination" of contacts.[15] This term refers to vaccination of all susceptible individuals in a prescribed area around an outbreak of an infectious disease: the concept is to form a buffer of immune individuals to prevent its spread. However, the early WHO global eradication policy and that of countries with endemic cases was to rely on mass vaccination with the expectation of 80% of the populations being vaccinated, thus disrupting the transmission of smallpox. The strategy did not work in densely populated countries such as India and Indonesia and would not work unless the 20% of unvaccinated persons were not randomly distributed throughout the population.[15] Therefore the strategy of the Smallpox Eradication Unit shifted to the intensive case-finding and ring vaccination approach, which has become known as "surveillance and containment," while maintaining an emphasis on mass primary vaccination. Eradication of smallpox was achieved in Indonesia in 1972, in Afghanistan and Pakistan in 1973 and 1974, respectively, and in the rest of the Indian subcontinent in 1975. Progress was steady in Africa so that by early 1976 Ethiopia remained the only endemic country in the world, with some cases imported to Somalia and Kenya from Ethiopia.[15] With the war between Ethiopia and Somalia, hundreds of thousands of refugees poured into Somalia and while the last case of smallpox occurred in Ethiopia in August, 1976, in September that year there was an epidemic in Mogadishu, the capital of Somalia.[15] The last case of endemic smallpox in the world was a hospital cook in the town of Merka, Somalia.[15]

A number of factors, some biological and some social, made the eradication of smallpox possible with a major effort of international collaboration; these are also relevant to the consideration of other potential eradication initiatives for comparable infectious diseases. The biological conditions were: the disease was severe with high mortality and serious side effects among survivors' there were few cases of subclinical infection, that is, if someone had the disease it could be diagnosed, cases became infectious at the time of the onset of a rash so the infectious period was evident, there was no recurrence of infectivity, there was only one serotype of the virus so new vaccines did not need to be developed over time, an effective and stable vaccine was developed that could be transported in many climatic conditions without loss of potency, and there was no animal reservoir for the virus. The social and political conditions were that earlier countrywide eradication showed that global eradication was attainable, there were no social or religious barriers to recognition of cases, the costs of quarantine and vaccination for travelers provided a financial incentive for wealthier countries to support the program, and the Intensified Smallpox Eradication Unit of the WHO had inspired and inspiring leaders and enlisted devoted public health workers. The program involved active participation of laboratory scientists (virologists), physicians, nurses, epidemiologists, biostatisticians, policy makers at local, national, and international levels. Thus, public health workers and health care providers worked as a global team over a long period to successfully implement an ambitious campaign to eradicate smallpox.

CASE STUDY—UNDERSTANDING THE LIFE CYCLE OF A VECTOR TO
DESIGN CONTROL MEASURES

Malaria

In 2006 there were an estimated 247 million cases of malaria among the 3.3 billion people at risk.[21, 22, 23,24] Approximately one million deaths occurred annually, mostly among children under 5 years of age.[21] In 2008 there were 109 countries endemic for malaria, 45 within the African region of the World Health Organization.[21]

Public health officials at the beginning of the twentieth century were divided among those who advocated mosquito control and those who called for eliminating the parasite within human hosts.[19, 20] Vector control programs focused on elimination of the breeding sites through drainage and by spreading oil on water surfaces to destroy larvae.[19, 20] Adult mosquitoes were killed with pyrethrum sprays.[20] Quinine was used to destroy parasites but, while effective in reducing symptoms of malaria and mortality, it did not eliminate the gametocytes that infect mosquitoes so did not reduce transmission.[20] Figure 2-2 shows the lifecycle of the malaria parasite.

In the United States during World War II, there was rapid development of synthetic chemical pesticides in order to support the health of military troops in tropical areas of the world.[19, 20] The most notable development for vector control was dichloro-diphenyl-trichloroethane (DDT).[20] DDT was first synthesized in 1874 by Othmar Zeidler, a German student, but the insecticidal properties were not described until 1939 by Swiss chemist Paul Muller.[19, 20] In 1942, the US Department of the Army began experimenting with DDT and discovered the immense military possibilities in controlling insects that impeded war efforts. The need to control lice, which carried typhus, and mosquito species that carried malaria, yellow fever and dengue was pressing. Having identified the

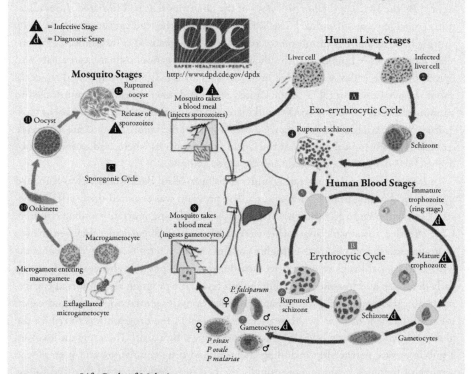

FIGURE 2-2 Life Cycle of Malaria.

Source: US Centers for Disease Control and Prevention, Parasitology Diagnostic Website (CDC-DPDx)

potential of DDT to control insects causing diseases among military personnel raised a demand for a production system that could produce large quantities of the synthetic compound. DDT retained its toxicity for months; therefore spraying only once every six months was required and when sprayed on walls sometimes only once a year. Human toxicity was very low so the compound was widely adopted. Allied forces reduced typhus and malaria among troops in the Pacific using DDT.[19]

During the 1955 Eighth World Health Assembly in Mexico City, the assembly was asked to ratify a proposal to use DDT to eradicate malaria by targeting killing female anopheline mosquitoes.[21] The program involved four strategies: (1) epidemiological study of the characteristics of the disease in order to develop an intervention plan; (2) indoor spraying of DDT on the walls of every house or hut in which humans slept based on the assumption that female anopheline mosquitoes fed primarily indoors while people were sleeping; (3) screening of infants and active case finding and treatment to eliminate remaining cases after the number of infective human carriers was zero or close to zero with continued surveillance for countries certified as free of malaria to prevent reintroduction from neighboring countries; and (4) continuation of the program until global eradication was achieved.[21]

By the early 1960s, elimination of malaria on all continents except Africa seemed in sight.[21] By the 1970s, a total of 26 (56%) of the countries that had initiated the eradication campaign were successful.[21] The WHO abandoned the eradication strategy in 1969, shifting back to a policy of mosquito control.[21] Widespread DDT resistance in anopheline mosquitoes led public health officials to turn to organophosphate, carbamate and pyrethroid insecticides, which were more costly than DDT.[21] Environmental concerns about the persistence of DDT in the United States and other developed countries led to banning use within country borders and increased the cost of insecticide control of mosquitoes.[21] Antimalarial drug resistance was also cited in the failure to eradicate malaria in tropical and subtropical regions of the world.[21] In countries where eradication had not been achieved, cases rebounded during the 1970s and 1980s.[17, 21]

In 1998, a new program operating under the slogan "Roll Back Malaria" was launched by the world public health community.[21] The program was centered on a series of specific interventions, largely shown to be effective in reducing mortality among children. Cost-effective, sustainable approaches were emphasized with particular focus on the use of insecticide-treated bed nets in highly endemic areas. Intermittent preventive therapy with antimalarial drugs to protect women during pregnancy was also endorsed, as was early detection and treatment of children with fever. The program also endorsed engagement of a wide range of government ministries (a multisectoral approach) and called for reinforcement of basic health services.[21] The goal of the program was to reduce the global burden of malaria by half by 2010 and by 75% by 2015.[21] The program involved a public-private partnership including chemical and drug companies, and it employed a range of methods (acquire and properly use bed nets, seek antenatal care and follow preventive regimens, recognize symptoms of malaria, and obtain medical care for children with fevers).[21]

The success of the program is being constantly monitored.[21] According to the World Malaria Report 2011, issued by the World Health Organization, malaria mortality rates have fallen by more than 25% globally since 2000, and by 33% in the WHO African Region.[24] The report states that progress is the result of a significant scaling-up of malaria prevention and control measures in the last decade, including the widespread use of bed nets, better diagnostics, and a wider availability of effective medicines to treat malaria.

CASE STUDY: BUILT ENVIRONMENT AND TRANSMISSION
OF AN INFECTIOUS AGENT

Legionnaire's Disease

In July, 1976 a common-source outbreak of pneumonia affected people attending the 58th annual convention of the American Legion, Department of Pennsylvania in Philadelphia.[25, 26] The epidemic was first recognized on August 2, 1976.[23] An epidemiologic investigation of the outbreak determined that the disease was most likely airborne and focused on one of the convention hotels, which subsequently closed because of defective air conditioning equipment, implicated in the investigation.[23] The specified period of time for this epidemic was July 22 to August 3, 1976.[23] Of 182 persons who became ill, 147 (81%) were hospitalized and 29 (16%, the case fatality rate) died.[23]

About six months later the etiologic agent, a Gram negative bacillus (*Legionella pneumophilia*) was identified for the first time, and the disease came to be known as Legionnaires' disease because of the association with the American Legion convention.[22] The source of the agent was a bacteria circulated throughout the hotel in the ventilation system.[22] Public concern about future outbreaks led to the closing of the hotel, which had been a landmark in Philadelphia.[22] Since that time, infection with Legionella spp. has become recognized as an important cause of community and hospital acquired pneumonia. Legionella spp. are ubiquitous and found in natural aquatic environments (streams, rivers, ponds, lakes, and thermal pools) in moist soil and mud.[22] They can survive chlorination and therefore enter water supply systems and grow in thermal habitats, including air conditioning cooling towers, hot water systems, shower heads, taps, whirlpool spas, and respirator ventilators.[22] Most cases of legionellosis can be traced to man-made aquatic environments and therefore Legionnaires' disease has become a major concern of public health professionals and individuals involved with the design, construction, or maintenance of water systems, including air-conditioning systems, circulating water systems, and cooling towers.[22] Prerequisites for infection include the presence of virulent bacteria in an aquatic environment, amplification of the bacterium to an unknown infectious dose, and transmission of the bacteria as an aerosol to a human host who is susceptible to infection.[22]

As a result of this multidisciplinary investigation, legionellosis is now considered a preventable disease though controlling or eliminating the bacterium in air conditioning reservoirs. Identification of the causal agent and mode of transmission required input from a wide range of scientists from the physicians who first diagnosed the cases to the epidemiologists who conducted the outbreak investigation to the laboratory scientists who worked to isolate the organism causing the disease. The work conducted to identify the other reservoirs of the organism included that of environmental scientists, and control of the organism today involves a wide range of public health workers, including engineers, to improve the design of heating and cooling systems. This example also illustrates the role of the economic environment in contributing to the outbreak, since the water cooling system used at the hotel was old and probably not well maintained due to financial constraints. In addition, it reflects the social environment: the outbreak occurred during a convention that brought people together from across a nation; this created conditions for widespread distribution of cases, which made tracking them more challenging.

CASE STUDY: CONTROLLING A TOXIC SUBSTANCE
ASSOCIATED WITH AN INDUSTRIAL SOURCE

Lead Levels in a Canadian Community—Local Example of a Global Issue

Preamble: Any child failing to reach full intellectual potential due to a preventable environmental cause such as exposure to toxic levels of lead is a tragic loss for the family and for society. Therefore, in many nations around the world, such environmental toxins are being brought steadily under control. For example, in 1999–2000 the US National Health and Nutrition Survey found that the mean blood lead level (BLL) for children 1–5 years in the United States was 2.2 µg/dl. Even so, over 2% of this age group still had BLL above 10 µg/dl, which translated into half a million children at risk of attributable learning disabilities and behavioral problems in the United States. The US government set a national goal of eliminating BLL >10 µg/dl among children 1–5 years by the year 2010.[27] Although the current level of concern for BLL in children is 10µg/dl, recent studies suggest that even lower levels can be associated with lower test scores.

Our story starts in 1971 in Canada with an investigation into horses with lead poisoning traced to contaminated pasture near the town of Trail, in the province of British Columbia.[28] Recognition of air pollution as an issue in Trail was not new, being the site of a major lead and zinc smelting operation for over 90 years. By the mid-1960s, the company operating the smelter had recognized air pollution as a significant concern to which it must respond.[29] As lead exposure, even at low levels, may impair intellectual development, especially early in life, a study of blood lead levels (BLLs) of children aged 1–3 years was carried out in 1975 by the provincial Ministry of Health and Health Canada, revealing elevated levels in Trail (average 22 µg/dl) that were attributed to smelter emissions; elevated levels were also identified from Vancouver and Nelson, in children living near major transportation routes.[30, 31] At this time, adding lead to gasoline was the norm for the petroleum industry.

Efforts to reduce lead emissions and exposures accelerated. In 1989, a team from the University of British Columbia sampled children living in Trail, aged 2 to 5 years: their average BLL was 13.8 µg/dl (range 4 to 30 µg/dl).[32] While 40% lower than in 1975, this was still much higher than other locations in Canada. Children with high levels tended to live in neighborhoods close to the smelter, and soil levels and house dust were the principal determinants. However, 39% of children had levels above 15 µg/dl, then defined by the US Environmental Protection Agency (EPA) as a "level of no concern" (later revised as reflected in the preamble). The purpose of the 1989 study was to define a basis for precautions and protection against future lead exposure. Recommendations called for implementing a comprehensive lead awareness and education campaign and provided the impetus for creating the Trail Community Lead Task Force.

The Task Force set two goals: at least 90% of children age 6 to 72 months in neighborhoods closest to the smelter should have blood lead levels less than 10 µg/dl by 2005, and at least 99% should have blood levels less than 15 µg/dl by 2005.[33] The Task Force comprised representatives from BC Ministries of Health and Environment, the City of Trail, Cominco Limited, the general public, the local School District, United Steelworkers of America Locals 480 and 9705, and a local network of environmental groups. The Trail Lead Program was the operational arm of the Trail Community Lead Task Force. The two BC ministries, Cominco and the City of Trail, shared responsibility for funding the program. This effort constitutes a case study of community action (see chapter 4) and an early example of public-private partnership in support of public health (see chapter 8).

From 1989 to 1996, blood lead levels in children 6–60 months fell slowly from an average of 13.8 µg/dl to 11.5 µg/dl, an overall rate of decline of 0.6 µg/dl/year.[34] Since 1991, the Task Force carried out BLL screening, case management, education programs targeted at early childhood groups and the general community, dust abatement, exposure pathway studies, and remedial trials. While some of the decline would have derived from phasing out leaded gasoline from which Trail children would have benefited (like all BC children), BLL improvement from 1989 to 1996 was attributed mainly to the community interventions, especially reducing exposure to contaminated soil and household dust.

From 1996, BLLs fell more rapidly to 5.9 µg/dl in 1999;[35] the average rate of decline tripled from 0.6 µg/dl per year (1989 to 1996) to 1.8 µg/dl per year (1997 to 1999). This accelerated reduction was attributed to the start-up in May 1997 of a new lead smelter using modern flash-smelting technology, following which mean air levels fell from 1.1 µg/m3 to 0.28 µg/m3 in 1998, and lead concentrations in outdoor dust-fall, street dust, and indoor dust-fall fell by 50%. Since 1998, yearly ambient lead levels have been substantially below guideline levels set by BC Pollution Control, US Environment Protection Agency, and the World Health Organization.[36] By 2007, the goals set by the Task Force were virtually achieved: 89% of children in neighborhoods closest to the smelter had levels of <10 µg/dl and 100% were <15 µg/dl. It may be concluded that the type of smelter technology used for so long in Trail was largely responsible for toxic levels of lead in children, and replacing this was the most important intervention.[37]

This ongoing intervention, and others, now comes under the auspices of the Trail Health & Environment Committee (THEC). In reviewing this story, which is steadily approaching success, it is important to recognize that *"averages" do not apply to the experience of individuals* whose BLLs fall within a range outside the mean. Given the current norm regarding 10 μg/dl as the level above which neurotoxicity can be clearly demonstrated, in the context of individual variability and susceptibility that apply in the real world, further reductions nonetheless must be achieved; as already noted, even lower levels can be associated with reduced developmental test scores. Thus, the THEC has concluded that BLL testing should be reevaluated and new scope and goals proposed.

It is noteworthy that THEC won a Premier's Innovation and Excellence Award for Partnership in 2011, recognizing excellence in public service in the areas of leadership, innovation, organizational and service excellence, partnership, and cross-governmental integration.

Note: See chapter 7 for more recent global developments regarding lead exposure.

CASE STUDY OF AN INDIRECT HEALTH EFFECT OF A GREENHOUSE GAS

Chlorinated Fluorocarbons (CFCs) and the Increase in Malignant Melanoma

The role of greenhouse gas (GHG) emissions on climate change and associated impacts on human health are discussed in chapter 9. Many of those impacts, serious as they are, such as the expanding global reach of disease vectors and the displacement of peoples due to rising seawater levels, can be viewed as indirect. However, despite their major importance to the environment and these indirect impacts, GHGs generally do not have a direct impact on human health, with one notable exception: chlorinated fluorocarbons (CFCs). These emissions are responsible for depleting the Earth's ozone layer.

The earth's stratospheric ozone layer protects humans from solar radiation, which is important because a causal relationship between sun exposure (particularly Ultra Violet-B radiation) and skin cancers is well-established.[38] Attention has been drawn also to the potential for ocular damage.[39] Trends in the incidence of melanoma (the most serious skin cancer for which good data are available) in Canada are presented in Figure 2-3, which reveals a steady increase in recent decades.[40] This continues to grow as a percentage of all male and female cancers. Other skin cancers, squamous cell carcinoma and basal cell carcinoma, are also associated with UV-B radiation.

The single most important factor affecting UV-B exposure is the amount of ozone in the atmosphere. CFCs are largely responsible for depleting this ozone layer: as much as a 2% increase in UV-B radiation may be expected for each 1% reduction in stratospheric ozone concentration. CFCs were used for decades as propellants in spray cans and as freon gas in refrigerators and air conditioners until a Canadian-led global moratorium on their manufacture and use was adopted in 1987 as The Montreal Protocol on Substances that Deplete the Ozone Layer. To celebrate the success of the first 20 years, countries gathered

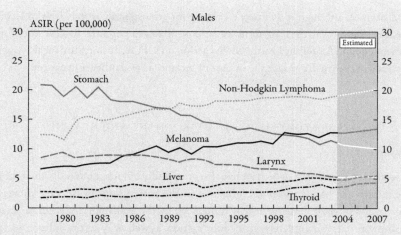

FIGURE 2-3 Age-Standardized Incidence Rates (ASIR) for Selected Cancers, Males, Canada, 1978–2007.

Note: Rates are Standardized to the age distribution of the 1991 Canadian population. Actual incidence data are available to 2004 except for Newfoundland and Labrador, Quebec, and Ontario, where 2004 incidence is estimated.

Source: Canadian Cancer Society's Steering Committee on Cancer Statistics. *Canadian Cancer Statistics,* 2007. Toronto, ON: Canadian Cancer Society; 2007.

in Montreal, Canada, in 2007, to recognize the broad coalition of governments, scientific researchers, and others who have developed smart, flexible, and innovative approaches to protecting human health and the global environment.[41]

Although the treaty has been a great success in curbing CFC emissions, unfortunately, as CFCs have a half-life of about 100 years, ozone depletion from existing CFC contamination will continue well into the twenty-second century.[42] A global increase in the incidence of skin cancers in recent decades has been attributed in part to this phenomenon, because of its role in increasing the intensity of UVB exposures.

The UB-V radiation dose for most individuals is a function of duration of sun exposure, which ranks high among lifestyle behaviors (e.g., sun bathing) occupational exposures (e.g., farming), and other outdoor pursuits (e.g., gardening, hiking). The *good news* is that most people have a choice in these aspects of the exposure they receive. For example, there is evidence from Australia for a birth-cohort effect consistent with variations in sun exposure and the use of protective measures (e.g., protective clothing, sun blocks).[43] According to the US National Cancer Institute, such preventive measures may outweigh the effects of decreases in stratospheric ozone.[44] Similarly, tanning beds and sunlamps have also been recognized as preventable risks in the causation of melanoma, as well as for other forms of skin cancer;[45] increasingly these are being regulated, especially to ensure that the main users (young adults) are advised of the risk and, in some jurisdictions, restricting access to persons under age.

On balance, although it will take a century for atmospheric ozone levels to stabilize, there is reason to view the long-term scenario positively: a potential success story for the environment and for public health. Global action on CFC emissions and local actions on lifestyles will eventually reduce the impact of melanoma and other skin cancer.

CASE STUDY—SOCIAL ENVIRONMENT AND HEALTH

Tobacco

The social environments in which we live also profoundly influence our individual choices; these in turn can have a profound influence on the patterns of disease. Our choices are usually made in environments heavily influenced by the availability of accurate, inaccurate, and sometimes completely wrong information, as well as by access, culture, and peer pressure. For example, where advertising targets specific groups of people, they are more likely to believe that using certain products will enhance their lives. Tobacco advertising is one such example.[46-51]

Worldwide, approximately 1.3 billion people currently smoke cigarettes or use other tobacco products.[43] The decline of smoking in developed countries, in response to health policy and promotion initiatives, and the increasingly aggressive marketing of tobacco products in the developing world, has shifted the geographic distribution of smoking toward developing countries.[43, 44] In 1995, more smokers lived in low and middle income countries (933 million) than in high income countries (209 million).[43, 44] An estimated 4.9 million smoking related deaths occurred in 2000, with a projection that in 2020 there will be more than nine million annual deaths, of which seven million will occur in developing countries. To address this pandemic of tobacco related diseases, in 2005 the World Health Organization (WHO) launched the Framework Convention on Tobacco Control.[43]

WHO also supports a tobacco free initiative that includes surveillance of the prevalence of its use, identifying its health and economic consequences, assessing social and cultural determinants of its use, identifying tobacco control policies, and monitoring actions of the tobacco industry.[45] The approach used to monitor the pandemic and evaluate the success of tobacco control programs implemented in different countries incorporates a broad vision of public health and cooperation at the global level.

Tobacco products are associated with numerous diseases, including cancers of the lung, esophagus, larynx, tongue, salivary glands, lip, mouth pharynx, urinary bladder, kidneys, uterine cervix, breast, pancreas and colon, heart disease, chronic obstructive pulmonary disease (chronic bronchitis and emphysema), and peripheral vascular disease (atherosclerosis).[43] Some evidence also suggests an association between cigarette smoking and osteoporosis, thyroid problems, and the onset of type-2 diabetes; there is strong evidence that smoking is one of the most powerful factors determining severity of outcomes for all forms of diabetes.[43] Smoking cessation programs traditionally targeted current smokers, ignoring the larger social context that encouraged and supported smoking through marketing.[45, 46]

Tobacco products, legal for mainly historical reasons, are the only consumer product that kills half of its regular users.[46, 47] The tobacco industry has used economic power, lobbying and marketing, and manipulation of the media to discredit scientific research and to influence governments to propagate the sale and distribution of its product.[47] The tobacco industry makes large philanthropic contributions to social programs worldwide, thereby creating a positive image; sponsorship of sports and cultural events also have been widely used by the industry to promote this false image.[47] Effective tobacco control is counter to the economic interests of the tobacco industry, associated industries, and stockholders.[47]

The primary goal of tobacco control is to prevent related diseases and premature death. To accomplish this goal programs are designed to prevent people from initiating tobacco use (primary prevention) and to assist current smokers in quitting (secondary prevention). Efforts to reduce exposure to second-hand smoke are included in control measures, with the most effective approach being the prohibition of smoking in public places.[45] Additional tobacco control efforts worldwide include prohibitions on advertising and on sponsorship of events, tax and price increases, labeling tobacco products as hazardous, and monitoring illicit trade of tobacco.[46]

Recognition of the social and cultural context of the populations involved has been a key component of successful control programs. For example, cultural sensitivity is a widely accepted principle in public health. To tailor tobacco prevention programs for specific populations requires acknowledgment that there are differences in prevalence of tobacco use across age, sex, racial, and ethnic groups.[48] But there are also different types of smoking patterns across such groups, thus requiring programs to be tailored to address the pattern differences. For example, African Americans are more likely to smoke menthol cigarettes than other groups, but they and Hispanics are less likely to be heavy smokers than whites.[48] Information such as this might be used to target programs, but tailoring programs requires focusing on the functional use of cigarettes within different populations.[48] Tobacco may be used for socialization in various ways such that peers may play a role different from parents' in different groups.[48] For example, peers have been reported in the United States to have a stronger role on initiation of smoking among whites and Hispanics compared with African Americans.[48] Therefore, while using peers as a means to influence behavior may be effective among white and Hispanic youth, it would be unlikely to be effective among African American youth.[48] Engaging parents and other adult role models may be a more effective way of designing intervention programs for African American youth.[48]

This closing case study of tobacco control illustrates why social and behavioral sciences have proven important to understanding such public health challenges and developing relevant and effective approaches to health promotion and disease prevention and control.

Public health services are part of the social fabric of nations. The values and beliefs of public health professional workers are as important as their scientific education and technical skills. Public health professionals should be able to make ethical decisions, and should have moral and philosophical insights that inform and justify their decisions and actions. This chapter presents some philosophical and moral perspectives and considers some ethical issues and problems that can arise in the course of decision making in public health. We illustrate with a few examples of situations where values and beliefs can complicate decision making.

3

PHILOSOPHICAL AND ETHICAL FOUNDATIONS

OF PUBLIC HEALTH

HUMANS ARE A gregarious species and find comfort and security in the company of others—family, friends, neighbors, communities defined in various ways, and aggregated into states and nations. We care for defenseless infants and small children, and in almost all societies we care for others who are unable to care for themselves, the infirm and the elderly. All human societies have certain taboos, behaviors considered unacceptable, including the incest taboo and proscription of crimes such as murder and infanticide—although there are exceptions in some societies and cultures. We are compassionate and care for others in distress or danger, even at risk to ourselves. This is illustrated in TV images from scenes of disaster where strangers do not stand idly by but come to the aid of those in danger from fallen masonry after an earthquake or at risk of drowning in floods. We do all we can to save them. Without the drama or publicity of TV cameras, public health specialists come to the aid of those afflicted by contagious disease epidemics, ensure the safety of water and food supplies, and do all the other things necessary to keep the people as healthy as possible. This is a simplistic philosophical explanation of why we expend tax dollars on public health infrastructure, staff salaries, and services. We do it because we belong to a society that cares about others. This is reinforced by the pragmatic recognition that certain threats to some of us—from infectious diseases or contaminated food, for instance—are threats to all of us; and as groups, communities, nations, we take the necessary actions designed to protect us all. As Steven Pinker demonstrates in *The Better Angels of Our Nature*, human societies have become less violent and more compassionate and caring over at least the past 500 years.[1]

Growing consciousness of the interdependence of human health and ecosystem health adds another dimension to this philosophical perspective of public health, and another ethical imperative: our actions must be compatible with global ecosystem sustainability. Here we may perceive an ethical dilemma. Our actions as public health professionals preserve the lives of infants and children who would otherwise die before growing up and having children of their own—thus leading to a population surge and increased stress on fragile life-supporting ecosystems. History reveals, however, that if there is a population surge when public health services are first established, it is transitory: parents soon observe that they don't need to give birth to six eight, or ten babies to ensure the survival of one or two who will provide for them in their old age, and therefore may accept available family planning services. A necessary prerequisite for understanding how to promote health and understand available options for family planning is literacy, especially for girls. That said, other problems can emerge: in European countries such as Italy, for example, the demographic transition has gone further. Birth rates have fallen well below replacement level, and many frail and infirm elderly people have insufficient fit and income-earning younger generations to provide and care for them. In China, an approaching demographic crisis will confront national planners as the birth cohorts of the one-child-per-couple policy reach old age.

Ethical Theory

Ethics guidelines and codes of conduct for public health workers provide rules on how to protect and enhance the right to health and well-being. The Greek philosopher Aristotle (384–322 BCE) compiled his book on ethics about 334 BCE. He discussed virtues required to achieve "happiness," which we can interpret in modern words as harmony between and among people, and contentment. Virtue-based ethics, probably the most pertinent philosophical foundation for public health ethics, derives from Aristotle. The relevant virtues include compassion, truthfulness, prudence, integrity, trustworthiness. Another quality that is often important is objectivity or impartiality, which helps us avoid conflicts of interest. The importance of these virtues to the good practice of public health is self-evident.

Two additional underlying ethical constructs have relevance for public health moral reasoning.[2] The first are Kantian (named after Immanuel Kant, a German philosopher 1724–1804) or deontological principles, which hold that people should not be treated as a means to an end and that there are actions that are inherently right or inherently wrong irrespective of their consequences.[3] For example, this leads to understanding that individuals involved in research must be protected from undue risk even if this slows the process of completing research studies. The other dominant theories (such as articulated by British philosopher John Stuart Mill1806–1873) are utilitarian and based on an effort to maximize beneficial consequences for the group: briefly stated, as long as the maximum benefit is derived for the good of the population, choices are justified on a moral basis. This principle can be invoked in public health to justify mass compulsory immunizations, speed limits on roads, fluoridation of public water supplies, and outbreak investigations that may be viewed by some people in particular settings as violating the rights of the individual to freedom of choice.

In some instances of applied ethics, one theory or another may provide a better grounding for decision making and some people prefer one theory over another. Public health is by nature an applied field and requires a general approach to policy making grounded in ethical guidelines.

The trials of the Nazi war criminals in Nuremberg (1947) after World War II disclosed shocking abuses by Nazi medical scientists who used humans as experimental animals. This led to the Nuremberg Code (see Box 3-1), which offered ten points for the conduct of experiments on humans. The first of these points is that the voluntary and fully informed consent of participants in research on humans is absolutely essential. (Although this first of the ten points remains valid, we now recognize a few exceptions). The year after the Nuremberg Code appeared, the United Nations Universal Declaration on Human Rights (1948) was published. The Universal Declaration of Human Rights (see Article 25) was adopted by the United Nations General Assembly on December 10, 1948. The committee that drafted the declaration included representatives from Australia, Canada, Chile, China, France, Lebanon, the United Kingdom, the United States, and the Union of Soviet Socialist Republics.[3] Contained in the document were statements that established health as a right of all people. This provides an important reference point for the role and obligations of public health professionals in that they are instrumental in ensuring this right is implemented. Soon there was much discussion of human rights, patients' rights, and the rights of persons recruited for experimental treatments and other interventions.

Universal Declaration of Human Rights: Article 25

1. Everyone has the right to a standard of living adequate for the health and well-being of himself and of his family, including food, clothing, housing, and medical care and necessary social services, and the right to security in the event of unemployment, sickness, disability, widowhood, old age, or lack of livelihood in circumstances beyond his control.

BOX 3-1

TEN POINTS OF THE NUREMBERG CODE

1. The voluntary consent of the human subject is absolutely essential.
2. The experiment should be such as to yield fruitful results for the good of society, unprocurable by other method or means of study, and not random and unnecessary in nature.
3. The experiment should be so conducted as to avoid all unnecessary physical and mental suffering and injury.
4. The experiment should be so designed and based on the results of animal experimentation and knowledge of the natural history of the disease or other problem under study that the anticipated results will justify the performance of the experiment.
5. No experiment should be conducted where is a prior reason to believe that death or disabling injury will occur; except, perhaps, in those experiments where the experimental physicians serve as subject.
6. The degree of risk to be taken should never exceed that determined by the humanitarian importance of the problem to be solved by the experiment.
7. Proper preparations should be made and adequate facilities provided to protect the experimental subject against even remote possibilities of injury, disability, or death.
8. The experiment should be conducted only by scientifically qualified persons. The highest degree of skill and care should be required through all stages of the experiment of those who conduct or engage in the experiment.
9. During the course of the experiment the human subject should be at liberty to bring the experiment to an end if he has reached the physical or mental state where continuation of the experiment seems to him to be impossible.
10. During the course of the experiment the scientist in charge must be prepared to terminate the experiment at any stage if he has probable cause to believe, in the exercise of the good faith, superior skill, and careful judgment required of him that the continuation of the experiment is likely to result in injury, disability, or death of the experimental subject.

2. Motherhood and childhood are entitled to special care and assistance. All children, whether born in or out of wedlock, shall enjoy the same social protection.[4]

The World Medical Association produced the Helsinki Declaration (1960 and subsequently); this dealt mainly with protection of patients from harm due to medical experiments. Ethicists and philosophers expounded on ethical approaches to medical care, especially matters such as trial of new therapeutic regimens, at meetings and in monographs.

The monograph by Tom Beauchamp and James Childress, *Principles of Biomedical Ethics* (1979),[5] led to the concept of principle-based ethics, which now dominates ethical theory and practice in clinical medicine and medical research but is not always the most suitable way to approach ethical problems in public health. The four principles are respect for autonomy, or the right to make one's own choices; doing good, or beneficence; not harming, or non-maleficence, which derives from Hippocrates' maxim, "First, do no harm"; and equity or justice, acting equally toward all, not singling out some for special attention while neglecting others. Application of these four principles works generally very well in clinical practice and in most aspects of biomedical research but is not always appropriate in public health practice, where virtue-based ethics often works much better.

Ethical Guidelines

Since the Nuremberg Code in 1947, it has been clearly understood that informed consent is a necessary prerequisite for all research involving human subjects. Codes of conduct, policy statements, and guidelines about ethical and unethical conduct of daily practice have been discussed and published by many subgroups within the health professions. In the professional groups that constitute the public health profession, discussions and published documents lagged behind those that were developed or revised from previously existing codes of conduct in fields of medical and nursing practice involving patient care. Among public health professionals, the first to define ethically acceptable and unacceptable conduct were actuaries, statisticians, and public record-keepers (concerned about privacy and confidentiality) and occupational health specialists (whose position is challenging because they are usually employed by management of an industrial corporation to whom they are answerable, but care for workers, not management). Questions about setting safety standards that have cost implications, and who owns and has access to confidential medical records about industrial injury or illness, therefore sometimes become ethically ambiguous. Public health nurses who work on contact-tracing in sexually transmitted disease clinics were also in the forefront in establishing rules regarding privacy and confidentiality.

Ethics guidelines for public health workers are just that: guidelines. They do *not* provide rules on how to protect and enhance the right to health and well-being. Each and every situation in which ethical concerns exist must be assessed on its merits, and if these concerns are sufficiently complex or troubling, a specially designated ethics review committee is charged with the responsibility for conducting the review and reaching a decision about the best ethical response. This commonly happens in research projects and programs but is less common in public health practice.

Public health measures that protect human health are often addressed by government regulations and legislation, and practitioners may invoke a legal mandate to enforce them. Such measures include mandatory reporting of selected communicable diseases by physicians or laboratories,[6] mandatory reporting to registries for surveillance of cancer, immunization programs, outbreak investigation to identify contacts to control transmissible diseases, screening for diseases, inspection of food preparation and the authority to close a restaurant or other food processing outlet found to be in violation, and treatment of water supplies to prevent enteric diseases. Applications of these and some of the ethical questions and unintended consequences that surround them are discussed later in this chapter (see Case Study—Ethical Lessons from a SARS Outbreak); core aspects of disease prevention and control are discussed in chapter 6.

Social responsibility is a central concern of public health professionals because of their role in making decisions and taking actions in complex situations involving advanced technology, high levels of specialization, overlapping areas of expertise, and having to work with decision makers from diverse educational, political, and social backgrounds.[7] Responsibility has many levels, including individual accountability for personal actions, community or organizational responsibility through a commitment to principles that focus on achieving valuable outcomes consistent with the fundamental aims of public health in preventing disease and promoting health, and reliable performance of tasks expected of public health professionals.[6]

Public health professionals are accountable to communities, other health professionals, and decision makers (e.g., politicians, regulators, administrators) for actions taken on their behalf. They also have a commitment to action in pursuit of achieving a social good as in ensuring the rights of all to health. Such action is sometimes termed "affirmative action" or "positive discrimination" or even "reverse discrimination," depending on the sociopolitical situation; it can be controversial even when driven by the ethical imperative of social justice. For example, understanding the link between poverty and educational attainment and poor health outcomes might lead some public health professionals to advocate for more support for school programs to increase school engagement of students from low-income families. When public health professionals teach or mentor students, they have additional ethical obligations. They are role models, so their behavior should be ethically impeccable. They should treat students as junior team members through acknowledging intellectual property and following standards that have been developed by most peer-reviewed publications on authorship and attribution.

Social responsibility includes striving for social justice. Social justice has been defined as the concept and implementation of equity. One philosophical justification for advances in public health is recognition that many disparities in health are caused by deprivation and that alleviation of these disparities requires correction of deprivation. The adverse impact on health was a powerful incentive to eliminate child labor, slavery, and racial segregation, to elevate the status of women in society, and in all other ways to aspire to a just and equitable society. These and related issues are explored further in chapter 4, including through a range of case studies.

In pursuing the aims of the discipline, public health professionals should perform their duties within a professional community of honesty, integrity, prudence, and self-effacement where excellence is the ultimate goal of reliable professional performance.[6] An example of this is the actions of public health scientists who have applied the results of their research to develop evidence-based interventions designed to promote health and prevent disease, including people like John Snow and Joseph Goldberger (chapter 1); they did not do this to seek awards or gain financially from their accomplishments. To the contrary, when prestige and financial gain become the driving forces behind motivation in the health sciences generally, the likelihood of scientific misconduct has been observed to increase.[8] Underlying the practices of those who have shown leadership in public health are motivations that are predominantly influenced by good character, formal training, and sound mentoring; these and commitment to virtue-based ethics are the bedrock of excellence in public health sciences and practices.

In order to provide a more practical understanding of the importance and complexity of ethical issues in public health, we now turn to particular areas of application for illustration.

Quarantine and Emergency Preparedness

In public health there is a delicate balance between protecting the rights of an individual to privacy and the need to protect the community from risk of exposure to diseases. As discussed in chapters 1 and 6, quarantine is one of the oldest known methods for controlling the spread of communicable diseases. The use of quarantine, in its strictest form, is a direct violation of individual freedom and is a clear example of the difficult decision making involved in protecting the health of the population while restricting the rights of an individual. This type of dilemma was highlighted in 2007 when a man from the state of Georgia who was infected with a drug-resistant form of tuberculosis disregarded doctors' advice and traveled from the United States to Europe to get married. Eight people who shared a flight with him filed a lawsuit in Canada seeking $1.3 million USD in damages.[9] He was detained in Denver, Colorado and quarantined in a hospital. He was the first American subjected to federal quarantine since 1963 and later filed a lawsuit against the Centers for Disease

Control and Prevention for unlawfully and unnecessarily revealing his private medical history. Initially doctors believed he had an extremely dangerous form of drug resistant tuberculosis (XDR-TB), but later tests revealed he had a less severe strain.

This is a classic example of the difficulty balancing protection of the community against the rights of an individual.[10] On the assumption that he had a severe and contagious form of tuberculosis officials detained him to reduce the potential spread of disease to others. This decision was made with the best information available at the time and, had it been correct, it would have seemed an appropriate action. Laboratory results take time and critical decisions sometimes must be made without complete information. Weighing the risks and benefits of having a deadly form of tuberculosis spread, the choice was made to reduce the risk to the general population. However, confidential medical information that identified him by name was made public, so what would normally have been his right to privacy was violated. There are laws that govern this situation in order to allow individual rights to be managed differently when there is potential for harm to the community as a result of disease in an individual.

Another example of this dilemma occurred during the 2009 pandemic of H1N1 influenza (also known as "swine flu"). In March and April of 2009, cases were reported in Mexico and the United States.[11] On June 11, 2009 WHO declared a global pandemic based on the number of countries reporting cases, not on the severity of the disease. At that time more than 70 countries had reported cases. China (and a number of other countries) took an aggressive approach to controlling spread of the disease from foreign visitors. Their public health staff began boarding airplanes, using pistol-grip thermometers to test passengers' temperatures.[12] The United States State Department issued a warning to travelers noting that 1800 Americans had been quarantined in hotels near the airport after being removed from airplanes for suspected swine flu; 200 had tested positive.[11] Most public health professionals did not believe these aggressive actions would do anything to reduce the spread of the disease.

Fever screening illustrates a classical dilemma of screening decision making: it has been used as an examination question to challenge students about the validity and reliability of mass screening. For example, not every infected person will exhibit fever: some may be incubating the virus, and become symptomatic within 24 to 48 hours; some may have other symptoms, but no fever; some may be taking antipyretics to ease symptoms or evade detection; and some may simply be asymptomatic carriers. Some individuals with fever may have another febrile condition unrelated to influenza. Screening results may also be confounded by factors such as consumption of hot beverages or alcohol, pregnancy, menstrual period, or hormonal treatments, all of which can increase skin temperature and cause false positives.

Conversely, lightly dressed persons coming off an aircraft might be cold due to low cabin temperatures; intense perspiration or heavy face make-up can also reduce measurable skin temperatures resulting in false negatives. However, such screening for early symptoms, even when nonspecific (fever), and isolation of suspected cases are standard public health practices in some countries. In the swine flu example, due to the high likelihood of false positives (people with fevers who did not have H1N1 influenza), a large number of people were held in quarantine. This situation caused serious disruption to international travel yet, for the most part, was viewed by public health authorities in many countries as an ineffective approach to reduce the spread of the virus.

Other ethical issues related to the H1N1 pandemic were raised in efforts to distribute and immunize high-risk populations in the United States and other nations. Taking the US example, first, there was a shortage of vaccine, therefore guidelines had to be provided to determine who should receive the vaccine first. Target groups for the H1N1 vaccine were pregnant women, people caring for children under 6 months of age, health care and emergency workers, followed by those aged 6 months to 24 years, and those 25–64 years with chronic conditions or compromised immune systems.[10] Exactly who was considered a health care worker? Would this include only those with direct patient contact (e.g., nurses, doctors) or would laboratory technicians, janitors, and food service workers also be immunized? In a hospital setting, in the presence of vaccine scarcity would high-risk patients be immunized first or the health care workers? If health care workers refused to be immunized should they be put on leave during the pandemic? All of these questions are evidence of the complexity of choices that face public health professionals. In the presence of an emergency such as the rapid spread of disease as in the pandemic described, there is no time to make these decisions in a reasoned manner, so it is important to take time after an outbreak to develop a process for emergency planning to assess what the critical questions were that had not been previously addressed and should be before the next emergency. Often, however, that is not accomplished because of pressures to return to more routine activities.

Ethics and Environmental Health

Fluoridation of community water supplies to prevent dental caries has been recognized as one of the 10 great public health achievements of the 20th century by the US Centers for Disease Control and Prevention.[13] However, fluoridation has also evoked intense opposition, using arguments such as the right of individuals to decide for themselves; objections to "mass medication"; and concerns of adverse health effects of fluoride ranging from skin rashes to weight gain to production of wrinkles to deterioration of ligaments, muscles, and tendons to cancers and immune system suppression to simply objecting to additives or contaminants in food.[13] The debate has been more political than one based in the scientific evidence that weighs risks and benefits. The use of public opinion and the media rather than scientific evidence raises a question about where public health decisions should be made. In the United States, political decisions regarding fluoridation have been made at the state and local levels. There are two methods by which such decisions are made: first, elected officials and policy makers may decide the fluoridation policy and, second, in many states voters determine such issues through direct ballot votes in the form of initiatives and referenda.[13] This scenario raises an issue of direct democracy versus representative democracy: should citizens make decisions about public health laws and regulations or should such decisions rest with experts and elected officials?

In the case of fluoridation of community water supplies, decision-making resulting from direct democracy has favored anti-fluoridationists, who have been extremely successful in removing fluoride from community water supplies.[13] In contrast, when elected officials at the local and state levels have made the decisions, fluoridation in the community water supplies has been supported.[13] Scientific evidence compiled for more than 6 decades has demonstrated that fluoridation is safe and provides a cost-effective intervention that benefits everyone consuming the water in the community without regard to financial status. Not fluoridating water that is fluoride deficient is likely to have a differential impact on the population, such that those least likely to be able to afford dental care will be at higher risk of dental caries in the absence of fluoride treatment of the water. This public health issue highlights the inherently political nature of decision making that influences public health policy and practice. Further, it points to the importance of communicating scientific information to the general public in a manner that is clear while also addressing issues such as distrust of government, environmental concerns, and other fears such as additives or contaminants in food that may influence the ability of people to respond favorability to scientific information if not presented in proper context.

The precautionary principle as an environmental policy is also a core principle for public health. Even though no standard definition of the principle has been agreed upon, the central concept is that if an action has a suspected risk of causing harm to people or the environment, even in the absence of scientific evidence that it is harmful, the burden of proof that it is *not* harmful falls on those taking the action. Endorsed by the United Nations Conference on Environment and Development in 1992,[14] this principle has been included subsequently in numerous international environmental agreements and has been incorporated in the legal framework of the

European Union, as well as within the domestic laws of many nations.[15] Regulating environmental risks has always involved precaution in the face of uncertainty, but the adoption of the precautionary principle makes that an explicit policy and may allow for more deliberative, transparent, and coherent decision making. Certainly there are numerous examples of initially underestimating the risk of an environmental contaminant that have resulted in harming the environment or humans, including DDT, asbestos, leaded gasoline, and other examples, as discussed in chapters 2, 7 and 9. Some proponents of the principle advocate for more precaution than in the past.

However, occasionally too much precaution may have been applied, such as with regard to the artificial sweetener saccharin and the public health response to swine flu in 1976. In the case of saccharine, animal studies in the 1970s demonstrated a relationship between bladder cancer and saccharine, and the US Congress accordingly mandated that food containing saccharine include a warning label.[16] Later studies demonstrated that the relationship was specific to rats, and human epidemiology studies revealed no consistent evidence of an association with bladder cancer incidence. The requirement for a warning label was repealed in 2000. In the case of the 1976 swine flu strain (Hsw1Nsw1), a small number of cases were reported at a military base in New Jersey.[17] Because swine flu caused major mortality in the 1918 pandemic, public health officials were concerned that the new strain may cause a similar epidemic, since it had not been seen since 1918 and few people would have immunity. A massive campaign to immunize the United States population was undertaken. The epidemic never occurred, but the vaccine itself was associated with Guillain-Barré syndrome (a serious though very low-frequency side effect), and a major criticism of the program was that no measures were put in place to halt the immunization campaign if the virus did not spread.

Determining the concerns that turn out to be false, or conversely those that were not taken seriously enough in the initial phase, is sometimes clear in retrospect but not always clear at the time a decision is made. The ethical dilemma is how to strike a balance between the cases of false negative and false positive decisions in order to provide an optimal balance for the purpose of regulation. Industry and government regulators may move too slowly in reducing harm when there is evidence of adverse effects or in imposing stronger premarket testing that may permit earlier detection of product risks.[14] Also there has been a call for stronger postmarketing surveillance of products once licensed, keeping in mind that trials are usually not large enough to detect rare but serious side effects.

However, when risks are unknown it is not clear how the precautionary principle should apply. Decisions are based on the current state of knowledge and, even in situations for which we believe we have made an informed decision, new scientific information may arise that calls into question what we currently believe to be true. An example of some difficulties related to arbitrary application of the precautionary principle is that of genetically modified (GM) foods by the European Union. The restriction of GM food was strongly advocated by organic growers despite safety tests that have been conducted and although there is still uncertainty about the safety for the environment and humans; to date the risks are more hypothetical than documented. In contrast, why are there not similar concerns about organic growers and food safety? Despite known cases of human diseases from contaminated organic lettuce, alfalfa sprouts, and apple juice, organic foods have not generally not been subjected to safety testing.[14] While there may be sound reasons for applying the precautionary principle to GM foods but not to organic foods, these need to be clearly articulated rather than based on arbitrary choices reflecting individual and group self-interests and biases.

Environmental Ethics

The field of environmental ethics as a subdiscipline developed almost simultaneously in three countries: Australia, Norway and the United States.[18] Its emergence reflected concern about population growth and serious environmental crises resulting from human activities. The field questions the assumption that humans are morally superior to other species. Species are viewed as having intrinsic value, more valuable than individuals, since total loss of a species represents the loss of genetic possibilities and deliberate destruction of a species would show disrespect for biological processes that lead to the emergence of individual living things.[18]

Here are some examples of questions addressed by environmental ethics:

Suppose that putting out natural fires, culling feral animals or destroying some individual members of overpopulated indigenous species is necessary for the protection of the integrity of a certain ecosystem. Will these actions be morally permissible or even required? Is it morally acceptable for farmers in non-industrial countries to practise slash and burn techniques to clear areas for agriculture? It is often said to be morally wrong for human beings to pollute and destroy parts of the natural environment and to consume a huge proportion of the planet's natural resources. If that is wrong, is it simply because a sustainable environment is essential to (present and future) human well-being? Or is such behavior also wrong because the natural environment and/or its various contents have certain values in their own right so that these values ought to be respected and protected in any case?[18]

Many of these questions are directly relevant to public health practitioners as they make choices in how to approach protecting human health and preventing disease. The focus of environmental ethics on population health for plants and animals, as well as humans, is important. Further the focus on maintaining intact ecosystems through natural resource conservation is also the purview of public health as it relates to future sustainable practices that are ultimately needed for the survival of all life forms on our planet.

Mandatory or Voluntary Consent for Newborn Screening

Newborn screening programs (chapter 6) were introduced in many Western countries in the 1960s. Now considered routine practice, newborn screening is widely protected by legislation. The first condition screened was phenylketonuria (PKU), a metabolic disorder that gives rise to early onset mental and developmental disabilities when left untreated.19 The test for PKU requires a heel stick to obtain blood, which is then stored on filter paper (a Guthrie card). Treatment requires avoiding foods with phenylalanine. Even at that time, not everyone supported mandatory testing; some suggested that there was insufficient evidence whereas others expressed concerns about government involvement in medical practice.[19] Following the introduction of PKU testing and further technological advances, other conditions have been steadily added to screening test panels.

From a public health perspective, the following criteria have been used to justify mandatory screening tests: (1) the disease or condition should be a significant health problem; (2) the natural history of the disease should be understood; (3) there should be a test that is suitable and acceptable to the general population; (4) there should be an accepted and acceptable treatment for the condition; and (5) there should be a policy about who would be treated.[19]

However, newborn screening in many jurisdictions now includes the identification of sickle cell carriers and carriers of other hemoglobin variants. In all other circumstances in which carriers are identified, consent is required. There is no apparent reason that newborn screening that has the potential to identify carriers should not require the same process. Still, there are issues to be addressed; for example, although the screened individual is the newborn, because sickle cell is an autosomal recessive disease both parents must carry a recessive version of the gene for an infant to have the disease. The parents' carrier state is therefore revealed by the testing and the implication is that they should be asked to provide consent before the test is done.

The rationale for voluntary rather than mandatory screening became stronger with the application of tandem mass spectrometry in the 1990s, which led to the identification of many metabolic conditions and variants. Some of these conditions are not treatable and some have unknown clinical significance, thus removing screening for them from the realm of a public health emergency.[19] A more troubling ethical aspect of the issue is the increasing interest in using the retained blood spots for research, a development that moves the discussion away from screening for treatment to involvement as a study participant. A cornerstone of research ethics is voluntary consent of the participant or, in the situation where the individual cannot give consent, that of a proxy. This example leads into the next topic of discussion—public health genomics.

Public Health Genomics

Biobanking is the storage of biological samples for clinical purposes (genetic diagnosis, transfusion, transplantation), research (testing for neurodegenerative disease, twin studies, and genetically isolated populations), and criminal investigation (police biobanks).[20] The hope that research in this area will lead to better treatment, diagnosis, recognition of genetic and environmental diseases, and identification of individual susceptibility and more personalized medical care (as discussed in chapter 6) has also contributed to the development of a new field within public health called public health genomics.

Public health genomics "is defined as the responsible and effective translation of genome-based knowledge and technologies for the benefit of population health."[21] It addresses the impact of gene interactions with behavior, diet, and the environment. International collaborations within the field have increased, and the need to develop a standard set of rules and practices to facilitate such collaborations is an ongoing conversation. Ethical issues that come into the discussion include the problem of obtaining informed consent (related to use in future studies, access for other scientists, use of samples from donors who have died or who were minors), the need to ensure privacy (how samples are stored, if the samples are obtained with identifying information or the degree of anonymous coding, protection of personal data), the right of individuals not to be informed if they are diagnosed with conditions coupled with the risk of discrimination if they are found to have certain genetic profiles, and the possibility of commercial use of samples and how donors should be compensated if their tissues and samples are used in a profit-making enterprise. However, many countries do not have a national approach to public health genomics. For example, in Canada decision making with regard to ethical issues has been made largely through institutional research ethics boards, although efforts have been undertaken to harmonize with the international community through the

Public Population Project in Genomics.[21,22] Issues that are of particular relevance for public health professionals relate to gaps in surveillance efforts, the lack of registries of conditions detectable at birth to facilitate evaluation of interventions, providing genetic services to First Nations and other vulnerable communities, lack of consistent quality assurance in laboratories, and lack of educational materials to provide information about the meaning of screening results.[21] Despite these shortcomings, there is increased availability of screening tests directly to consumers or professionals from for-profit companies that may provide misleading information, a situation that calls for the development of regulatory oversight.[22]

Moral and Political Responsibility for Childhood Obesity

Public health approaches to childhood obesity have focused on improving diet and increasing physical activity primarily through information, education, and awareness activities.[23] The acknowledgment of the vulnerable, dependent role of young people and the unique rights and entitlements they should be afforded have largely been ignored. According to the *Convention on the Rights of the Child,*[24] children have the right to attain high standard of health, and all states, agencies, and families should consider the interests of children as a primary concern, particularly with regard to their safety and health. Public health activities designed to reduce childhood obesity therefore should be undertaken at many societal levels.

The conflict between individual rights to free choice and the greater good provides a backdrop for understanding the challenge of developing more effective programs to reduce the childhood obesity epidemic that now affects many countries. This challenge is complicated by the traditional view that parents and families should be the primary caregivers of children: in this view, the individual rights of the child are overshadowed by the rights of the family and parents. Thus, for most children, food choices are family decisions rather than personal ones. In families without adequate resources to provide healthy and nutritious food for their children, the children's health may be compromised by familial disadvantage.

Public health programs have not done an adequate job addressing this type of disparity through developing social programs specifically addressing this need. Further, there has been minimal focus on regulation of direct marketing of unhealthy foods to children, industry standards for food sold directly to children (e.g., soft drinks, candy). and the built environment to promote safety and physical activity. In effect, government response has not focused sufficiently on the needs of the children in developing regulations to combat obesity. The focus has been on programs and policies that are more in line with traditional values that emphasize personal responsibility and will be supported by the food industry.[24] Although some have argued that restricting children's food choices through regulation infringes on their right to free choice, this ignores the fact that children's free choices are already restricted by the family choice's and by the social environment in which they live.

The role of the family serves to convert the needs of children into a private rather than a public responsibility and provides a setting where the needs of children are not considered on an equal basis to those of adults.[24] Therefore, as feminists have long argued, the privacy afforded the family masks injustices that would not be accepted in the public sphere.[24] In developing countries, this has been manifested in reduced food intake for different family members, for example especially girl children in Asia (see chapter 5 for a relevant case study), whereas in North America it may be reflected in providing children with fast food meals that adults in the family would not themselves eat. With few possibilities made available for children to develop healthy food preferences apart from the family and the marketing that we have allowed to be targeted at them while neglecting to provide adequate protection through regulation of unhealthy foods, we have created a situation that promotes the childhood epidemic of obesity.

Triage in Public Health Emergencies

A public health emergency exists when an event (earthquake, flood, rapid migration or displacement of the population, pandemic disease) occurs and overwhelms the community's capacity to respond.[25] During disasters, medical services are typically inadequate, and experience worldwide has demonstrated the need for more systematic planning. Topics that have been addressed by national and local communities include procedures for rapidly handling medical emergencies, protocols for interagency cooperation, and mechanisms for allocating limited resources. These activities have required priority setting, rationing, and triage.

The concept of triage is fundamentally at odds with biomedical ethics, whereby the medical care of an individual is balanced against the autonomy of the individual and is delivered within a unique relationship between the individual patient and the physician. Medical ethics is based on the Hippocratic Oath, which requires making decisions based on the best interest of the patient. By contrast, triage requires that the best interests of some patients are superseded by the needs of others, thereby representing the interests of the group rather than the interest of the individual. Triage requires rapid, accurate, objective decision making to ensure that the objectives of public health disaster planning are met. These are to protect life and health, respect human rights, promote justice, and build civic capacity to increase the resilience of community response and recovery.[25]

In triage during disaster, the fact that some people are more likely than others to survive their wounds confers advantage to those individuals and therefore neither equal shares of medical care nor equal opportunity for medical care are provided.[25] Within the discussion of ethics there is one aspect that emphasizes human dignity in general rather than individual autonomy and emphasizes precaution (the precautionary principle discussed previously) and solidarity of humankind. Within this framework there is an opportunity to address those in need of support who have the highest likelihood of survival, and triage can be framed as an action needed to address public health risks that begins with the pursuit of human solidarity. Human solidarity occurs when a group of people is committed to collective decision making to reach a desired outcome and where special attention is given to people with serious conditions even when there may be significant personal cost in terms of losing loved ones who have more serious injuries.[25]

In the setting of disaster triage, the decision to treat patients may be made according to likelihood of survival and ability to contribute to greater good (human solidarity), for example a physician or a nurse may be treated before someone else, and in some cases individuals will not receive treatment at all. The elements that solidarity provides that can be useful in decision making are attentiveness to the needs of others, responsibility to duties according to professional values and beliefs, and competence needed to provide the appropriate care. These values were also addressed previously. In the context of disaster triage, here are some general principles that may help:[25]

- Intervention must be necessary and effective.
- Intervention should be the least restrictive alternative.
- There should be procedural due process that offers the right to appeal.
- Benefits and burdens of intervention should be fairly distributed.
- Public health officials should make decisions in an open and accountable manner.

Conclusion

Ethical guidelines and codes of practice are general rules to assist in making public health decisions in many different settings. They cannot provide specific guidance for specific circumstances because there are often times when needed scientific information is not available quickly enough for a response in a crisis situation. Individual public health practitioners have to assume responsibility for their role in ensuring ethical decisions they make in terms of individual virtues and values and their role in the larger society. As technology advances there may be added pressure to develop new approaches to ensure that the values and goals of public health have been incorporated into policies, regulations, and practices.

CASE STUDY—ETHICAL LESSONS FROM A SARS OUTBREAK: TORONTO, 2003

In October 2002, an outbreak of a previously unknown severe acute respiratory syndrome (SARS) was reported from Guangdong Province, China. Within months it spread to over 30 countries. The experience of Toronto, Canada (where it appeared in February 2003) has been analyzed and reviewed regarding decisions involving competing ethical values.[26, 27]

Ethics of Quarantine: Because of evidence of person-to-person transmission, it was considered to be in the public interest to quarantine those who may have been exposed. Associated ethical issues included duty to protect the public from harm that may arise through contact with someone in an infectious state, restrictions on personal liberty, the need to exercise proportionality (the least restrictive measures to achieve this measure without discrimination), transparency (all stakeholders informed), and that quarantined persons receive care and not suffer financial loss.[26]

Privacy versus the Public Need to Know: Normally, individuals have a right to privacy about their health: this protects them from the stigma of public scrutiny. However, this right can be overridden for the perceived greater good. When such action is taken, the public benefit must be balanced against risks to the individual. Believing these conditions to be met, early in the outbreak, authorities named the woman who carried SARS from China to Canada, with her family's consent.[26] However, given the limited understanding of transmission among the general public and health professionals, this resulted in an unintended consequence: widespread stigmatization of Chinese people and others who had recently traveled in China.

"Fear of the unknown" became widespread among callers to radio talk-shows; ethnic Chinese were stigmatized, their businesses suffering heavy financial losses. When WHO issued a travel advisory warning people to avoid Toronto (probably not necessary), meetings and conventions were canceled, trade and commerce were curtailed. Estimated financial losses to the city were $35M/day. The SARS outbreak demonstrated that attitudes and reactions to poorly understood life-threatening epidemic disease could occur in the 21st century just as in mediaeval times.

Duty of Care: Frontline health care providers were facing a potentially deadly infectious disease for which there was no known effective treatment. How were they to protect themselves and their families against the disease while fulfilling their duty to care for others? These considerations are linked: providers also must maintain their own health in order to provide care for others.[26] A decade later, there remains lack of agreement regarding how much exposure health care providers are professionally obliged to accept. Further consultation is required to reach consensus on the issue of exposure and to what extent institutions can fulfill their duty of reciprocity by providing protection, stress management, risk acknowledgement, and plans for emergency situations.

Collateral Damage: In addition to the direct effects, thousands of other patients were adversely affected by restrictions placed on hospital admissions. Individuals with varying afflictions, some life-threatening, were confronted with serious delays and barriers to care.

Those admitted faced loss of contact and emotional support from family and friends. Weighing the benefits of health protection against these costs also presents an ethical challenge. Risks, benefits, and opportunity costs must be weighed to determine which services to maintain under such circumstances.[26]

Global Implications: The experience of SARS illustrates the necessity for communications and cooperation among nations so as to achieve mutual protection against such threats. It is neither ethical nor acceptable to conceal health information that can protect others.[26, 27] Had China stepped forward earlier with information about the disease and its origins, the global spread of SARS may have been reduced.

Envoi: The causal organism, identified only after the epidemic subsided, was a coronavirus that appears to have jumped from wild civet cats to humans and was then transmitted person-to-person by close personal contact. In retrospect, the disease has made only a tiny impact on public health globally, although the lessons loom large. By providing a test of the capacity of health systems (including the adequacy of investment in public health capacities), including national, provincial, local, and hospital responses, the world may now be better prepared (or at least forewarned) for the anticipated next pandemic infectious disease.[28] The take-away message for those working in public health at all levels: tell the truth calmly, engage responsible media to disseminate the facts and best advice to the public, avoid blaming or stigmatizing identifiable groups or individuals.

This chapter examines the central role of communities in their citizens'
health and why public health decision makers and practitioners must
be fluent in this role in order to be effective. The key to involvement of
communities lies in the participation of people in processes that affect their
health. While top-down policy initiatives are often essential, much of what
makes a difference happens in communities: leadership, intersectoral action,
and change management "from the ground up." Thus we explore community
development, health promotion, and primary health care as frameworks
that underpin and mutually reinforce the health of populations, primarily
through their impact on community health. Case studies are utilized, and
the social-ecological model introduced, as ways of appreciating how humans
relate through family and community to the larger society and how this
relationship is a key to effective interventions. We consider the mantra "think
globally, act locally" and its converse "think locally, act globally": what
they mean, how we know when they apply, and how then to proceed. This
brings us to conclude with an examination of the challenges of "scaling up"
and sustainability.

4

COMMUNITY FOUNDATIONS OF PUBLIC HEALTH

FOR MILLENNIA, LONG before governments accepted any responsibility for environmental and health conditions, people came together to protect the habitat that supported them and to care for one another. This tradition still exists in most parts of the world, however imperfectly, and is even upheld as a democratic ideal. Because such commitment is found mostly at local level, led primarily by volunteers, it is often referred to as grassroots.

What Are Communities?

A community is a human population with characteristics that confer a basis for people feeling that they belong, such as common ethnic, religious, or cultural features or economic cooperation requiring interdependence. Communities tend to have belief systems and shared insights or wisdom, and they may create knowledge and become a source of learning. These characteristics may be applicable or not to society as a whole. The qualities of a community may extend from situation-specific to globally generalizable. There is usually a belief in mutual welfare and often a system for identifying leadership, which may or may not include a governance system, for example, councils (elected or otherwise) capable of making decisions on behalf of the community.

There is no necessary size or geographic area for a community, and communities may overlap with one another. Individuals may belong to more than one community: in numerous countries, especially in urban settings, many individuals do not belong to a single, distinct community, but maintain membership in several based on commonalities of location, culture, religion, language, occupation, social, and leisure interests.

Functional communities are able to combine outside assistance with local self-determination and effort. They achieve goals that are both *material* (e.g., a new health center) and *non-material* (e.g., healthier lifestyles). Viewed thus as a *unit of action* with some capacity for self-determination, it follows that ideas, innovations, and actions that promote or protect health may commence at community level and not necessarily wait for centrally determined decisions (e.g., national or state/ provincial policies). A well-balanced health system should have strong elements of community involvement within a more centrally determined framework.

Once types of community are defined, "community" can be utilized as a *unit of analysis* for research and development and for planning. Valuable insights can be gained by observing and learning from what happens in particular communities that are achieving success or otherwise, and (when this experience is generalizable) it is sometimes desirable and feasible to apply these lessons for the benefit of others. For example, initiatives may be tested by one community, then scaled-up so as to benefit other communities or society as a whole; we examine the feasibility of this later in the chapter.

Why "Community Health"?

From Africa to America, it is now well established that health is mostly made in households and communities.[1] It is at the community level that the interplay of actions that promote health with those which deal with ill-health after it occurs is best understood—in how people live, in what control they may have over their health conditions, and how this is facilitated. According to the Institute of Medicine, "there is strong evidence that behavior and environment are responsible for over 70% of avoidable mortality, and health care is just one of several determinants."[2] The formal health system needs to be appraised in this light: for example, while launching a new health facility may be cause for local pride and even a ribbon cutting ceremony with political gains (just like a new road or a bridge may be), what goes on in the facility, and in the community itself, are more important than the facility. As urban philosopher Jane Jacobs (1916–2006) famously said: "old ideas can sometimes use new buildings, but new ideas must use old buildings"[3] This idea is best understood, not only as relevant to physical structures in the context of urban renewal, but also as a metaphor for community living and working with communities: drawing from wisdom, skills, and other resources that communities possess is empowering, building upon rather than displacing or reinventing a capacity that already exists. Community efforts in promoting healthy lives for all people at all ages make the difference in health outcomes in the long term.

How to work effectively with communities, tailor interventions to local settings, and scale up to large populations offers a rich source of ideas for public health systems research and development.[4] Community-based research is required for defining needs and identifying workable solutions in challenging urban and rural settings. For example, impoverished inner-city communities, areas with high immigrant and refugee populations, just like remote rural communities and indigenous minority populations, cannot be assumed to fit the pattern that applies to urban or rural populations as a whole. Such communities have unique experiences, perspectives, and challenges and may require solutions that are different from those that are applicable to mainstream society.

Consider, for example, the situation of colonized racial, cultural, and religious minorities throughout the world. Nested within powerful societies, these colonized minorities are mostly organized and/or viewed as distinct communities: the Uyghurs and Tibetans in China, the Ainu of Japan, the Dalits of India, Amerindian enclaves in the Caribbean, tribal minorities in Africa, Boznian Muslims in former Yugoslavia, the Kurds of Iraq, and others in all continents and among the Pacific islands. All these groups suffer systematic disadvantages ranging historically from benign neglect to extreme prejudice. For example, in Australia, Canada, New Zealand, and the United States (all former colonies of the United Kingdom), "the legacies of colonial dispossession, land alienation, forcible relocation, suppression of indigenous cultural practices, values and beliefs, loss of language, disruption of families, violations of indigenous inherent sovereignty and right to self-determination, treaties, international law and indigenous cultural law, and other factors, have resulted in indigenous peoples experiencing a deplorable health status compared to non-indigenous settlers."[5] Such situations cannot be approached with a one-size-fits-all mindset. Indigenous leadership and community participation are required for issues to be resolved, along with genuine partnership from the larger society; learning from these situations may also help avert other conflicts now and in the future.

At this stage it will be clear to the reader that population health research and actions appropriate to the larger society (e.g., epidemiological and sociological) may not translate well to all communities and settings. For this reason, in large-scale surveys it is important to ensure that communities with particular needs are represented and sometimes critically important to develop more locally appropriate research methods, such as *community-based participatory research* (chapter 2); actions intended to improve health at community level must take local realities fully into account.

How Does Community Health Differ from Public Health and Hospital Services?

In its contribution to the health system, community health, *as a subdiscipline of public health*, is built upon *community development principles* and requires participatory approaches at all stages from defining the issues to designing solutions. The key principle is that a community's ownership of the issues and its rightful role in local leadership and participation in problem analysis and problem solving are often essential ingredients in determining whether locally effective action is taken and for this action to be sustainable.

Community health thereby differs from, and complements, other public health initiatives, which approach populations in a jurisdictional manner (e.g., country, province/state, district/county) and those that emphasize entitlements (e.g., universal childhood immunization). It differs from the modus operandi of hospitals, which plan services around catchment areas (a market concept geographically defined in terms of distance, transport routes, ease of travel, and relevance to their own referral networks). When hospitals or public health agencies conduct community outreach activities, these are usually developed in relation to their jurisdictional boundaries and catchment areas, and do not always enlist community participation in their design. This said, both mainstream public health and hospital services can also benefit from application of community development principles, applying these to become more locally relevant and effective.

Although formal responsibility for public health is shared across levels of government (see chapter 8 for comparative organization and function), with delegation of policy, planning, and operational decisions within this hierarchy, unfortunately this process often does not involve people in the communities that are intended to benefit. Too often, senior managers and professionals in centrally based agencies tend to assume that, even without training in community development or local experience, they "know best" what communities need and how to lead change. All too often, technically well-trained individuals with good intentions identify problems and arrive in a community with problem statement and solution already in hand. Or in some instances, they may formulate social policy interventions that are assumed to be universally relevant and effective but are not. However, if instead the situation analysis is done with the affected communities, both sets of stakeholders will better understand the problem, and for the community this is a vital element in owning the solution and its sustainability. Not taking this approach may reflect a deficiency in professional training. Stated another way, technical know-how is not enough: public health professionals need skills in community development so as to involve community representatives as partners.

Nongovernmental Organizations and Voluntarism as a Community Force

Ultimately community health is about the right of people to self-determination: to act in their own self-interest and to organize solutions in a manner responsive to locally perceived needs, especially if these are not adequately met by society as a whole. This right is recognized in the *United Nations Covenant on Economic, Social and Cultural Rights* (1966).[6] As more societies move toward democratic futures, the balance will shift toward increasing and sustaining community involvement in solving health challenges. The involvement of communities in their health therefore rests on democratic principles. If locally perceived needs are not recognized or met by jurisdictionally designed services, communities may organize their own responses, often through community-based organizations (CBOs), or become of legitimate interest to other nongovernmental organizations (NGOs) that share similar priorities or agendas. Ideally, community health planning should involve all relevant parties, but especially the communities presumed to be beneficiaries and that will be affected by the resulting decisions.

All this leads us to examining the role of NGOs. What does this term mean? Paradoxically, by referring only to what NGOs are not (i.e., they are "not" governmental) this term fails to define such organizations for what they really are, and (if taken literally) lumps together everything from the corporate sector to local community groups. In a more positive sense, NGOs are organizations that represent visible public support for particular causes and constitute an organized response to perceived needs.[7] As distinct from spatial communities, these may be viewed as communities of interest (people coming together due to a common bond). Most NGOs are locally based, others are national, and some are international in scope. Although many types of NGOs make contributions to health, it is mainly the voluntary "not-for-profit" organizations that represent grassroots commitment. Although larger NGOs often have paid staff (which may enhance their effectiveness), their leadership and membership remain voluntary.

Through such voluntary nongovernmental organizations, objectives are achieved on a person-to-person basis, more so than for government agencies whose first mandate is to carry out tasks set for them under legislation. Voluntary organizations have a sociology that includes a high degree of loyalty to the group and an ability to network that cannot be achieved by governments or private enterprise because of the bureaucratic requirements of official agencies or obsession with the bottom line of profit-and-loss statements. Voluntary organizations have the potential to be much more flexible than governments, big labor, big professions, or big business. Characteristically, such organizations are smaller and potentially more able to respond to community needs as they arise, mostly because people can change faster than institutions. In the face of global political and economic challenges, the increasingly important role of voluntary organizations constitutes a powerful social movement that must be reckoned with and may be indispensable to social and economic development in all countries. The spirit of voluntarism empowers people and gives them a sense of belonging and of purpose; because this process is voluntary, they feel good about themselves and their contributions to society. This process is essentially spontaneous, not statutory, and surely represents enormous potential for the promotion of health and social development.[7]

Each successful NGO requires leadership from within the group and mechanisms for ensuring effective succession and sustainability. To be effective it must have a capacity for communications and access to resources. Underlying NGO initiatives one may find bold aspirational thinking, not always matched by operational capacity. To become fully effective in pursuing their strategic vision, many NGOs need to be strengthened in such areas as governance, planning, and management skills. If this is achieved, they may become more politically potent and operationally effective as they scale up from local to national levels, depending on whether their focus is primarily local or more broadly based, requiring mutually reinforcing actions at several levels. When voluntary initiatives incorporate national health goals within community agendas, they illustrate a vital source of collaboration with government for the common good and often bring with them unique capacities, resources, and motivation to get things done. A network of internationally active NGOs (as addressed in chapter 8) recently adopted a Code of Conduct for Health Systems Strengthening, which reflects this move toward improved working practices.[8]

Community-Based Health Services

Community-based health services are an essential component of health care delivery, especially with regard to the critical elements of accessibility and utilization. For example, control of many communicable diseases—whether through vaccines, diagnostic tests, drugs, or environmental controls—depends largely on such measures being incorporated within functional community-based systems and participatory approaches.

It is a common fallacy to view community-based services simply as low-cost alternatives to institutional services (e.g., hospital based outpatient or social service departments); along with primary health care, they are much more appropriately viewed as a platform from which a comprehensive health system may be developed. Even when a service must be delivered in whole or in part from an institutional base, community involvement in designing, developing, and operating systems can result in approaches more responsive to the needs of local culture and priorities. Health reforms are more likely to succeed if those whose health is at stake "own" the reforms (or at least have been meaningfully consulted during their formulation). Developing participation therefore has become a key step for enlightened planners and decision makers, based on greater awareness and sensitivity to the social complexity of community-based programs.[9]

The active involvement of community-based organizations within public health systems is an increasingly used strategy, especially in resource-challenged settings (a form of resource mobilization). As governments increasingly recognize this as a potentially competent and well-motivated resource for health and social development (often in response to advocacy by such groups) and the related necessity for new ways of working (participatory rather than outmoded "command and control" approaches), they can also consider using the tools of government to help this process along, such as innovative tax policies and grants that promote self-help and community development. For example, Canada's federal tax system has several disability-related programs dealing with income support and tax relief and with promoting independent community living, education, employment, family support, and care-giving. The personal income tax system has become a frequent instrument for disability policy making because of court decisions and sustained lobbying efforts by disability groups, among others.[10]

Health advisory boards of government agencies active at the community level also benefit from the participation of community members; the challenge here is to ensure that this input is as authentic and representative as it needs to be to truly reflect community interests, as distinct from vested interests. To ensure such representation, as well as competence regarding the community, it is sometimes desirable to have several representatives on such boards to reflect a range of diverse and legitimate perspectives. Technical expertise can be added, depending on the nature of the issues at hand, but this properly should be viewed as an input rather than the key to effective decision making.

Planning and developing the community component requires mainstream public health organizations to have on their staff people with the skills to cross traditional organizational boundaries, such as by coalition building and the formation of public-private partnerships (sometimes referred to as P3s, these may include both nonprofit and commercial enterprises, which may also embody a social purpose in their mission), and the insight and humility to recognize that it is often the partner organizations who have the greater knowledge, skills, and values required for successful intervention. (Note: public-private partnerships are discussed more fully in chapter 8.)

To illustrate the uniquely helpful yet mainstream roles that such participants can play, consider for example Meals on Wheels, a program active in Australia, Canada, the United States, and the United Kingdom, run by nonprofit community organizations and typically supported by local hospitals and restaurants. Sometimes assisted by government grants, these initiatives supply meals delivered by volunteers to seniors and others less able to fend for themselves through ill health or disability. Another example is the provision of food to homeless and low-income families by community-organized food banks—these, too, operate outside the defined roles of local and state/provincial public health agencies. Similarly, domestic violence shelters operate as independent nonprofit organizations and may offer health education and counseling programs to reduce related issues (e.g., drug abuse). Once organized, persons affected by particular conditions, and their allies, have been a major force in motivating more appropriate responses from the health system and play potent partnership roles, such as diabetes associations, HIV/AIDS organizations, and organizations advocating for improved mental health services, among others.

The ability of community organizations to make a difference in people's lives is even more critical in emerging economies because the capacities of their formal health systems are often underdeveloped. For example, *malaria control* in South India improved with the adoption of a community participation strategy involving committees in program design and implementation.[11] Bangladesh revealed that collaboration between government and nongovernment organizations improved access to and quality of *tuberculosis services*.[12] Similar principles have been applied successfully in the World Health Organization (WHO) Integrated Management of Childhood Infections (IMCI) protocol, involving health workers and family members in complementary roles.[13] Shelters for *homeless* people in communities worldwide are provided by philanthropic and faith-based groups.

By these examples, it is clear that community-based health and social sector initiatives are active in all countries: people helping people. Exploring the roles of community organizations through site visits, projects, and actual involvement in their work, as well as documentation (e.g., term papers based on field assignments, practicums, and electives), is an excellent mode of learning for all students of public health.

New Trends in Organizational Forms and Functions—Shifting Sands

As the 21st century unfolds, it is timely to alert readers to the way in which long-standing assumptions, rules, and practices regarding how organizations were supposed to work have been shifting, increasingly over the past decade. The lines demarcating public and private sector domains, and even the nature and roles of the voluntary sector in a variety of forms, are becoming blurred. To place this in context, consider the following observations regarding the conflicts confronting traditional organizations:

- Private companies have always had to strike a balance between achieving the largest possible profits for shareholders and retaining trust and contact with their other stakeholders: the local community, consumers, subcontractors, and advocacy groups. However, it is clear from the global financial crisis in 2008 that some companies are "too big to fail." Despite mismanagement, to avoid serious impacts on national economies, often with global implications, several financial institutions and motor vehicle manufacturers have been rescued in North America and Europe, bailed out by governments, that is, the public sector.
- The public sector in many nations is simultaneously facing political pressure to downsize and to privatize various functions. However, the action of the European Union since 2011 in bailing out Greece reveals that when a nation mismanages public finances, it may be rescued (if deemed too politically important to fail) by other governments to avoid "financial contagion"—global default on interest payments on government bonds.
- Due to fierce competition from other voluntary organizations and reduced state financing, voluntary organizations, including public health and international development groups (sometimes under political pressure) are having to generate independent income (e.g., sale of products and services) in order to stay solvent. These activities can be in conflict (potential or real) with their mission and goals.

The emergent outcome of these trends is that many public and voluntary organizations no longer operate in the "pure" manner implied. Increasingly public enterprises compete with the private sector, while the voluntary sector has become commercially astute. For example, the success of many not-for-profit organizations today is due to a fully funded core staff, supplemented by contract income, thus able to build "working capital funds," while remaining eligible for government grants (competitive advantage retained). In effect, such NGOs have become a good "business model" (now accepted terminology). Meanwhile, many public sector entities (including some public health agencies) have become so depleted that they must hire private contractors to deliver the expertise that actually belongs with their public mandate. In addition to consulting firms, much of this is now obtained from universities, themselves having become "hybrid" organizations.[14] Faculty engaged in consulting generate substantial overhead income for the institution. Even publicly funded universities now engage in industry partnerships while receiving government financing and simultaneously contracting out services to government.[15]

The Emergence of Fourth Sector Organizations: Out of this complex scenario, in which the neat role relationships that once separated traditional organizational forms seem to be breaking down, "fourth sector organizations" are emerging. Operating outside the world of grants (for which they are mostly ineligible under existing rules) and inside the reality of surviving as a business, their mission is one of social purpose. This new class of organization, also known as "for benefit" enterprises, has the potential to become a force for community health, as it is for other social enterprises.[16] In a rapidly changing world, as a new paradigm in organizational design it aims to link two concepts traditionally portrayed as juxtaposed (even as a conflict of interest): private interest and public benefit. Like it or not, the lines separating these concepts are already blurred at the highest levels of government, commerce, and even academia, such that they represent a false dichotomy.

The recognition, comparative assessment, and documentation of all forms of enterprise that benefit community health now constitute a legitimate and valuable learning opportunity for students of public health, with potential for broader application.

Community Health as a Vital Ingredient in Health Reform

In reforming the health sector, well-planned and implemented community-based systems are a critical ingredient. They enhance the impact and sustainability of interventions owing to advantages of local cultural acceptability, accessibility, and utilization. Unfortunately, despite the appropriateness of this approach and its potential cost-effectiveness (it usually embodies greater commitment to prevention and community support), more emphasis continues to be placed by more centrally located decision makers on curative and hospital-based technologies located in institutional settings. This reveals a perception of market demand that, in part, reflects powerful advocacy from institutional and related interests (including the mostly institutionally based health care professions themselves), and that is still a more potent consideration at policy level. Nonetheless, achieving the right mix of investments across the health service spectrum is important to meeting population health needs, and this usually requires more investment at community level.

In particular, community-based programs require resources for public education and mobilization, and for training leaders. From an investment standpoint, this is not simply a lower-cost option; rather it is a more effective platform for high impact and broadly based interventions. Where the command-and-control model dominates, public sector managers tend to lack expertise in community participation methods, which is one reason for weak community health systems in many countries. Such skills are more often found in the nongovernmental and private sectors, thus reinforcing the case for strengthening P3s. For government to move further in this direction, in consultation and with participation of the private sector, it must evolve the policy framework to foster an enabling environment so as to nurture those synergies that will improve health outcomes, for example through the creative use of incentives. Monitoring and evaluation will be necessary; along with information sharing at all levels so that lessons learned will benefit all concerned. (Note: Health sector reform is dealt with more comprehensively in chapter 8.)

Primary Health Care as a Community-Centered Activity: Although primary health care (PHC) is often defined as health or medical care that begins at the time of first contact between a physician or other health professional and a person seeking advice or treatment for an illness or an injury, this is a "profession-centered" definition. It ignores the role of family members as first-line caregivers and accords no role to communities in addressing health issues. By contrast, the World Health Organization offers a broader definition of PHC that applies to the health system as a whole and recognizes the role of public health while respecting the need to involve communities in their health.

Primary Health Care: PHC means essential health care made accessible at a cost that a country can afford, with methods that are practical, scientifically sound, and socially acceptable. Everyone should have access to it and be involved in it, as should other sectors of society. It should include community participation and education on prevalent health problems, health promotion and disease prevention, provision of adequate food and nutrition, safe water, basic sanitation, maternal and child health care, family planning, prevention and control of endemic diseases, immunization against vaccine-preventable diseases, appropriate treatment of common diseases and injuries, and provision of essential drugs.[17]

This broader concept of PHC grew out of an international conference in 1978 hosted by WHO and the United Nations Children's Fund (UNICEF), at which 134 countries were represented, and that issued the Alma Ata Declaration on Primary Health Care.[18] However, while the role of medical care was well appreciated, public health was less understood and how to work at community level even less so. If higher priority had been given to promoting leadership skills, developing countries might have progressed both in public health and in making basic medical care accessible, particularly for rural and disadvantaged communities. But this did not happen largely because a group of "global experts" questioned the feasibility of PHC and started a countermovement, curiously named "selective PHC" as an interim strategy for disease control in developing countries. Their principle was to apply, in a vertically integrated manner, modern technical approaches (surveillance-based) to control infectious diseases, selected from a global list of 23. Both approaches were genuine attempts to strengthen public health in developing countries, but the ensuing decades witnessed at least partial failure of both.[19] Local communities failed to develop integrated models of PHC and in many instances had to compete for priority and resources with vertically driven disease control strategies heavily supported by external donors. Although the success of some disease-specific initiatives is a matter of record (see chapters 2 and 6) more basic health provisions such as clean water, food security, and attending to locally prevalent conditions fell by the wayside, with little change in overall health status. If instead communities had been supported to develop local health systems, then so-called "vertical approaches" would likely have been more effective and sustainable. With benefit of hindsight, this deficiency is now widely acknowledged, and efforts are under way in some countries to enable communities to participate in defining their needs and solutions, thus approaching health systems development in a more respectful manner.

The People's Health Movement: Out of frustration with the heavy emphasis on selective disease control programs in the virtual absence of locally integrated health systems development, and fears regarding the powerful forces of economic globalization perceived to be submerging local health and social agendas, along with persistence of a heavy burden of ill health associated with endemic poverty, a People's Health Assembly was convened in Dhaka, Bangladesh in 2000. A movement mostly of NGO, faith-based and academic delegates from 113 countries, the Assembly issued a People's Charter of Health. This expressed disappointment over the Alma Ata Declaration's unrealized goals, which were perceived to have been distorted and disowned by major international players.[19] The Charter called for a return to the broader concept of PHC and appropriate public health programs, emphasizing the social and economic roots of ill health and poverty and their mutual linkages. In echoing the slogan issued at the time of the Alma Ata Declaration of "Health for All by the Year 2000," this called for "Health for All, Now."[20] Interestingly, also in 2000, a United Nations heads of government meeting issued the Millennium Development Goals (see chapter 5).[21] It seemed that the people and their governments were expressing similar concerns and aspirations for workable solutions;

however, while limited progress has been made so far toward achieving the goals, the global economic crisis has reversed development gains in some countries and appears to have undermined Goal 8 (which deals with international support).[22] Still holding governments to account however, the People's Health Movement held a second Assembly in 2005, this time in Cuenca, Ecuador. The movement deserves recognition as it shows how nongovernmental, faith-based, and other community groups (together representing what is also referred to as "civil society") can align as an international voice advocating health worldwide. The People's Charter for Health is the most widely endorsed consensus document on health since the Alma Ata Declaration.

The Bangkok Charter of Health Promotion in a Globalized World: Also released in 2005, this WHO Charter highlights the changing context of global health and challenges faced in achieving its aims.[23] It examines the health effects of globalization such as widening inequities, rapid urbanization, and the degradation of environments. Building on the Ottawa Charter for Health Promotion (described next), the Bangkok Charter adds value to health promotion practice worldwide. Commitments were identified: to make the promotion of health central to the global development agenda, a core responsibility for all of government, a key focus of communities and civil society and a requirement for good corporate practices.[24] The Bangkok Charter thereby complements and builds upon the values, principles, and action strategies of health promotion established by the Ottawa Charter and the recommendations of subsequent global health promotion conferences as confirmed by Member States through the World Health Assembly. It calls for policy coherence, investment, and partnering across governments, international organizations, civil society, and the private sector. We cite it here because of the increased emphasis given to the roles of community, civil society, and the private sector and also because it highlights the need for global leadership to address the effects of trade and marketing strategies where these are harmful. It calls for health promotion to become an integral part of domestic and foreign policy and international relations, including situations of war and conflict. Its advocates have concluded that action centered on empowered and capable communities, in synergistic collaboration with other key players, may be the most powerful instrument available for the future of health promotion in a globalized world.[25]

The Ottawa Charter on Health Promotion: The core principles of the contemporary health promotion movement were first laid out at the 1st International Conference on Health Promotion, November 21, 1986. The definition of health promotion, as defined in this formative Ottawa Charter, now follows:

Health promotion is the process of enabling people to increase control over, and to improve, their health. To reach a state of complete physical, mental and social well-being, an individual or group must be able to identify and to realize aspirations, to satisfy needs, and to change or cope with the environment. Health is, therefore, seen as a resource for everyday life, not the objective of living. Health is a positive concept emphasizing social and personal resources, as well as physical capacities. Therefore, health promotion is not just the responsibility of the health sector, but goes beyond healthy life-styles to well-being.[26]

The Charter recognized three broad strategies for health promotion: *advocacy* to create the essential conditions for health; *enabling* all people to achieve their full health potential; and *mediating* between different interests in society in the pursuit of health. In support of these strategies, five priority action areas were identified: (1) build healthy public policy; (2) create supportive environments for health; (3) strengthen community action for health; (4) develop personal skills; and (5) reorient health services. These actions were incorporated in a logo (Figure 4-1),

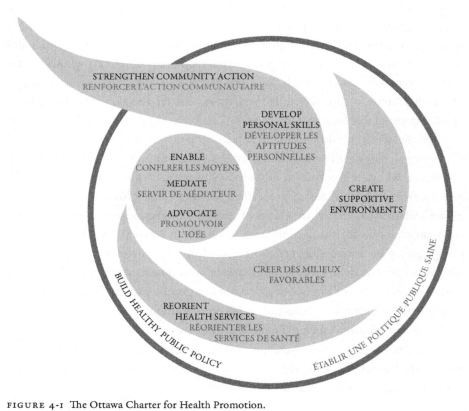

FIGURE 4-1 The Ottawa Charter for Health Promotion.

Logo showing the operational elements.

Acknowledgment: Reprinted with permission of the Canadian Public Health Association.

first developed at the conference and later adapted by WHO as its symbol for the health promotion effort globally.

Health promotion thus represents a comprehensive social and political process. It embraces actions directed at strengthening the skills and capabilities of individuals, but also actions directed toward changing social, environmental, and economic conditions so as to alleviate their impact on public and individual health.[27]

Because it laid out important principles that require action at the community foundation of the public health enterprise, it is particularly useful to examine the third action listed in the Ottawa Charter. Important references are made here to community action and community development. This section, entitled "Strengthen Community Actions," states: [26]

Health promotion works through concrete and effective community action in setting priorities, making decisions, planning strategies, and implementing them to achieve better health. At the heart of this process is the empowerment of communities—their ownership and control of their own endeavours and destinies. Community development draws on existing human and material resources in the community to enhance self-help and social support, and to develop flexible systems for strengthening public participation in and direction of health matters. This requires full and continuous access to information, learning opportunities for health, as well as funding support.

The roles of health promotion in public policy and in disease prevention and control are examined in chapters 8 and 6. For a comprehensive discussion of health promotion as a challenging and evolving public health discipline, we recommend the reference cited.[27]

Fundamentals of Community Health—A Synthesis

Taking into account the foregoing discussions, we have selected ten observations to support the case for increasing the involvement of communities in their health:

1. There is a difference between designing policies and programs and taking them to the people versus asking people first what their needs are and then working with them.
2. Where public health is driven by centrally mandated policies or donor priorities, formal programs may overlook health issues important to local communities.

3. Policies and programs developed with community involvement are likely to enjoy enhanced levels of acceptability, accessibility, utilization and sustainability.

4. Public health needs and initiatives often have local beginnings, may lack recognition at central levels, and their proponents may be actively discouraged.

5. Externally or internally conceived initiatives are more likely to be adopted, supported and sustained if linked to their perceived importance to the community.

6. Communities themselves are often uniquely able to shape solutions around locally recognized realities, assets, opportunities and resources.

7. Community groups should have an active role in defining the scope of their health needs and solutions: filling gaps in formally mandated public health programs.

8. Community participation is more effective when the need for it is recognized and facilitated by leaders, managers and professionals in formal public health services.

9. The importance of community participation is supported by findings from participatory action research and widely recognized: the Alma Ata Declaration (1978), the Ottawa Charter on Health Promotion (1986), the People's Charter of Health (2000), the Bangkok Charter for Health Promotion (2005) (among others).

10. All elements of an integrated health system, from family and community to non-governmental organization to government ministries and the private sector are interdependent, and must work together to achieve a healthy population.

Planning to Involve Communities

In light of the foregoing, public health professionals need to better understand and be able to apply community development principles to health from the "ground up." There is a need for sensitivity to all who make up a community, including not only the established interests that have always influenced decision making, but also others who represent interests that have often been excluded from this process. To facilitate this desirable broader participation, public health professionals must be prepared to build capacity for leadership and teamwork from within the community itself, drawing as appropriate from the full spectrum of age, gender, and minority groups; of equal importance they must enable communities to take credit for what they achieve and are able to sustain.

Effective community initiatives require strategic thinking and an evidence-based approach to planning. In chapter 8 we introduce four questions that represent a logical planning sequence: *Where are we? Where do we want to be? How do we get there? How do we know we are getting there?* Community participation in answering these questions is a critical success factor for successful initiatives at community level.[28] Whenever this element of participation is lacking, health development projects aimed at the community level do not fulfill their potential. Along with *communication* and *participation, leadership, advocacy* and *mobilization* are also key elements for success. However, even with these essential elements, such efforts may still not succeed if they do not result in an operational plan and the mobilization of sufficient resources to carry out that plan.

Mobilization strategies such as team-building can simultaneously foster leadership and support roles in community groups. The likelihood of success is enhanced when the initiative is owned and led by the community group and seen as their success. To achieve this requires that health practitioners serve as *mentors,* and to the extent that this may be leadership in itself (like coaching), it is "leadership from the sidelines." To organize effectively, community mobilizers are often recruited. If they are drawn from the community itself, they often know the area and the issues better than outsiders, may be better accepted, and can work more freely. They are also more likely to have a sense of ownership and thereby foster this sense among community members.

Preparing a community for change is an investment in people. This can be a challenging process which may delay short term results. However, it is an investment that must be made to achieve lasting success. Unfortunately, some health professionals, community participants and funding partners (e.g., governments with 4-year election cycles—too short to achieve long term change, and donor agencies working within such constraints) are often more obsessed with short term results and pay little attention to the slower processes of behavior and attitudinal changes, and the time required for the development of leadership and management skills. Such capacity-building can be lengthy and may not deliver expected results quickly. Health problems that have taken decades to emerge cannot be swept away within unrealistic timeframes.

Facilitating health innovations at community level is usually a slow and steady process, requiring willingness to invest in building partnerships and other working relationships locally. The likelihood of success can be enhanced by promoting a learning culture which enables all players to reflect on where they are coming from, where they are, and to analyze progress and share lessons in a participatory manner on a regular basis.

The Social-Ecological Model of Relationships

Before we move to examine a selection of case studies whereby communities have been involved in addressing their health, with varying success, it is timely to introduce

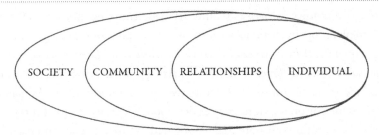

FIGURE 4-2 The Social-Ecological Model.

the "social-ecological model" as a way of appreciating how humans relate through family and community relationships to the larger society (Figure 4-2). Relationships can become disturbed to the extent that they are not aligned and mutually reinforcing; and the extent to which this occurs may enable understanding of the social and other pathologies that may arise. Conversely, the model can serve as an analytical framework through which prevention strategies (chapter 6) may be designed, implemented, monitored and evaluated. Regardless of complexity, all variations of this model are conceptually similar, reflecting an evolving synthesis of epidemiology with social and behavioral sciences.[29]

For example, the US Centers for Disease Control and Prevention (CDC) uses this type of model in its approach to violence prevention.[30] Prevention requires understanding the factors that influence violence.[31] The model considers the complex interplay between individual, relationship, community, and societal factors, and helps to identify those which put people at risk for experiencing or perpetrating violence. Prevention strategies should include a continuum of activities that address multiple levels of the model. They should be developmentally appropriate across the lifespan. This approach is more likely to sustain prevention efforts over time than any single intervention. The following are descriptions of what may be relevant at each level, adapted from the CDC example cited.

Individual: The first level identifies biological and personal history factors that influence the likelihood of becoming a victim or perpetrator of violence. Some of these factors are age, education, income, substance use, or history of abuse. Prevention strategies at this level are often designed to promote attitudes, beliefs, and behaviors that ultimately prevent violence. Specific approaches may include education and life skills training.

Relationships: The second level examines close relationships that may increase or reduce the risk of experiencing violence as a victim or perpetrator. A person's closest social circle (peers, partners, family members) influences their behavior and contributes to their range of experience. Prevention strategies at this level may include mentoring and peer programs designed to reduce conflict, foster problem solving skills, and promote healthy relationships.

Community: The third level explores settings, such as schools, workplaces, and neighborhoods, in which social relationships occur, and seeks to identify characteristics of these settings that are associated with becoming victims or perpetrators of violence. Prevention strategies at this level are typically designed to impact the context, processes, and policies in a given system. Social norm and social marketing campaigns are often used to foster community climates that promote healthy relationships.

Society: The fourth level looks at broad societal factors that help create a climate in which violence is encouraged or inhibited. These factors include social and cultural norms. Other large societal factors include the health, economic, educational and social policies that help to maintain economic or social inequalities between groups in society.

In summary, the essence of the "social-ecological model" is that, while individuals are often viewed as responsible for what they do, their behavior is determined largely by their social environment e.g., community norms and values, regulations, and policies. Barriers to healthy behaviors are often shared across their community, even society as a whole; as these are lowered or removed, behavior change becomes more achievable and sustainable. The optimal approach to promoting healthy behaviors therefore may be a combination that reinforces efforts at all levels—individual, interpersonal, organizational, community, and public policy. The "social-ecological model" is also relevant to some disease prevention and control applications, and therefore discussed again in chapter 6.

Involving Communities in Their Health—Selected Case Studies

We now present a series of community health case studies illustrating a diversity of experience from developing and developed countries. Lessons from these examples have global significance: an opportunity for mutual learning across this spectrum.

As you consider these examples, note the universal principles underlying them, and the elements of broad strategic thinking: 1. Social development, 2. Healthy public policy, 3. Systems development for health and social policy and related programming. They all require leadership within a political context, and each could be defended as a public health priority. They all followed an evidence-based approach to planning: *1. Where are we? 2. Where do we want to be? 3. How are we going to get there? 4. How will we know we are getting there?* Community participation is a key success factor for all of them.[1]

The Work of AMREF with the Masaai: Our first story is of the African Medical and Research Foundation (AMREF): in 1957, three men of vision launched the Flying Doctor Service in Kenya. From this emerged the African Medical and Research Foundation, Africa's largest indigenous health NGO. While their first two decades focused on service delivery, AMREF came to realize that episodic clinical visits were neither effective nor efficient, and that community-based approaches were vital. AMREF's Mission today reflects this recognition: "*... In creating vibrant networks of informed communities that work with empowered health workers in stronger health systems, we aim to ensure every African has access to the good health which is theirs by right*"[32]

AMREF evolved from those beginnings to become a health systems development agency for many countries. Its operations reflect disease burdens at the grassroots: malaria, HIV, school health, water, sanitation and hygiene. Its success in promoting primary health care builds on partnerships. It finds ways to improve people's health by examining the determinants: environment, culture, economics, micro-financing, politics, leadership and other ingredients. Supported by operational research, many AMREF initiatives become health systems models for Africa, influencing policies and practices across the continent. AMREF is committed to evidence-based community health: an example for the world.

Moving from its origins to an example of AMREF in action: Kenya's plains offer little water and swarms of flies, and trachoma persists among the Masaai. In traditional culture, each wife shares a one-room home with her children and newborn animals, preparing meals on a contaminated floor. To tackle this leading infectious cause of blindness, AMREF applies WHO's "SAFE" protocol: *S*urgery to treat end-stage disease, *A*ntibiotics to reduce the reservoir of infection, *F*acial cleanliness and *E*nvironmental improvements, for example: "leaky tin technology" (a tin-can with a hole plugged by a thorn allows clean water to remain uncontaminated and used sparingly) to reduce transmission.

A recent report on AMREF's work in the Rift Valley reveals that the SAFE protocol reduced active disease within 3 years in children from 47% to 16.0%, while potentially blinding trachoma declined 4.5% to 1.7%. The proportion of faces with many flies fell over 4 years from 48% to 6%.[33] The strategy is sustainable and has advanced eye care policy globally, boding well for WHO's goal of elimination by 2020 (GET 2020).[34]

AKU's Approach to Community Health Development in Pakistan: Turning now to the Aga Khan University's community health field sites in Pakistan, AKU's mandate emphasizes "*training... young people for leadership in addressing the health problems of the people... (and)... development of prototypes of health services that are effective and affordable.*" Beyond improving local conditions and outcomes in urban and rural settings, these initiatives have contributed to health systems developments that resonate nation-wide.[35] For example, during an initial 10-year period, AKU's urban health interventions in Karachi's squatter settlements more than halved infant and maternal mortality, as recognized in a *"Commonwealth Award of Excellence... in Women's Health."* Other institutions followed suit, shifting Pakistan's earlier model of institution-based education toward one more integrated with primary health care. This model of community health development, using locally-recruited health workers and basic health information systems augmented by surveys to assess health status and intervention impacts, contributed to the Family Health Program in Sindh province, provincial and national School Nutrition Programs, and Pakistan's Lady Health Workers program.[36, 37]

AKU's community health model recognizes social development as the core determinant of health outcomes and commits to evidence in designing and evaluating interventions. Specific interventions include: iron supplementation in pregnancy, access to emergency obstetric care, water quality technologies, hygiene education and contraceptive choices. Participation lies at the heart of governance and delivery of services in all sites, achieved through community health management teams comprised of active and influential members e.g., teachers, entrepreneurs, religious leaders, volunteers. A critical emphasis is to promote the role of women in leadership and decision making.

The benefits are mutual: field sites help communities organize to address their needs, while the communities help AKU to strengthen its teaching and research.[38] Being part of the Aga Khan Development Network, AKU achieves a multiplier effect through translation and dissemination of its experience throughout South Asia and East Africa.

As an example, stimulated by an enlightened government policy requiring resource companies to contribute up to 5% of their profits toward local development, a Rural Community Development Project was launched in 1996 as a collaborative venture between Lasmo Oil Company and AKU. A baseline assessment was carried out by AKU in Jangara, a poverty afflicted rural area: home deliveries comprised 92% of all births, infant mortality was 67/1000, and childhood immunization coverage (age7<C;5) was 8%, clearly establishing maternal and child health as priorities.[39]

Forward now to a 2002 report by the International Finance Corporation, a private-sector lending arm of the World Bank, which applies environmental and social standards to projects it supports. Their review of Lasmo operations states: *"the most successful effort is a Maternal and Child Health Center in Jangara, equipped with a laboratory, maternity ward, examination room, and ambulance serving local communities 24 hour a day. The center is staffed largely by women and includes a woman doctor, two lab assistants, one midwife, and a traditional birth attendant. Established in 1998, patients have increased from an initial monthly total of less than 200 to 800. The center sends four mobile clinics to remote villages every month to provide direct health services.*[40] The project also addressed water, sanitation and hygiene, primary education and income generation. AKU's role phased out in 2002–3, with transition to local NGO management.

The Health Policy Initiatives of Mauritius: Now turning to an island in the Indian Ocean, with 1.3 million people, Mauritius is a "community" that has shown impressive global leadership. In the late 1980s chronic diseases accounted for almost half their disease burden with an upward trend. Accordingly they set as a national priority "the reduction of non-communicable diseases"[41].[42] Using legislative and fiscal measures, community-level health promotion, and mass media support, they adopted as goals: healthy nutrition, exercise, smoking cessation, and reduced alcohol intake. They applied taxation and advertising bans to diminish sales of tobacco and alcohol, and subsidized a transition from palm oil (high in saturated fats) to soybean oil for cooking. Within 5 years, favorable changes were observed in lipid levels, blood pressure, smoking, alcohol use, and physical activity. The mean number of risk factors for women and men declined, although overweight and obesity increased. They succeeded in reducing the risk of heart disease and cancer, although the prevalence of type 2 diabetes continued to increase.[43]

In 2001, the initiative gained new support from the African Development Bank, using a goal setting exercise: by 2010, using health promotion methods, life expectancy would be increased from 66.7 to 69.5 years for men, and from 74.5 to 77.5 years for women.[44] By 2005 they had almost met the life expectancy target for men (69.2 years) and were fast closing the gap for women (75.7 years).[45]

The experience of Mauritius encourages other middle and lower income countries to develop similar initiatives, setting quantifiable targets within a health policy framework.

The North Karelia Project, Finland and its Global Impact:

This decades-long initiative is a global benchmark for population health that contains strong community components. Launched in 1972, within two decades, the incidence of ischemic heart disease was more than halved in both sexes in this Finnish province.[46] Intersectoral policy initiatives were joined with community action, medical intervention and public-private partnerships. The North Karelia Project (NKP) was from inception a "big tent" intervention that shows how many community elements can be successfully combined in a public health intervention.

More operational details from this experience are presented in chapter 6, where we revisit this as a model for integrated noncommunicable disease (NCD) prevention and control. However, focusing now on its community foundations, NKP showcases the potent role of a locally based demonstration project that eventually scaled up to global level. First, it was extended to Finland as a whole, then (impressed with its effectiveness) was emulated by many other countries. Among European countries that launched initiatives, 22 are now linked within the CINDI network.[47] The acronym stands for Countrywide Integrated Non-Communicable Disease Intervention. This movement was emulated by the Pan American Health Organization in initiating the CARMEN network of projects in 1995,[48] starting with Chile.[49] The two networks actively collaborate.

Community Interventions for Health (CIH) Initiative: CIH operates under the umbrella of the Oxford Health Alliance,[50] a new global network to promote NCD interventions that can provide evidence of the effectiveness of local action in diverse countries (e.g., China, India, Mexico, England), which can then be adapted to other settings. Each country project consists of an intervention site and a control site, so that intervention effects may be compared. CIH is an example of "global-local" partnership.

The CIH project in India has been showcased by the Commonwealth Secretariat as a good practice case study.[51] Centered on Trivandrum (capital of Kerala state) it aims to intervene on diet, physical activity, and tobacco use in schools; health care centers, workplaces, and rural villages. Similar to the CINDI-CARMEN model of leading with a baseline survey, such a survey was completed in 2009 that assessed, for example, the location of food shops, parks, and schools and population health data such as BMI and blood pressure. Responding to the first question in evidence-based planning (*Where are we?*), this is the key step by which demonstration projects add scientific value: enabling rational targets, monitoring, and evaluation. Intervention activities include tobacco initiatives (e.g., advocating for stricter enforcement of a 2003 Tobacco Control Act by which hospitals and schools should be tobacco-free); promoting healthy food choices in hospital and workplace canteens (e.g., to reduce salt and sugar and to improve the range of healthy snacks); and physical activity (e.g., bicycle training for schools girls, and sports equipment distributed to schools, health centers, clubs, and selected worksites).

The project engaged the participation of a variety of local people and organizations: teachers, the local education department, employers in local industry, local health directors and health professionals, local government, and community leaders. It has also faced challenges (e.g., the belief that being overweight is a sign of good health, or that traditional healthy foods are not seen as attractive compared with many processed foods).

As the results of ongoing monitoring surveys become available from Trivandrum and other CIH sites, much will be learned about how to impact health behavior and eventually health outcomes at the community level; what works and what doesn't.

The Healthy Cities—Healthy Communities Movement: A historically important WHO-associated initiative that remains in the vanguard of urban health development, the Healthy Cities—Healthy Communities movement, offers considerable global learning. Sponsored initially by WHO's European Regional Office, it aims to enhance quality of life by making communities more conducive to healthy living: providing resources and facilities for recreation; easy access to settings for exercise, sport, and physical activity; and designing dwellings amenable to good living. Like CINDI-CARMEN, this approach emphasizes sustainability and requires long-term commitment. Success in Düsseldorf, Toronto, Dakar, and other pioneer cities encouraged expansion to cities in over 50 countries and stimulated similar initiatives for rural and island communities.[52] The Strong Rural Communities Initiative in Wisconsin, whose purpose is to improve health indicators by promoting prevention, illustrates application of this model to rural areas.[53]

To the extent that distinctions exist between CINDI-CARMEN and Healthy Communities, the former is explicitly focused on leading causes of morbidity and mortality and their risk factors, and it requires quantitative evaluation of outcomes. By contrast, the Healthy Communities movement gives more attention to process indicators, reflecting a greater emphasis on determinants and intersectoral interventions. CINDI-CARMEN initiatives are nationally endorsed and operate at state or provincial level with local demonstration areas, usually with Ministry of Health leadership, while Healthy Communities are driven more by urban planning principles and centered on municipalities. Although each has a distinct philosophy and tends to have operated separately, more could be achieved by combining elements from both models.[54]

Gun Control—Community Work in Progress in the United States: Gun violence is a significant public health problem in the United States. Despite public support for stricter gun control, most Americans uphold their right to own a gun, sustaining what is often referred to as a "gun culture." A National Firearms Survey in 2004 revealed that the population continues to hold at least one firearm for every adult.[55] Long guns are the most prevalent type and handguns also are widespread: 38% of households and 26% of individuals reported owning at least one firearm. This translates to 42 million households with firearms, and 57 million adult gun owners. Almost half (48%) of individual gun owners reported owning 4 or more firearms: 45% of men stated that they personally owned at least one firearm, compared with 11% for women.

In all countries, violence reflects underlying social and mental health issues that impact communities. In 2000, an estimated 1.6 million people died as a result of violence globally; many more suffered injury. Of the deaths, nearly half were suicides, almost a third were homicide, and about a fifth were war related.[56] Of all forms of violence, gun violence is among the most lethal. It is the most frequent method of homicide and suicide in the United States; the United States leads the developed world in deaths due to homicide.

In the United States, although many community groups and NGOs concerned with health and safety advocate for stricter gun control laws, pro-gun groups such as the National Rifle Association (NRA) are often politically effective in opposing laws restricting firearm manufacture, ownership, and use.[57] The minimal success of gun control advocacy is largely due to the work of pro-gun lobby groups at community level, sustained by support from an effective synergy across industrial, financial, and political interests. However, the divisions go even deeper than this in the sense that there is as much a community-based anti–gun control constituency as there is a pro–gun control constituency: the former takes its energy mostly from the veneration of firearms as an intrinsic part of American frontier mythology and a particular interpretation of rights under the US Constitution. To change this self-destructive aspect of American culture is as large a challenge as, for examples, the historic gains in reproductive rights for women (which remain under constant threat) and the acceptance of universal health care.

There has been some progress, largely due to the efforts of people who have suffered loss due to senseless gun violence. The most prominent example is The Brady Handgun Violence Prevention Act that initiated federal background checks on firearm purchasers, signed into law by President Clinton in 1993, implemented in1994. The Act was named after James Brady who was shot during an attempted assassination of President Regan on March 30, 1981. The same James Brady has since been a force behind the Brain Injury Association of America, a national advocacy group with state and local affiliates.

Most victims of gun violence are ordinary people living everyday lives. However, even disasters such as school shootings (the large majority globally take place in the United States), have not moved elected representatives to take effective action, especially in the face of "Second Amendment Rights" under the US Constitution: the "right to keep and bear arms," adopted in 1791, eight years after the close of the American War of Independence. Every election cycle, the NRA heavily subsidizes elected officials and challengers who believe that the Second Amendment provides an absolute right to bear arms. The meaning of this amendment in the 21st century is a current focus of national debate. It has also had an adverse impact on international efforts at small arms control.

Gun control advocates enjoy only lukewarm support from their own public health system: in 2002, the Task Force on Community Preventive Services, reporting through the US Centers for Disease Control and Prevention, conducted a systematic review of scientific evidence regarding the effectiveness of firearms laws in preventing violence, including violent crimes, suicide, and unintentional injury.[58] Although the ready availability of guns in the United States is a major factor in their use in violence, the review found insufficient evidence to determine the effectiveness of any existing firearms laws or combination of laws on violent outcomes. The Task Force did note that insufficient evidence to determine effectiveness should not be interpreted as evidence of ineffectiveness. Clearly there is a need to update this assessment as new studies come to light, just as there is a need to design more effective strategies to reduce the problem. In the meantime gun control advocates lean more than they would like on moral reasoning and testimonials from persons affected by gun violence.

Clearly, therefore, the "precautionary principle" is not applied as rigorously to gun control in the United States as it is to other areas of regulation designed to protect public health and safety. In this ambiguous situation it is unclear what constitutes effective policy advocacy and how advocacy organizations can strengthen their efforts.[57] As the situation reflects ingrained cultural beliefs, as well as financial and political interests that invest in "wedge politics" (designing strategies to pit different groups against one another rather than trying to reach consensus), effective gun control is an elusive goal for affected communities. There is a clear need to build on promising initiatives such as the Brady Campaign to Prevent Gun Violence, the Coalition to Stop Gun Violence, and Mayors Against Illegal Guns. Consistent with cultural realities: a "third way" is now being sought that calls for balance between gun rights and responsibilities.[59] This is a work in progress.

Mothers Against Drunk Driving (MADD): Compared with gun control in the United States, MADD illustrates a much more successful community-based advocacy effort in that country and elsewhere. Founded by a mother who lost a child to a "hit and run" drunk driver whose record involved four prior arrests for drinking under the influence (DUI), MADD's success in defining DUI as a public health problem reflects the power of capturing the attention of media and policy makers by projecting personal tragedies of loved ones lost through the irresponsible behavior of others. In turn, the political effectiveness of local and state/provincial MADD chapters in successfully advocating state/provincial legislation against DUI reflects the power of victim-based leadership and membership. The success of this approach over the past 25 years has been attributed to the following factors:[60]

Highly Visible and Focused Consumer Group. Since the late 1970s, this organization, which started in California, grew to several hundred chapters across the United States, Canada, and Mexico. MADD not only fought for harsher penalties against drunk drivers, but also developed a range of programs to assist victims in coping with their loss.

Legislative Agenda. Since inception, MADD has successfully lobbied legislators; this effort has been influential in the enactment of over 1000 new laws at local and national levels in the United States and Canada, including minimum drinking age, server liability laws, and sobriety checks. Also effective was MADD's production and dissemination of an annual inter-jurisdictional "Rating of the States/Provinces," which has the effect of generating peer pressure across political jurisdictions. An evaluation of the impact of these measures in Ontario, Canada, revealed that formation of MADD was associated with a subsequent decline in DUI fatalities from 1982 to 1996 of approximately 20%.[61]

Victim Services. Grief resulting from a drunk driving crash is not unlike that in which a family member is murdered: the loss is sudden and unanticipated, the death violent, and the crime senseless. MADD membership fulfills the survivors' compelling desire "to do something," often after a draining courtroom experience. MADD chapters have provided opportunities to participate in a victim impact panel as part of DUI offenders programs; however, when compared with simpler informational approaches, results are equivocal.[62]

Influencing Social Norms. Youth and community programs promoted by MADD have been widespread. Their message has been taken up by others, such as by government departments (e.g., health, education, transportation, and even by the beverage industry in the form of "responsible drinking" campaigns). These efforts have resulted in a substantial shift in social norms, which in turn has led to reductions in alcohol-related collisions.[61] Drunk-driving "accidents" have thereby become "crashes due to criminal negligence," reflecting a new collective moral mentality. In turn, random breath testing has led to the promotion of "designated drivers": a person who volunteers not to drink at an event so as to provide safe transportation for others. This type of health promotion involves increasing mass media visibility around times of public celebration and has resulted in reducing the occurrence of drivers who drink over the prescribed limit.

Availability of Valid and Reliable Monitoring Data. Alcohol being a legal substance in many countries allows for the quantitative monitoring (virtually by definition this is lacking for the study of illegal psychoactive substances). Surveillance of drunk-driving statistics thereby enables ongoing assessment of impacts influenced by changes in the alcohol control measures, including the efforts of MADD on the DUI environment.[60]

In summary, MADD is a showcase of what a grassroots organization can do to promote improved social norms to achieve enormous benefits for the health and safety of families and communities. There are lessons here for other community advocacy groups.

Canada's Aboriginal Peoples—A Case Study of Failed Public Policy: Policies flowing from cultural ignorance and prejudice can damage communities. Examples may be found in many countries, but here we focus on how five generations of enforced residential schooling in Canada destroyed many indigenous families and broke up communities.

Throughout much of Canada's history, the official policy of the Canadian government was to assimilate aboriginal people into the dominant (colonizing) society by educating children away from their parents' and their community's culture. In 1879 the federal government adopted the American model of Indian residential schools, with the proviso that these schools be operated by Christian denominations. In 1920 the Indian Act was amended to make school attendance compulsory for all children between 7 and 15 years of age. Indian and Inuit residential schools operated in Canada for nearly 150 years. Education administered by the church (Roman Catholic, Presbyterian, Anglican, and the United Church of Canada) became an essential tool in a policy of assimilation.[63]

Looking back on this era, as described in a submission to The Royal Commission on Aboriginal Peoples (1996):

> *Aboriginal knowledge and skills had enabled the newcomers to find their way, to survive and to prosper. But they were now merely historic; they were not to be any part of the future as Canadians pictured it at the founding of their new nation in 1867. That future was one of settlement, agriculture, manufacturing, order, lawfulness and Christianity. In the view of politicians and civil servants in Ottawa whose gaze was fixed upon the horizon of national development, Aboriginal knowledge and skills were neither necessary or desirable in a land that was to be dominated by European industry and, therefore, by Europeans and their culture.[64]*

In residential schools, missionaries thus taught Western culture to Indian children. Yet these same people (priests, brothers and nuns) lived on the fringe of their own society, denying sex, marriage, and family. They knew little of the indigenous culture and did not value it. The consequences, designed to "Christianize and civilize," were disastrous. For as long as five generations, children thus were removed from their homes, families, culture, and language to be immersed far away for long periods. Referred to as "inmates," many were separated from siblings, tortured for speaking their mother tongue, and forbidden to honor their traditions. Scores died from disease; others were emotionally and spiritually destroyed by the harsh discipline and living conditions. Grievous sexual abuse occurred for some, as well as physical abuse.

Deaths due to abuse and neglect were concealed; had the schools been held accountable they would be guilty of serious criminal offences. Some communities were completely depopulated of children from ages 5 to 20. Traditional education and parenting methods were lost. Many extended families were destroyed. Generations were alienated from their past, often confused and frustrated, unable to readjust to their own families and communities. Languages were nearly wiped out; traditions lost. Due to inferior education, with no attempt by the government or the churches to draw upon the indigenous cultures, they were alienated from their own families, communities, and cultures yet poorly prepared to join mainstream society.[65]

By creating the policy in the first place, and for financing and regulating this system of schooling, the Government of Canada bears ultimate responsibility for this deplorable situation, ignored for so long. The last residential school closed as recently as 1996. During the 1990s, apologies were issued by the Catholic, Anglican, United, and Presbyterian churches and by the Minister of Indian Affairs and Northern Development for the federal government; a Prime Ministerial apology came in 2008. The Government of Canada proposed to work with First Nations, Inuit and Métis people, the Churches, and other parties to resolve the long-standing issues that must be addressed. A Truth and Reconciliation Commission, part of the court-approved Residential Schools Settlement Agreement that was negotiated between legal counsel for former students, legal counsel for the churches, the government of Canada, the Assembly of First Nations, and other aboriginal organizations has been established to assist individuals and communities in dealing with the consequences of this policy failure. The ultimate purpose of the commission is to encourage reconciliation between aboriginals and nonaboriginal Canadians, intended as a form of restorative justice. This differs from the customary adversarial or retributive justice, which aims to find fault and punish the guilty. By contrast, restorative justice aims to heal relationships between offenders, victims, and the community in which an offence takes place; the commission seeks to uncover facts and distinguish truth from lies to allow for acknowledgement, appropriate public mourning, forgiveness, and healing.[65] This remains a work in progress.

The Importance of Leadership

Perhaps the most essential ingredient in the successful initiatives, whether innovative or restorative, is leadership or "the capacity to influence others to work together to achieve a common purpose." To achieve success, leadership must exist or be developed and reinforced at several levels (consistent with the social-ecological model). Leadership development is not done solely to improve the skills of individuals, but is also a core component of developing organizational capacity. Leadership itself is often an outcome of processes that take place in complex social and organizational environments; it can develop out of personal experience and may also be mentored. It is in the interests of health at community level to enhance the potential for effective leadership to emerge.

Health leadership frameworks are useful in fostering effective leadership for public health organizations and community health initiatives; attention can be given to this in educational and training settings. One such framework speaks to five elements: leading self (self-motivation), engaging others, achieving results, developing coalitions, and transforming systems.[66] These components link strongly with the other critical ingredient for successful interventions: community participation. If these principles were to be applied actively, we would be more successful in addressing not only community health needs but also those of health care systems as a whole.

Scaling Up: When Does It Apply, and How Can We Do It?

Just as we consider the mantra "think globally, act locally," urging people to consider the health of the entire planet and to take action in their own communities, we can also consider alternative formulations, such as "think locally, act globally." The latter points to the potential for "scaling-up" locally successful interventions to impact larger populations. However, while this is often appealing, it may sometimes miss the point: some situations and solutions are uniquely local. And though other scenarios may have potential for scaling-up, this does not necessarily imply that the latter are more important than the former. Indeed, there may be a greater need for locally designed solutions fitted to the needs of particular communities.

The notion that locally successful interventions (wherever carried out) might justify wider implementation requires caution. Contexts become more complex as one moves from local to national levels; more so if one strives to cross cultures or attempts global application.[67] Although it is important to consider whether lessons may be translated to locations where similar opportunities exist, it is not sufficient to know "that" an intervention worked in a particular setting, one must also know "how" it was achieved.[1]

Frameworks for assessing the potential for scaling up initiatives are only recently emerging. When viewed globally, success seems dependent on several ingredients already addressed in this chapter. Community health interventions must be scientifically sound and managerially feasible. Strong leadership and governance and the active engagement of community organizations appears to be critical; in fact, such initiatives are likely to fail unless they engage local implementers and the recipient community itself. Flexibility is important in fitting the initiative to particular settings, that is, avoid one-size-fits-all assumptions. It is relevant to consider incorporating a research component, at least at the level of monitoring and evaluation. This will help implementers better understand how contextual factors, such as politics, sociocultural norms and beliefs, and the fiscal environment, can influence everything from replicability and adaptation to potential success of scaling-up.[68] This will also enable the lessons learned to be translated to other locations where similar opportunities may exist. Because of the inevitable lag between evidence and action, all too often decision makers are not well versed in new approaches. It is therefore important to encourage dissemination of research findings in ways that are policy-relevant. Another reality is that as health systems evolve they retain the seeds of inertia: powerful entrenched stakeholders can produce inequitable internal competition for future resources. Timing is a key factor: for example, political considerations or financing may be more critical to the decision than the technical merits of the proposal.

Sustainable Communities

Intrinsic to the ecological foundations of human settlements, the concept of sustainable communities embraces the economic, social, political, and cultural means by which they evolve in ways that are socially and environmentally sustainable.[69] A sustainable community has capacities essential to being able to adjust to changing social and economic circumstances, thereby to survive and thrive while preserving the environment that supports it. How this plays out varies across time and place depending on local actions and circumstances, even as external geopolitical and economic forces influence prospects. For a community to be sustainable requires effective leadership operating within a vibrant civil society. It follows that where these qualities are deficient, they must either be developed or strengthened, a work in progress everywhere. The concept of sustainable communities lies at the core of the Healthy Cities/Communities movement (case study previously discussed).[69]

Viewed globally, the ideal of sustainable communities is challenged by dynamic forces, many of which are not amenable to local control. In many countries enormous sociodemographic shifts are taking place, such as rural-urban migration contributing to the decline of many rural communities and the emergence of urban slums and squatter settlements. Overdependence on obsolescent technologies and nonrenewable resources places resource-dependent communities at risk of losing their economic livelihoods. For example, this may apply to communities dependent on production of fuel-inefficient vehicles just as it has done for single-industry towns (e.g., mining, specialized manufacturing) that continue to be eclipsed as their resource runs out or markets fade. Global shifts in the balance of economic and political power are resulting in economic stresses on communities in most countries. These are not new phenomena: threats to the sustainability of communities have been a fact of life since the industrial revolution, which started in Western Europe in the nineteenth century, giving rise to major upheavals that continue to have profound socioeconomic and cultural impacts around the world.

Actions to promote sustainable communities in developed countries include measures such as forming car cooperatives to reduce the cost and necessity of car ownership; creating public investment in energy conservation and audits; encouraging manufacturers to develop environmentally friendly products through research and development assistance; increasing affordable housing supply through zoning codes that promote a variety of housing types, including smaller and multifamily homes; experimenting with local self-reliance by establishing closed-loop, self-sustaining economic networks; developing community support of agriculture to preserve farmland and help farmers, while making fresh fruits and vegetables available in city neighborhoods; supporting local exchange trading systems and local ownership development with a revolving loan fund (microfinance); and encouraging employee-owned businesses and those likely to hire, train, and promote local residents.[70]

In developing countries, there are many parallels to the approaches just described. However, sustainable community development in these countries is more obviously linked to the most intractable global challenges of our times—to eradicate poverty and meet the world's development needs in a way that does not destroy the environment. For example, improving access of the world's poor people to clean water, sanitation, and safe household energy sources would have a huge effect on the main killers of young children (pneumonia and diarrhea). Utilizing sustainable development principles, the Grameen Bank in Bangladesh launched the modern practice of micro-credit that has motivated women and men in urban squatter and impoverished rural settlements to form their own community-based organizations, initiate cottage industry projects, invest in girls' education and skill-building projects, and advocate with local authorities for clean water and sanitation.[71]

The aspirational challenge of sustainable communities brings us full circle to the theme of this chapter. Ultimately, it is the extent of genuine participation and a community's sense of ownership that are the foundations of sustainable development for a healthy people. Action on these principles of sustainable community development, in all countries, will help put the planet back on a healthy and sustainable path.[72]

Acknowledging Community Development—a Legacy

In closing this overview of the role of community in public health, it is important to acknowledge the foundation laid decades ago by exponents of community development.

In fact, the Ottawa Charter for Health Promotion drew heavily from this foundation when addressing *strengthening community action* as one of its strategies.[27] In deference to this discipline, we therefore close with the definition of community development as stated at the International Association for Community Development meeting in Budapest (2004):[73]

Community Development is a way of strengthening civil society by prioritizing the actions of communities, and their perspectives in the development of social, economic and environmental policy. It seeks the empowerment of local communities, taken to mean both geographic communities, communities of interest or identity and communities organizing around specific themes of policy initiatives. It strengthens the capacity of people as active citizens through their community groups, organizations and networks; and the capacity of institutions and agencies (public, private and non-governmental) to work in dialogue with citizens to shape and determine change in their communities. It plays a crucial role in supporting active democratic life by promoting the autonomous voice of disadvantaged and vulnerable communities. It has a set of core values/social principles covering human rights, social inclusion, equality and respect for diversity; and a specific skills and knowledge base.

Building especially on scientific and community foundations, this chapter introduces the role of demography in public health. Beyond contributing data that describe population structures and providing denominators for epidemiological measures such as incidence and prevalence, demographers make direct contributions to our understanding of population health, illustrated here with case studies. After examining demographic transition theory, the chapter proceeds to explore two main approaches to assessing the health of populations: health situation analysis and public health surveillance.

5

ASSESSING POPULATION HEALTH

Demography, Health Situation Analysis, and Public Health Surveillance

AS A FOCUS of inquiry, the term *population health* refers to the health of human populations as measured by health indicators, taking into account considerations such as social, economic, and physical environments, personal health practices, individual capacity and coping skills, human biology, early childhood development, health services, and, not least, population dynamics (demographic forces that shape the composition of populations). While populations are traditionally defined by geographic boundaries (place), there is also a long-standing practice of identifying particular groups as populations so as to target health services or interventions in accordance with shared attributes such as age, gender, language, ethnicity, circumstances, health risk status, and other indicators of need.[1] As a discipline, population health refers to the use of health statistical indicators and related techniques to characterize the health of a population, track trends over time, and contrast different populations within or across defined geographical areas.

A *health indicator* is a directly measurable variable that reflects the health status of the population and includes, for example, infant and perinatal mortality rates, incidence rates of notifiable diseases, sickness absence from school or work, cancer incidence as recorded by a cancer registry, records of selected prescribed medications, records of causes of death, and others. Some health indicators also may be measured in terms of their presence or absence, for instance related legislation (e.g., statutory entitlements such as maternity leave) and universality of medical and hospital insurance.

The *aim* of population health as a discipline is virtually synonymous with public health: to maintain and improve the health of a defined human population, correct deviations from good health, and reduce health inequalities across population groups.[2] This is achieved by examining conditions and behaviors that influence people over their lives, identifying systematic variations in their patterns of occurrence and how these may be interrelated, then applying the resulting knowledge to develop and implement policies and actions to improve health.[3] Population health is an inherently flexible approach to public health, practiced by individuals and organizations committed first to measurement and the evidence base. It commences as systematic enquiry, then transforms into action by selecting from a spectrum of potential interventions that range from broadly based community health and health promotion strategies (chapter 4) to more specific disease prevention and control initiatives (chapter 6), or it may enlist other capacities of the health care system (chapter 8) or combine elements of all these frameworks. In other words, population health is an evidence-based approach to public health that makes explicit all relevant contextual issues as a basis for selecting from an array of intervention options.[4]

Role of Demography in Population Health

Before we examine applications, we must first understand the central concept of *population dynamics*: the process by which changes occur in the composition of a population through births, deaths, migrations, and related observable socioeconomic changes. *Demography*, as the study of the dynamics and resulting characteristics of populations, measures such phenomena as fertility, mortality, migration, distribution, density, growth, size, distribution, age and sex structure, and vital statistics and how these interact with social and economic conditions. In turn, population health assessment continues where demography leaves off: taking into account these dynamics, it examines their health consequences while also taking into account other inputs from the full range of disciplines that underpin public health.

Demography plays a critical role in understanding population and public health, as we now illustrate with two examples: very old people and very young people. The number of very old people in a population depends on the number of births 8 or 9 decades earlier and risks of death at successive ages throughout the intervening years.[5] In contrast, the number of preschool children depends in part on the number of mothers born two to three decades earlier but is also strongly influenced by the current fertility rate in this group, which in most societies is now a function of child spacing and family size expectations. However, in addition to the absolute size of these groups, for health planning purposes, we also need to know their proportion in relation to society as a whole: for this simple calculation, the absolute number becomes the numerator, while the total population size is the denominator. Again, demography makes this disciplinary contribution: the denominator itself is also a function of reproductive behavior, and the starting point in its assessment can be a census or a projection or alternative technique, as described next:

A Census: A census is a periodic enumeration of the population (carried out in most countries every ten years), primarily intended to collect information to identify eligible voters, tax payers, and many other useful facts (e.g., housing conditions). Depending on its design and content, this tool may provide data on particular characteristics of interest, and is virtually indispensable in providing numerical input for valid denominators on which basis rates can be reliably calculated, thereby facilitating objective comparisons of areas or social groups within a country. The term *census* also implies total enumeration of a population, at least with regard to core data such as identities of all persons in every place of residence, birthdates, sex, occupation, national origin, language, marital status, income, and relationships to head of household. Censuses have important roles: they are often the only source of data for small areas or particular groups (e.g., minorities); they are valuable in guiding economic development; they provide a sampling frame from which surveys can be designed and validated. For data less critical to core applications, for intercensus estimates, or for population subsets where there exist particular data needs, samples are also used.

The United Nations recommends that censuses be conducted decennially. Nonetheless, conducting a census is a challenging task: the goal of unbiased data necessitates that participation is required by law in many countries, which can be controversial. Also, complete enumeration is expensive, and some countries are moving away from this practice as other data sources become available and are perceived to fill the gap (e.g., registries, specialized surveys). However, in some instances this has pitted short-term political and financial considerations against best statistical practice in the longer term: alternative data sources are often biased, and it remains to be seen whether countries moving in this direction (e.g., Canada) will make the necessary investment to ensure data quality in the alternative systems they are developing.

For other concepts and terms commonly used in demography, refer to Appendix A at the end of this chapter.

Population Pyramids

The power of *fertility* and *mortality* (defined in Appendix A) in determining the relative size of age-sex groups in populations can be readily appreciated by comparing the demographic structures of developing and developed countries (Figure 5-1). It is

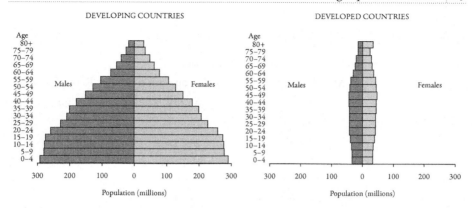

FIGURE 5-1 Populations by age and sex 2008.

Source: United Nations Population Division, *World Population Prospects: The 2006 Revision.*

Acknowledgment: Pyramid diagrams reproduced with permission from the Population Reference Bureau.

apparent that both the higher fertility and mortality of the former largely explain why the demographic structures of those countries are more like an actual pyramid (broad base, reducing upward to a peak) than those of the latter (which tend to have a more columnar shape due to low fertility and little mortality until older ages). The other variable that influences the shape of pyramids is *migration*, a powerful modifier of the demographic structures of populations that either gain or lose people through migration, especially considering that migration is almost never equally distributed across all age-sex groups.

To illustrate the power of migration, consider the United Arab Emirates (UAE), which reveals a major excess of young males (see Sex Ratio column in Table 5-1; also known as the Male:Female Ratio or M:F). These are mostly unskilled immigrant laborers from rural areas of South and Southeast Asia where employment prospects are unfavorable due to adverse economic conditions in their own communities. Without these people (now comprising >80% of the UAE population) the economy of this Gulf state would not be viable. Remittances from these migrant workers are an important source of income for their countries of origin and therefore are encouraged by those countries. Demographically, depending on the size of the exodus and preexisting sex ratios (case study), there can be a converse impact on the communities from which they came; some become depleted of males. For both host and guest populations in the UAE and other Gulf states that also depend on migrant workers, serious social and political consequences are emerging, reflecting major underlying human rights issues.[6]

As a demographic exercise, readers may convert the data in Table 5-1 into the population pyramid for the United Arab Emirates. The US Census Bureau

TABLE 5-1

United Arab Emirates 2011

Age-specific male and female populations and sex ratio.

Age	Male Population	Female Population	Sex Ratio (Sr) M:F
0–4	211,308	202,375	1.04
5–9	183,931	176,438	1.03
10–14	142,686	134,759	1.06
15–19	150,225	125,800	1.19
20–24	280,758	169,602	1.66
25–29	553,067	209,723	2.64
30–34	589,861	191,120	3.09
35–39	495,770	147,735	3.36
40–44	381,599	99,887	3.82
45–49	252,550	62,057	4.07
50–54	148,033	38,880	3.81
55–59	79,146	23,142	3.42
60–64	37,949	12,771	2.97
65–69	15,788	7403	2.13
70–74	7951	4333	1.83
75–79	4029	2841	1.42
80–84	1906	1591	1.20
85–89	578	585	0.98
90–94	162	229	0.71
95–99	29	57	0.51
100 +	3	7	0.42
Total (All Ages)	3,537,329	1,611,335	2.20

Source: US Census Bureau International Database. http://www.census.gov/population/international/data/idb/informationGateway.php Accessed Nov 24, 2011.

International Database also provides pyramids, as an online service, for every country in the world.

By examining population pyramids and their underlying data, as just illustrated, one can visualize that less developed nations have more young people relative to elderly, while more developed nations have fewer young relative to elderly. One can also identify imbalances between age-sex groups. It is almost intuitive from such observations that the relative magnitude of human needs, and the potential for related sociopolitical and health issues to arise, will reflect in part the age-sex distribution of a country's population.

Similar kinds of contrasts and observations can also be made within a country. For example, within the United States, Alaska has a younger age structure than Arizona, a difference largely explained by the movement of young people north for employment in resource industries (e.g., oil, gas, fishing, forest products), while older people tend to move south and west in search of gentler climates more conducive to retirement. Of course there is more to health planning than eyeballing demographic pyramids, but this is an important starting point for all population health applications.

Global Perspectives: On October 31st, 2011, the global population reached 7 billion, accompanied by a call to world leaders to meet the challenges that a growing population poses, from ensuring adequate food and clean water to guaranteeing equal access to security and justice.[7] "Today, we welcome baby 7 billion. In doing so we must recognize our moral and pragmatic obligation to do the right thing," Secretary-General Ban Ki-moon said at an event to mark the milestone. We return to this challenge in chapter 9.

Consider this milestone in the context of world population growth (Table 5-2).

By the middle of the 21st century, the world population is projected to exceed 9 billion, with most of the expansion taking place in less developed countries (Figure 5-2).[8] This differentiation between developed and developing countries is sometimes referred to as the "demographic divide": consider Table 5-3, comparing Canada with Uganda. The former reflects the situation of wealthy countries with low birth rates and rapid aging, while Uganda is typical of poor countries with high birth rates and low life expectancies. Whether this type of demographic contrast will become more or less stark over coming decades depends to a large extent on whether fertility continues to decline (as it has in recent decades in virtually all countries),

TABLE 5-2

Exponential human population growth[64]

Billions	Time Required	Date Achieved
1st Billion	All Prior Human History	Circa 1800
2nd Billion	130 years	1930
3rd Billion	30 years	1960
4th Billion	14 years	1974
5th Billion	13 years	1987
6th Billion	12 years	1999
7th Billion	12 years	2011
8th Billion	12 years	2023?

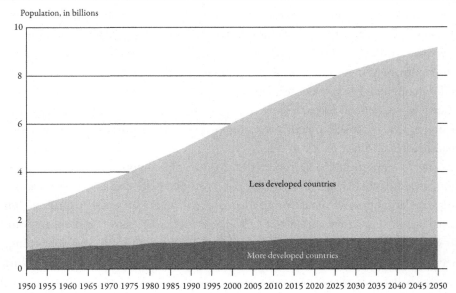

Population, in billions

FIGURE 5-2 World population growth, 1950–2050.

Acknowledgment: Diagram reproduced with permission from the Population Reference Bureau.

which in turn depends mostly on global convergence of expectations regarding birth spacing and family size, and access to family planning. Critical to this are the underlying determinants of inequalities within and between countries. To change this picture requires action on such issues as literacy, status of women, poverty alleviation, land and tax reform, public investment in education and technology, fair trade practices, and economic development.[9]

TABLE 5-3

The "demographic divide": Canada and Uganda 2009[65]

Key Demographic Indicators	Canada	Uganda
2009 Population	34 million	31 million
2050 Population (Projected)	42 million	96 million
Percent of Population Below Age 15	17%	49%
Percent of Population Age 65 and Older	14%	3%
Percent of Population Ages 15 to 24	13%	20%
Annual Births	371,000	1.4 million
Lifetime Births per Woman	1.6	6.7
Annual Infant Deaths	1900	110,000
Life Expectancy at Birth	78 years	50 years

Selected Demographic Case Studies

To illustrate the usefulness of demographic analysis in elucidating social trends, now consider two case studies: sex ratios in Asia and ethnic composition in the United States.

CASE STUDY #1: SHIFTS IN SEX RATIOS IN ASIA

What Is the Sex Ratio (SR)? As already illustrated in Table 5-1, this refers to the ratio of males to females (M:F) in a population and may be calculated for specific age bands, as well as at birth. Due to higher female life expectancy in most populations, SRs tend to decline across adult age groups. Values for the world population are overall 1.01; at birth 1.06; under 5 years 1.06; 15–64 = 1.03; and >65 years = 0.79.

What Is Happening in Asia? Sex ratios throughout much of Asia reflect long-standing cultural preferences and social practices favoring the birth and survival of one sex over the other (favoring males). The *sex ratio at birth* (SRB) began to increase in East Asia between 1980 and 1985, and in South-Central Asia between 1985 and 1990, while elsewhere in Asia the ratio remained relatively stable.[10] There are also variations within countries and between religious, ethnic, and socioeconomic groups. In some settings, it exceeds 1.30 (e.g., Guangdong and Hainan in China). The growing contribution of younger generations to the SR imbalance has offset the converse progress in SR being made by adults, among whom mortality improvements have particularly benefited the female population. Other factors also influence the sex ratio: changing ethnic and racial composition, violent conflicts, large-scale migration (e.g., male laborers unable to travel with their families), and gender-related health trends.

Why the Change in Sex Ratios in Asia? This trend is strongly linked to the increasing availability of prenatal sex selection in many Asian countries following the introduction of ultrasound and amniocentesis technologies in the late 1970s; this affects primarily the SRB. The deeply rooted preference for sons stems from numerous demand factors: social customs, marriage costs, and old-age support, motivating parents across cultures and locations to decide against allowing a girl to live, even before birth. Indeed, if the continent's overall SR was the same as elsewhere in the world, Asia's 2005 population would now include 163 million more women and girls.

What are the Consequences? While men of marriageable age are now finding a dramatic shortage of potential brides, girls and women of all ages experience the full brunt of this phenomenon: increases in gender-based violence, trafficking, discrimination, and general vulnerability. The ramifications will continue for decades.

What Has Been Done So Far? In India, decades of policy efforts have achieved no favorable change, and worsening ratios indicate a deteriorating situation.[11] Most policies regarding son preference have focused on reducing sex-selective abortion, but underlying motivations have not been adequately addressed. In China, tough measures are pledged: people who illegally test the gender of fetuses and perform sex-selective abortions or who kill, abandon, or injure infant girls or ill-treat their mothers are to be severely punished.[12] Medical procedures using ultrasound to check fetal health are to be closely supervised. A "Care for Girls" campaign was launched nationwide in 2000 to promote gender equality. Cash incentives are offered to girl-only rural families. Authorities pledged to continue the 33-year-old family planning policy, as China still faces huge challenges from a growing population; formulated in the early 1970s, the policy encourages late marriages and late child-bearing, limiting most urban couples to one child and most rural couples to two. It is credited with preventing 400 million births but faces a challenge in rural regions, where traditional preference for male heirs has not changed. To complete the picture, it is relevant to note that the long-term consequences of this policy include not only gender imbalance due to son preference, but China will steadily become demographically old compared with most other nations and thereby dependent on a proportionally small active workforce; in other words it is destined to achieve a high *Aged Dependency Ratio* (See Appendix A for discussion of this term).

A Way Forward: Although many factors influence sex ratios, women's education is the most powerful: educated women are less likely to prefer sons over daughters; highly educated women even less so. Women's exposure to primary-level schooling reduces son preference; higher education is even more potent. How many women are educated matters: women in villages with higher levels of female literacy are less likely to prefer sons than women in villages where most women are illiterate. Greater exposure to media is associated with weaker son preference, even after controlling for education and wealth. One important source for policy inspiration may be to better understand the motivations and social norms of women and communities who do not express son preference. There is also a need for research on what is happening to surviving girls, that is, nutritional deprivation and other forms of discrimination; sole surviving girls may be more vulnerable than girls with older sisters.

Eliminating sex selection must be made a priority wherever it is occurring; not only in the settings just noted, but also in immigrant communities in recipient countries like Canada.[13] There is a global need to monitor SR trends and underlying behaviors; coordinate research on motivations, interventions, and impacts; and a related need to develop strategies for engagement and accountability by men and boys in confronting violence against women (including sex selection) and to promote gender equality and sexual and reproductive health and rights. Policy experiences need to be shared locally and globally.

CASE STUDY #2: CHANGING ETHNIC COMPOSITION IN THE UNITED STATES

Population Growth in the United States: Demographic projections reveal that the United States is growing much faster than other developed countries.[14] This is true even when compared with countries where immigration accounts for proportionally much higher growth than in the United States; for example, Australia (3-fold higher immigration), Canada (2.3-fold higher). US growth projections for the 80 year period 1970–2050 reveal a more than doubling of population size, culminating in 439 million people by mid-century. For 2008 to 2050, the increase is 44%, compared to 32% for Australia, 26% each for Canada and the United Kingdom, 13% for France, 12% for Sweden, and 3% for Italy. During this period, the populations of Spain, Germany, Russia and Japan are projected to decline by 6%, 13%, 22%, and 25% respectively, all (by definition) below zero population growth (ZPG). As a whole, developed countries will average only 5% growth during this 42 year period, compared with 47% for less developed countries, and 109% for a category of least developed countries (as defined by the United Nations). The net population growth for the world is an enormous 39%, representing a 2.5 billion more people for this period; but this is smaller proportionally than the projected increase of the US population (44%).

What Are the Trends in Make-up of the US Population? The United States is becoming increasingly more racially and ethnically diverse (Table 5-4). By 2008, 10% of US counties had achieved what is referred to as "majority-minority" status: in other words, in these counties, nonwhites are now in the majority. And minorities in 2008 comprised at least 50% of the youth population among 1 in 7 counties. This is clearly a "cohort phenomenon": older populations are less diverse than the progressively younger ones replacing them. By 2040, approximately half the US population will be nonwhite; beyond that year, the majority will be nonwhite.

Why Is This Happening? This reflects two major phenomena: migration patterns (mostly in the past) and differential fertility rates across racial and ethnic groups. The future population is mostly determined by the fertility of present population groups; and fertility rates are much higher for Hispanics and people of mixed race, resulting in a steadily more diverse population.

What Are Some of the Implications? The emergence of a more racially and ethnically diverse population in a society, while enriching it culturally, poses significant challenges to the status quo in virtually every domain, from the adequacy of political representation (all levels from local to state and federal) to access to opportunity in

TABLE 5-4

Percent of US population by race and ethnicity—from 2007 to 2039[66]

	2007 300 Million	2039 400 Million
White Alone*	66	51
Black or African American Alone*	12	12
Asian, Native Hawaiian, and Other Pacific Islanders Alone*	5	7
American Indian and Alaska Native Alone*	1	1
Two or More Races	1	3
Hispanic (of any race)	15	26
TOTAL	100	100

*Excludes Hispanics

education, employment, health, and housing. And race and ethnicity are only two of the domains by which diversity is assessed; in addition, there is increasing diversity in relation to religious expression, sexual orientation, and so on. In each domain are found differences of opinion, vested interests, new opportunities, and potential for conflict. Demographic analyses, therefore, such as presented, serve as a useful point of departure from which one may address the extent to which the principles upon which a nation is founded, or upholds, are actually observed in its operations, from its leadership and political practices to the conditions of everyday living.

Are There Implications for Other Countries? Many other countries are also experiencing increasing diversity: some know it, some don't, and some (possibly) don't want to know. The underlying problem is that not all countries are collecting data that will enable them to generate the information needed to guide related policy development.[15] Take Latin America for example: outside of Brazil, data on Afro descendants are scarce. Nicaragua, Panama, Peru, and Uruguay lack census data for their Afro-descendant populations; Costa Rica and Ecuador collected these statistics for the first time in 2000, and Honduras in 2001. Only a few countries regularly collect data on race in household surveys. Even where race and ethnic data are collected, they usually are not sufficient to measure progress toward health targets. For example, data on infant mortality, maternal mortality, and access to potable water are rarely disaggregated by race. Yet available data suggest that Afro-descendant and indigenous populations in Latin America are far more likely than citizens of European origin to live in poverty, be illiterate, die younger, reside in substandard housing, and suffer from police abuse. Most observers agree that racial discrimination is a major cause of these disparities, but more research is needed to differentiate the factors fostering these inequalities.[18]

Global Demographic and Population Health Resources Online

Several organizations offer reliable demographic data online. Some websites facilitate customized searches to answer questions about particular nations or world regions and queries about economic, health, and social conditions. The following summarizes what these organizations are about and the data available from their websites (Table 5-5).

UNDP Human Development Indices: The United Nations Development Programme (UNDP) aims to advance living conditions around the world by working with governments to address critical needs such as governance, human rights, and poverty. UNDP maintains the world's most comprehensive database for social, economic, and health statistics. Their site also links to other resources on human development issues.

WHO Global Health Observatory (GHO): The World Health Organization (WHO) is the leading United Nations (UN) health agency, which works alongside national Ministries of Health in addressing national, international and global health needs. To sustain its role in evidence-based priority setting, planning, and systems development, WHO maintains a global population health database. From this site, the following information is accessible: core health indicators (time series for 193 countries); world health statistics (approx 50 indicators); statistics by topic, country, and global regions; burden of disease estimates; disease classifications; service availability mapping; demographic and socioeconomic statistics.

TABLE 5-5

Selected demography and population health resources online

UNDP Human Development Indices	http://hdr.undp.org/en/statistics/
WHO Global Health Observatory (GHO)	http://www.who.int/gho/en/
US Census Bureau International Database	http://www.census.gov/population/ international/data/idb/ informationGateway.php
Population Reference Bureau Data-Finder	http://www.prb.org/DataFinder.aspx
WHO Global Health Atlas	http://apps.who.int/globalatlas/
The Global Social Change Research Project	http://gsociology.icaap.org/data.htm
The Kaiser Family Foundation	http://www.globalhealthfacts.org

US Census Bureau International Database: In addition to population and health data for the United States, this US government agency maintains sociodemographic statistics for most countries, utilizing data from UN agencies and from national census and surveys. Data characteristics include temporal (1950 to present, projections to 2050); spatial (227 countries and areas); and subnational resolution (e.g., urban/rural, age, sex). Population pyramids, and their component data, are available for virtually all countries.

Population Reference Bureau Data-Finder: This site offers data on a larger set of sociodemographic and related health variables for most countries. The data are drawn mostly from UN agency sources (e.g., UNFPA), augmented by data from individual countries. The characteristics included are population trends, education, employment, environment, and a range of global health concerns: HIV/AIDS, reproductive health, youth, and other.

WHO Global Health Atlas: For persons interested in communicable diseases, this offers updated static maps and related documents, as well as capacities for interactive mapping and data queries. In addition to specific disease mapping, some selective program mapping is available (e.g., IMCI—Integrated Management of Childhood Infections).

Interest in global data of many kinds is increasing exponentially. However, searching the web can be challenging due to the vast number of sites of variable quality. The following additional websites are recommended as supplementary sources:

The Global Social Change Research Project: This site offers data on political, economic, social, criminal, conflict, peace, happiness and other important trends.

The Kaiser Family Foundation: This provides country-level indicators across a range of areas and topics, including Global Fund Priorities (HIV, TB Malaria). Data displayed in tables, charts, and color-coded maps can be downloaded for custom analyses.

Decoding Global Health Patterns: Population Transition Theories

The term *demographic transition* refers to the theory of how countries transition from high to low fertility (and mortality) rates. Historically associated with technologic change and industrialization, the process is now considered more directly related to the social forces of improved female literacy, status of women, and to evolving expectations than to other factors. The term *epidemiological transition* is a theory postulated by Egyptian demographer Abdel Omran in 1971 that associates phases in the demographic transition with particular patterns of morbidity and mortality: the "age of pestilence and famine," the "age of receding pandemics," and the "age of degenerative and manmade diseases," three generalizations based on the history of epidemics in Western civilization over the past 1000 years. As this general theory did not fit all situations, Omran then developed variants that offer lucid explanations for how the transition plays out in different times and places. A four-stage framework developed to depict how the general theory plays out, is shown in Figure 5-3.[16]

In the pretransition stage, both fertility and mortality rates are high. During early transition, the death rate plummets while the birth rate remains high. Fertility decline occurs in the late transition stage. The decline in fertility is followed roughly in parallel by secondary declines in infant and child mortality rates. The result is a reduced proportion of children and young adults and a steady increase in the proportion of older persons in the population; these changes are reflected in the transformation of population pyramids, as discussed earlier. Finally, in the posttransition stage, fertility rates converge with mortality rates, and the near-equilibrium between birth and death rates that occurred in the pretransition stage is restored. These therefore are the dynamics that underlie the contrasts presented earlier in Figure 5-1 and Table 5-3, which can also be viewed as broadly representing pretransition and posttransition societies.

Bringing transition theory fully into the present, and closely related to demographic and epidemiologic transitions, is a "nutrition transition."[17] Large shifts in cultural diet and physical activity, especially over the past three decades, appear to be converging on diets high in saturated fats, sugar, and refined foods but low in fiber (the so-called "Western diet") and more sedentary lifestyles. These changes are reflected in nutritional outcomes, such as changes in average stature, body composition, and morbidity. Despite the persistence of famine and undernutrition that still affects hundreds of millions of people, this trend is simultaneously resulting in a pandemic of overweight and obesity.

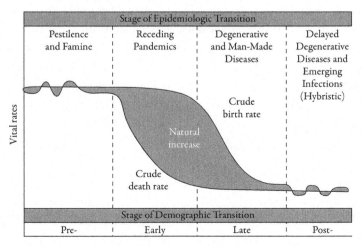

FIGURE 5-3 *Acknowledgment: Transition diagram reproduced with permission from the Population Reference Bureau.*

We return to epidemiological transition theory in chapter 6, emphasizing variants that help to explain global disease patterns and the prospects for prevention and control.

While demography is a discipline in its own right, the overview just presented serves to illustrate how critical it is to understanding population characteristics from other perspectives, including implications for health policies, interventions, and services. Population and public health depend on demography in a manner comparable to how they require epidemiology and biostatistics. These related population sciences share a need for data sources and have overlapping methods of analysis. In the context of health situation analysis and public health surveillance, we return to data sources later in this chapter.

The Health of Populations: Moving from Assessment to Action

Assessing the health of a population for the purpose of improving it is not a new idea: the history of such efforts goes back hundreds, even thousands of years in some cultures (chapter 1). This process continues today with progressively more scientific and strategic applications. Having positioned demography as a critical link in this process, we now examine how to characterize the health of populations at two specific levels: health situation analysis, emphasizing health policy planning and evaluation applications, and public health surveillance, focusing on disease prevention and control applications.

Situation analysis is the study of a situation that may require improvement, or that may offer valuable lessons for future application: it begins by defining the focus (a challenge, a problem, another view of reality, even a favorable situation), followed by measuring its extent, intensity, causes, and impacts upon the community, and then by an appraisal of how this relates to the existing system or way of doing things, including an assessment of its performance and environmental considerations. By contrast, *surveillance* refers to systematic ongoing collection, collation, and analysis of data and the timely dissemination of information to those who need to know so that action can be taken. Surveillance is a core feature of epidemiological practice, and it is applicable to both health and disease. A more elaborate definition is given later in this chapter.

Before delving into these applications, it is relevant to note a couple of examples dealt with in other chapters. One of the best known efforts in health situation analysis (HSA), and deriving action plans from this, is Healthy People 2020 (see chapter 8), a US Department of Health and Human Services rolling framework that uses a ten year cycle that identifies preventable threats to health and sets national goals and objectives to reduce these threats.[18] Similarly, already presented in chapter 2, among the best historical examples of surveillance is how this function guided smallpox eradication. In other words, HSA and surveillance capacities are critical to successful public health initiatives.

Health Situation Analysis

Assessing the health of a population requires examining its demographic composition and socioeconomic profile; its morbidity, mortality, and health behavior patterns; its political dynamics; and its organizational structures and how they work, not only within the health sector, but also in all areas of public policy that impinge on health. Assessing population health in this broad sense is integral not only to identifying its health characteristics, but also to its prospects and challenges. Such an exercise also requires the ability to integrate this information in a manner that enables its health problems to be addressed through contextually relevant and feasible interventions. Ultimately, HSA serves as a platform for well-planned interventions: from health promoting policy initiatives and social marketing strategies to programmatic actions that support disease prevention and control.

Five categories of information are usually needed for systematic analysis:[19]

- General information (history, geographic structures, and political characteristics; infra-structural aspects including policies, programs, and resources)
- Population information (demographic data, including the age-sex pyramid, fertility trends, and knowledge of internal and external migration patterns)
- Socioeconomic information (distributions by occupation, employment, and income)
- Health status information (morbidity, mortality, and behavioral risk factor patterns derived from surveys, monitoring, and surveillance systems)
- Health services information (structure and programs, service utilization data)

HSA may be carried out within a broad social framework and involve comprehensive national health surveys, or may deal with particular groups within that framework. To illustrate the latter, The Chief Public Health Officer's Report on The State of Public Health in Canada for 2009 presented a national overview of child health.[20] The same focus taken globally by UNICEF's is the basis of its annual report on the State of the World's Children.[21] Other agencies focus on particular diseases (e.g., malaria,[22] diabetes).[23]

HSA carried out by public health services at a local or district level is sometimes referred to as *community diagnosis*. This time-honored term[24] helps bring public health practice closer to the role of clinical colleagues who deal mainly with individuals and families. An active working relationship should be fostered between public health and primary care practitioners. However, the role of public health in this collaboration includes defining community health problems in a manner that facilitates remedial action beyond what individual practitioners can do: by addressing "upstream" issues such as modifiable environmental, social, and behavioral determinants and "downstream" ones too. To illustrate *upstream* factors: improving water quality may be the action needed in underserved communities where clinicians are dealing with a high incidence of diarrhea; enhancing childhood immunization coverage may be the critical ingredient in lower income settings where clinicians are seeing an elevated incidence of vaccine preventable diseases; promoting physical fitness and healthier nutrition may be called for where overweight and obesity are endemic. *Downstream*, the public health challenge might be to facilitate provision of community services, such as addiction counseling in urban areas where clinicians may be confronted with a high prevalence of drug abuse, while home care services may be applicable for settings with many dependent elderly and disabled.

At all levels from global to local, the availability of valid, reliable data will always be an essential condition for objective analysis and assessment of the health situation and for the related evidence-based decision making for health policies and programs.[25] In virtually all settings, the scope and relevance of information needs must be steadily updated in light of changing patterns of health and disease and program requirements. Where such data are not available, new sources must be generated. As the process increasingly utilizes information technologies, the emerging field of *public health informatics* concerns itself with supporting the programmatic needs of agencies, improving the quality of population-based information upon which public health policy is based, and expanding the range of disease prevention, health promotion, and health threat assessment capability at every level of public health, from local to global.[26]

HSA involves synthesizing relevant data into useful information on population health: only when the strengths and limitations of available data are understood and interpreted in light of actual needs does it become useful information for policies and programs.

Data Sources for Health Situation Analysis

In HSA, most of the basic data can usually be derived from existing sources. These sources include population censuses and surveys, vital statistics, disease registries, and health care utilization records, other health information systems that have been put in place to serve programmatic needs, and other sources pertinent to the question at hand, for example, social, environmental, and geographical. Special surveys and other forms of new enquiry may also be conducted to augment what can be gleaned from more routinely available data. Major data sources for the purpose of HSA are summarized in Table 5-6.

Regarding *the use of routinely available data*, there are both advantages and limitations.[27] Among the *advantages* are relatively low cost (the data have already been captured, usually for other purposes); the size of the database (by virtue of their large size, national and regional databases offer less potential for sampling error and selection bias); population coverage (some routinely collected data may include an entire population, which means that statistical calculations can be "exact" and not estimates); time period coverage (much routine data have been collected for many years, facilitating the analysis of trends); breadth and diversity (many large databases contain information collected for other purposes, which may enrich a health analysis application); in some jurisdictions, the capacity exists for records linkage across large databases which can enable more sophisticated questions to be posed and more complex analyses carried out.

Disadvantages of routinely collected data also must be recognized: when data are collected for a particular application then used for another, it may not be ideal. Various factors can affect data quality, such as the rigor of definitions used and the training and quality control over data collection procedures. Completeness of ascertainment is likely to be higher if multiple sources are used; for example, surveillance based on physician notification alone is well recognized for the risk of underreporting. Issues may also arise with regard to the qualities of sensitivity, reliability, and specificity (defined below).

Judgments must be made about the suitability of routinely collected data for the purpose of HSA; if not sufficient for the task, then new data may have to be developed through more purpose-designed data collection or simulation activities (e.g., surveys, mathematical modeling). Issues of *confidentiality* and *privacy* might also arise, such that some HSA applications may need to undergo ethical review, although a considerable amount of HSA is achievable through the use of data already in the public domain that has already met such requirements. However, as in the case of research, data quality issues may arise at any stage in the HSA process, from data collection to interpretation; this requires staying alert to the need for quality control and related operational research.

Most experts would agree that a *census* (described earlier in this chapter, and historically in chapter 1), and projections made from it, constitutes the most useful tool for the construction of any population profile and that census data are virtually indispensable for population health applications. Aside from providing essential

TABLE 5-6

Major types of data for health situation analysis, the information they produce, and their sources (examples)

Type of Data	Information	Source
Census	Population distributions by age, sex, locations, socioeconomic status and other group characteristics e.g., race, language; population pyramids; denominators for health and vital statistics, disease rates, and health status estimates; life tables.	Decennial census, inter-census estimates, related surveys, and projections.
Mortality statistics	Distribution of death rates according to age, sex, location, cause, etc Derived statistics include expectation of life at various ages, life tables	Death certificates
Natality statistics	Age, parity, duration of pregnancy, birth weight, type of birth (single, twin, etc)	Birth certificates
Hospital discharge statistics	Length of stay, outcome in relation to diagnosis, service, procedure, etc	Hospital charts (summary or abstract)
Notifiable disease statistics – Communicable – Occupational – Other conditions can also be made notifiable under public health legislation	Incidence of communicable, occupational diseases, others e.g., birth defects, animal diseases of interest	Notifications under public health legislation; worker's compensation claims; pathology reports; police reports of violence etc

(continued)

TABLE 5-6 (Continued)

Type of Data	Information	Source
Health care utilization statistics	Frequency of patient contacts with health care system, use of prescribed and over-the-counter drugs	Health insurance claims data, economic statistics on drugs, school health reports, etc
Health status indicators	Frequency of symptoms, complaints, impairments, disabilities	Community health surveys; statistics from specialized agencies e.g., for disabled etc
Responses to questionnaires	Symptoms, complaints, impairments	Health surveys, Insurance claims
Pension statistics etc	Disabilities, handicaps (prevalence)	Agencies for disabled
Behavioral data	Sales of alcohol, tobacco, etc	Economic and financial records
	Healthy and unhealthy behavior, as determined by surveys (prevalence).	Behavioral risk factor surveys
Unobtrusive data	Health behavior, patient and provider satisfaction	Traffic violations, etc. Graffiti; false fire alarms
	Risk taking behavior	
	Antisocial behavior	

data for vital and health statistics, including disease rates and health status estimates, censuses also provide direct information that is critical to public health services, for example, identifying proportions of single-parent mother-led families, and localities with high proportions of isolated old people living alone, who may be at high risk of poor health. Public health nursing and other services then can be assigned to the vulnerable people who live in such localities. In some countries record linkage systems and privacy laws permit relating census data to hospital discharge and death certificate data, providing a useful additional tool for health policy and epidemiological research studies. A census population can be broken down into geographically identifiable units for the purpose of analysis of issues relevant to population health (e.g., access to food, transportation, public services, and recreation).

Health Indicators: Variables that carry significant information value for a health situation analysis are usually termed *health indicators*. By definition these must be amenable to measurement, are usually constructed so as to allow comparison across persons, places, and times, and together reflect the overall health situation, or, if the HSA is specific to a particular condition or defined population group, they must be designed to reflect that situation. Commonly used indicators used in assessing large populations (e.g., country, state or province) include infant, child, and maternal mortality measures; morbidity and disability measures; statistics on nonbiological determinants (e.g., access to services, quality of care, living conditions, cultural, social, behavioral, and environmental factors). Although, as shown in Table 5-7, many indicators are standard vital and health statistical measures whose application is straightforward, some can be considered health status indicators per se, and others are more directly reflective of underlying risk factors and determinants. Sometimes more complex indicators are required to enable more refined analyses, such as the Gini Coefficient and Disability Adjusted Life Years (DALYs) (defined below). It is fully legitimate and indeed desirable to include an array of measures, from health determinants to outcomes, in a health situation analysis.

The quality and usefulness of an indicator are defined by its *validity* (effectively measures what it attempts to measure) and *reliability* (repeated measurements in similar conditions produce the same results). Additional attributes to ensure quality are its *specificity* (measures only the phenomena that it is meant to measure), *sensitivity* (has the capacity to measure changes in the phenomena that it is meant to measure), *measurability* (is based on available or easy to obtain data), *policy-relevance* (is capable of providing clear responses to key policy issues), and *cost-effectiveness* (results justify the investment in time and other resources). Indicators must also be easy to use and interpret by analysts and readily understandable to information users, such as managers and decision makers.[28]

Gini Coefficient: A measure of income disparity in a population, the coefficient ranges between 0 and 1, with 0 signifying complete income equality (everyone receives the same income) and 1 signifying complete inequality (one person receives all income). While evidence linking income inequality and health outcomes has been inconsistent, a recent meta-analysis supports an association with mortality and self-rated health.[28] This study also supports a "threshold effect" when the Gini rises above 0.3, where disparities in health outcomes are seen to emerge. Most countries in Europe have relatively stable coefficients of about 0.3, while the value for the USA is increasing and approaching 0.4. Income inequality is believed to damage health through various pathways, for example: an unequal society usually means that many live in poverty, a proven determinant of poor health outcomes; societies with high coefficients are hypothesized to experience psychosocial stress from associated loss of social cohesion, such as from the effects of income-segregated communities.[29] Researchers in this field caution that inequality by income is but one form, and that other forms such as unequal distribution of wealth, political power, cultural assets, social assets, honorific status (to name a few), could also be important health determinants.[30] Given the global economic crisis and emerging inequalities, this topic is likely to attract increasing attention in the foreseeable future.

Disability Adjusted Life Years (DALYs): This "burden of disease" measure was first developed at Harvard University for the World Bank, then later more fully developed by the World Health Organization. DALYs for a disease or health condition are calculated as the sum of the Years of Life Lost (YLL) due to premature mortality in the population and the Years Lost due to Disability (YLD) for incident cases of the health condition. One DALY can be thought of as one lost year of "healthy" life. The sum of these DALYs across a population, or the burden of disease, can be thought of as a measurement of the gap between current health status and an ideal situation where the entire population lives to an advanced age, free of disease and disability. Using DALYs, one may compare the burden of diseases that cause early death but little disability (e.g., drowning or measles) to that of diseases that do not cause death but do cause disability (e.g., cataract causing blindness). DALYs can be used to compare different regions or countries and for tracking trends. For example, in chapter 6, DALYs are used to rank the leading causes of diseases in low, middle, and high-income countries and for the world as a whole. For further details on methodology and various applications of DALYs and other measures, one may consult the website of the Global Burden of Disease (GBD) project at WHO.[31]

New Disability Indicators: All health indicators have their strengths and limitations. For example, the DALY approach is not sensitive to changes in people's functional status resulting from interventions that do not change an underlying medical diagnosis. For this reason, other indicators—for example, the Activity Limitation Score (ALS) and the Participation Restriction Score (PRS —have been advocated for assessing the impact of interventions on the lives of disabled people.[32]

Newer Indicator Technologies: Beyond the use of routinely or specially collected or constructed data, new technologies are also being applied at the cutting edge of HSA today. In particular, Geographic Information Systems (GIS) is a tool of increasing usefulness. GIS refers to a computerized system for collecting, storing, representing, and manipulating spatial data. Before GIS became available, assembly and analysis of spatial data was a painstaking task; for example, working manually with area maps and plotting individual cases or exposure zones in a two-dimensional manner. Now that GIS technology applications are available, such data can be more accurately collected due to satellite technology (global positioning), digitally uploaded, and analyzed to investigate a full range of epidemiological and health service issues at population level. GIS assists health studies across diverse areas, including mapping, monitoring, and modeling infectious and chronic diseases; disease surveillance and outbreak detection; exposure and risk factor assessment; emergency preparedness; and targeting intervention and health promotion initiatives; as well as examining health outcomes and related health care provisions. However, just as remains true of the use of routinely available data, users of GIS tools must remain on guard for issues of data availability and quality and understand the methodological limitations of these techniques. Information technology in itself, just as is true for advanced statistical methods, is no substitute for rigor at the level of data collection and consolidation. Further discussion of GIS applications can be found in many newer epidemiology textbooks and published papers.[33, 34, 35, 36]

Linking Health Situation Analysis to Public Health Action

The conduct of HSA as a baseline assessment prior to introducing health interventions is considered "good public health practice" and increasingly essential to attracting and sustaining funding support. In this context, it responds in particular to the first element in the classical planning sequence: *Where are we? Where do we want to be? How do we get there? How do we know we are getting there?* When HSA is conducted periodically throughout an intervention, it addresses the fourth element, thereby contributing to monitoring and evaluation (M&E) of the intervention process and progressively to the achievement of short, intermediate, and long-term outcomes. Ultimately, a fifth step is taken, which is in essence the same as the first step: *Where are we now?* This simple description of an ongoing process helps introduce how HSA fits within a cycle of health program planning and implementation, a topic that is presented more fully in chapter 8.

Several of the case studies presented in chapter 4 are now worth revisiting briefly to reflect on the usefulness of HSA for initiatives oriented toward well-defined populations: AMREF's work in the Rift Valley revealed that the SAFE protocol for the prevention and control of trachoma reduced active disease within 3 years in children from 47% to 16.0%, and potentially blinding infection declined 4.5% to 1.7%. The proportion of faces with many flies fell over 4 years from 48% to 6%.[37] Implicitly, neither documentation of the initial health problem nor these measures of success would have been possible without baseline and follow-up data; this well measured strategy has advanced eye care policy globally.[38] AKU's approach to community health development in Pakistan, as illustrated by its Rural Community Development Project in partnership with an international energy company, was guided by a baseline assessment of health conditions and needs in a poverty-afflicted area;[39] follow-up assessment 6 years later by the World Bank was able to document attributable improvements.[40] The Health Policy Initiatives of Mauritius were similarly based

TABLE 5-7

Examples of indicators of health determinants and status

Health Determinants	Health Status
Demographic	**Perceived Health**
Population distributions and trends by age and sex, race and ethnicity, fertility, urban and rural populations, life expectancy at birth and at other ages, dependency ratios, sex ratios	• Population % who perceive themselves in excellent, good, fair or poor health; • Measures of family/community support vs isolation • Perceived access to health care • Satisfaction with care received
Environmental population % with: • acceptable water analysis • access to potable water • access to sewage disposal levels of specified contaminants in water • e.g., arsenic, mercury, cadmium, lead access to quality and affordable housing access to transportation options e.g., road, rail, paths access to communications e.g., telephone, radio, TV	**Objective Health** • Mortality indicators: maternal, infant, age-sex-cause specific; age-standardized etc • Morbidity indicators: incidence of vaccine preventable diseases; other priority conditions for the setting e.g., HIV/AIDS, dengue fever,
Socioeconomic Adult literacy rates by gender; educational attainment; annual GDP growth rate; unemployment rates; poverty rates; measures of food security e.g., food bank use; working conditions e.g., occupational health & safety; social safety nets e.g., pensions, workers compensation, income support systems: government investment in social sector (health, education, social services); income % required for housing, food, clothing; income distribution measures e.g., Gini Coefficient (see text)	• Prevalence of morbidity e.g., metabolic syndrome, overweight & obesity, hypertension, type 2 diabetes, cancer (especially preventable forms), anxiety and depression, dental health e.g., DMF Index etc • Prevalence of impairment, disability, handicap; aids to independent living, etc • Related population measures: average number of days per year lost to school, work, and other social roles for a defined population • Disability Adjusted Life Years (DALYs) (see text)

(*continued*)

TABLE 5-7 (Continued)

Health Determinants	Health Status
Behavioral	**Other:**
• Measures of health literacy	Extent to which these indicators vary
• Proportion of regular smokers	as a function of age, gender, race,
• Proportion who take regular exercise	ethnic or immigration status
• Patterns of drinking e.g., drunk driving	*Note:* As is common in most attempts
Health Services	to create two groups of variables,
• Access to primary health care	some may equally well fit in either
• Distribution of health human resources	column, depending on context.
• % births attended by trained personnel	
• Contraception prevalence rates	
• Immunization coverage rates (age specific)	
• Growth charting (height and weight for age)	
• Early childhood development	
• Provisions for disabilities	
• Extent to which essential health services are universal vs barriers to access and use	
• Extent of use of informal care practitioners	
Other:	
• presence of war, civil conflict, crime, violence	

on a prior HSA exercise,[41] forming an evidence base for monitoring and evaluating goals and objectives that were ultimately achieved with sustained support from the African Development Bank.[42] The conduct of baseline and follow up HSA exercises is explicit in all CINDI-CARMEN protocols (adopted by numerous countries),[43] inspired by the success of the North Karelia Project, Finland. Similarly, the more recently launched Community Interventions for Health (CIH) Initiative depends on baseline and follow-up HSAs to define the challenge, design the interventions, and monitor progress and evaluation outcomes in a rigorous manner that can provide valuable lessons so that comparable initiatives may be adapted elsewhere in the world.[44, 45]

Beyond Health Situation Analysis, these examples also reveal the importance of taking political and financial contexts into account when proposing population health interventions. Without political will and financial support, needed interventions, however desirable (even obvious in the minds of some health professionals), may be neither feasible nor sustainable. Putting forward effective proposals requires relevant data.

Moving from Assessment to Action—Global Perspective

The health of populations has been well addressed at global level by the WHO Commission on the Social Determinants of Health (2008).[46] Extrapolating from population health statistical data, the Commission drew attention to the extreme nature of health inequities, for example, such contrasts as: "A girl in Lesotho is likely to live 42 years less than another in Japan. In Sweden, the risk of a woman dying during pregnancy and childbirth is 1 in 17,400; in Afghanistan, the odds are 1 in 8." Within countries, the Commission also noted numerous examples of inequity, among them: "Life expectancy for indigenous Australian males is shorter by 17 years than all other Australian males. Maternal mortality is 3–4 times higher among the poor compared to the rich in Indonesia. The difference in adult mortality between least and most deprived neighborhoods in the UK is more than 2.5 times. Child mortality in the slums of Nairobi is 2.5 times higher than in other parts of the city. A baby born to a Bolivian mother with no education has a 10% chance of dying, while one born to a woman with at least secondary education has a 0.4% chance. In the USA, 886,202 deaths would have been averted between 1991 and 2000 if mortality rates between white and African Americans were equalized." Whether between or within countries, such differences arise predominantly from the social environment where people are born and how they live, grow, work, and age. They are a reflection of the degree to which social justice exists between and within societies and are amenable to corrective actions that may range from policy interventions to program development. This has policy implications for all nations.

THE MILLENNIUM DEVELOPMENT GOALS

The inequities of the human condition within and between countries elicited a call for action to correct such injustice. At a United Nations conference in 2000, member nations pronounced the Millennium Development Goals (MDGs), to be achieved by 2015. Health and social conditions around the world were examined. Responding to the calls of civil society (for example, Peoples Health Movement, chapter 4), eight goals were constructed, reflecting the main challenges globally.[47]

Within these goals there are 18 operational targets, complemented by 48 measurable indicators to measure progress toward the MDGs.

Goal 1: Halve Proportion of People in Extreme Poverty and Hunger
Goal 2: Achieve Universal Primary Education
Goal 3: Promote Gender Equality and Empower Women
Goal 4: Reduce Child Mortality by 2/3
Goal 5: Reduce Maternal Mortality by 3/4
Goal 6: Combat HIV/AIDS, Malaria, and Other Diseases
Goal 7: Ensure Environmental Sustainability
Goal 8: Develop a Global Partnership of Development

The MDGs are ambitious: for example, the first goal is to cut poverty by half by 2015. The actual target set was to reduce by half the proportion of people living on less than a dollar a day (later adjusted to $1.25 per day). Three MDGs focus directly on health: covering maternal mortality, child mortality, HIV/AIDS, malaria, and tuberculosis. Other MDGs address issues closely related to health, such as gender equity, nutrition, water and sanitation, universal primary education, and the environment. While the task is enormous and unprecedented, if the global community could work effectively toward an end to poverty, the benefits in terms of health and well-being would be enormous.[48] For public health organizations, this is a call to respond to unfinished agendas such as the provision of potable water, sanitation, and hygiene education while taking on newer challenges such as the expanding burden of noncommunicable diseases (not addressed in the MDGs although now the leading cause of death in all regions except Sub-Saharan Africa) and lack of universal access to health care in many nations. The need to redress inequities applies to all countries without exception, although some more than others. Set against this are the challenges of political and social inertia, the crisis in the world economic order, leadership deficits, and issues of self-interest that produce resistance to change.

Nonetheless, it is important to note that unprecedented amounts of development assistance have been pledged, amounting to many tens of billions of dollars in aid targeted toward the MDGs. Although the track record of developed countries on keeping their aid commitments is not impressive (especially the G8 group of nations),[49] there is cautious optimism that most will honor these commitments, at least to some extent. Figure 5-4 lays out progress and deficits towards six of the MDGs circa 2010.[50] However, this graph also reveals that some countries are unable to measure their progress due to lack of data in some domains and implies that these nations do not have the capacity to analyze their health situations such as set out in this chapter. Equally important, in relation to Goal 8 (Develop a Global Partnership

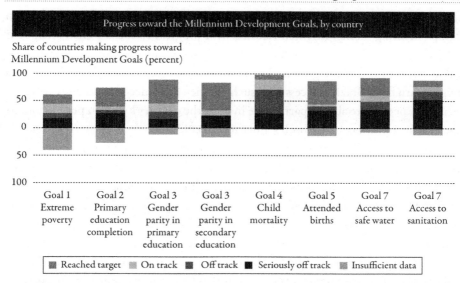

FIGURE 5-4 *Acknowledgement: Reproduced from Figure 1a in reference #53 with permission from The World Bank.*

of Development; not shown in the figure), without more reliable support from developed countries, several Goals are likely to be missed in many developing ones.[51] Regarding the 6th goal, monitoring and evaluation comes within the remit of a "Global Fund to fight AIDS, Tuberculosis and Malaria"; this goal is discussed elsewhere (chapter 6). Tragically, in November 2011, several European Union entities (Germany, Ireland, Sweden, and the European Commission), ostensibly in response to fraud in 4 nations (there are 120 recipient countries), but also in the midst of their own economic crises, drastically reduced their funding support with the effect that the Global Fund will be unable to take on new commitments for a 3-year period. In May 2012, some of this lost funding was restored thanks to the emergence of new donors and support from existing donors in the form of advanced payments and other arrangements. It is clear that global political support is a key factor in the success of the Global Fund.

Although encouragement may be taken from *initial* success in poverty reduction in some countries, success might take longer in some settings than in others, and how it should be measured might also differ. For example, a World Bank study of Brazil, China, and India revealed that all three achieved falling poverty during recent reform periods but to varying degrees and for different reasons. China had favorable initial conditions for rapid poverty reduction through market-led economic growth; at the outset there were ample distortions to remove and relatively low inequality in access to opportunities so created, though inequality has risen markedly since. By contrast, in Brazil and India, by concentrating such opportunities in the hands of the better off, prior inequalities handicapped poverty reduction. Brazil's success in complementing market-oriented reforms with progressive social policies helped it achieve more rapid poverty reduction than India, although Brazil is less successful in terms of economic growth. In the wake of its steep rise in inequality, China might learn from Brazil's success with such policies. India needs to do more to assure that poor people are able to participate in both the country's growth process and its social policies: lessons from both China and Brazil.[52]

Translating success in poverty reduction into measurable improvement in health equity is not a foregone conclusion. As the WHO Commission on the Social Determinants of Health points out,[49] enough is known for policy makers to initiate action. However, in literally all countries, there is a great need for training policy makers, health workers, and workers in other sectors to understand the need for action on social determinants, as well as on specific evidence-based public health and medical interventions. The feasibility of action is indicated in changes that are already occurring: Egypt achieved a major drop in child mortality from 235 to 33 per 1000 over 30 years; Greece and Portugal reduced their child mortality from 50 per 1000 births to levels nearly as low as Japan, Sweden, and Iceland; Cuba achieved over 99% coverage for its child development services in 2000. Such gains are no accident: they are the outcome of strategic policies and effective programming, guided by health situation analysis and public health surveillance.

A Summary of Health Situation Analysis: Recognizing assets, deficits, inequities, and opportunities in the health of populations first requires analysis of the existing situation. To achieve effective and lasting improvement in population health status then requires designing public health interventions; these in turn must be subjected to monitoring and evaluation to ensure that there is movement toward the desired new health situation.

Public Health Surveillance

Public health surveillance is a form of HSA carried out continually and focused mainly on health protection and disease control as *information for action*. As a process, it is defined as ongoing, systematic collection, analysis, interpretation, and dissemination of data regarding health-related events for use in public health actions to reduce morbidity and mortality and to improve health.[53] Operationally, surveillance is purposely designed to meet disease prevention and control and related health protection needs. Like other forms of HSA, public health surveillance data may also be useful for program planning and evaluation, formulating research hypotheses, and providing cases for epidemiological investigations such as case-control studies.

It may also contribute to other population health applications, such as health promotion, program planning, and evaluation.

Historically, surveillance has been focused on diseases of public health importance, initially focusing on communicable diseases,[54] often encoded in Acts and Regulations prescribing particular actions in the event of disease. Over the years, the focus broadened to address similar needs for toxic hazards, injury prevention, noncommunicable diseases, and other health threats.[55] Reflecting the contemporary emphasis on *results-based management,* public health surveillance today includes a broad array of goal-related activities and techniques that reflect "smart" principles: specific, measurable, action-oriented, realistic, and timeframe specified. Surveillance pays attention to current context, such as emerging public concerns and the more immediate underlying social and environmental determinants. Applications are numerous: infectious disease control, prevention of occupational and environmental hazards and exposures, injury prevention, and behavioral risk factor surveillance relevant to noncommunicable diseases.

Early detection of threats or events largely relies on health professionals working at primary care level: those who see clinical cases have a front line opportunity to recognize unusual patterns. In this respect, all clinicians are participants in the public health effort as they are obliged to notify unusual cases or events to the attention of public health officials, who will then manage the situation or call for support. In line of duty, the public health officer must analyze, interpret, and communicate ongoing results of the surveillance effort, so as to alert professionals, program managers, and decision makers to emerging trends. These might be local, such as a foodborne outbreak related to a community event, or may have potential to spread, such as meningococcal disease in a sports team that could be transmitted to other teams in the same league. Thus there exists a wide diversity of incidents that may require surveillance, some with mostly local potential and others with far reaching implications (keeping in mind that pandemic conditions always have their start in local settings, e.g., severe acute respiratory syndrome—SARS). Consider for example, the implications of a toxic hazard that has extended from an industrial site (e.g., a leak of toxic fluid into a watercourse or a gas emission that could have trans-boundary implications). The threat of terrorism and high-threat disease outbreaks has increased recognition that surveillance must have the operational capacity for early detection; this threat has renewed interest in surveillance development and upgraded the priority of this aspect of public health practice.

Timeliness and *relevance* are of particular concern when dealing with health threats, emerging diseases, and complex health trends. It is long recognized that depending on primary care health professionals for reports of unusual cases or events is a "passive" approach, and that relying on this alone results in relatively incomplete and inaccurate data, especially for widely prevalent diseases. More generally, data from most single sources suffer from varying levels of bias, due to differentials in diagnostic ascertainment, access to laboratory confirmation, and reporting variations across relevant levels: socioeconomic, geographic, and jurisdictional. Using multiple sources of data helps reduce this risk to the quality of the surveillance effort. It is essential therefore for public health agencies to stimulate such single-source systems to achieve more timely and complete information and to augment this with "active" forms of surveillance, more purpose-designed, also reflecting the *multi-factorial ecology* of health and disease.

In addition to health databases, other information systems are also tapped for public health surveillance purposes. Creative use of data collected for other purposes is not a new idea, as surveillance did start with and continues to make use of death certifications and hospital and clinic records (primarily designed for patient management and institutional administration) have been used for decades. However, in addition to such vital and health statistical data sources, contemporary surveillance makes use of data as diverse as travel and immigration trends, weather reports, and trends in literacy, income, poverty, unemployment, and crime, among others. In surveillance analyses, such data sets are often linked at aggregate level through such geographic commonalities as census districts and postal codes. In some instances direct *linkage* of individual records may be possible, with ethical protections for privacy and confidentiality.

In developing surveillance systems, it is useful to construct a *pathway analysis* of existing and proposed information flow to identify key points where flow may be impeded and to spot opportunities for new pathways and potential short-circuits using decision rules to achieve the goal of surveillance as *"information for action."* To paraphrase a principle from the management sciences: *If a step in a process does not add value, take it out.* Conversely, *if a new step may add value, modify the flowchart accordingly.*

To illustrate the utility of pathway analysis in the surveillance context, we show a flowchart developed by the US Centers for Disease Control and Prevention to improve the timeliness of early detection of outbreaks (Figure 5-5). Specifically, we draw attention to the use of *lateral arrows*, as well as vertical and diagonal ones. The figure thereby illustrates the use of "real-time data for early outbreak detection" and "automated analyses to signal something unusual noted," while higher-order functions are located further down the chain.[56] The *inversion of the authority hierarchy* (when compared with organograms which traditionally show information flowing "up" to senior decision makers at the top) is instructive: symbolically and operationally, it places at the top actions that have greater immediate impact at the local level (information in this depiction flows "down").

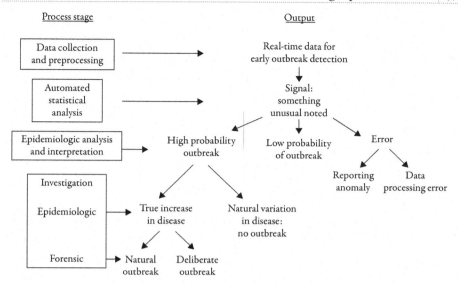

FIGURE 5-5 Surveillance process model—outbreak detection.

Source: Reproduced from Figure 1, US Centers for Disease Control and Prevention: reference #59.

Not shown in Figure 5-5 is the subsequent flow of information to policy level, which also must take place. The implication is that public health professionals at a local level should be trained and empowered to take action to address local events, without having to "ask" for authority to be delegated from a higher level (which has other duties, responsibilities, and priorities). This model moves us away from an era in which some public health systems were frozen from action due to antiquated decision rules (which still exist in some settings and remain a risk to others depending on the quality of leadership). The logic also implies that data flow with related lateral and vertical actions applies at all responsible levels (e.g., local, state/provincial, federal/national, international).

Extending these principles to the international level is required for global public health surveillance. Historically, the principle of countries reporting health events internationally has not always been honored: some have not understood the purpose or believed in its utility (e.g., a perception that this is simply for compiling statistical information with no benefit); others have been more preoccupied about the adverse impacts on trade and tourism than on protecting public health (in many countries the health portfolio is accorded low political priority).

As a result of this legacy, the International Health Regulations (IHRs) were revised in 2005. The new regulations emphasize protection against the global spread of public health emergencies without unnecessary interference with international travel and trade. They require member states to develop national surveillance and

response systems and describe how international health emergencies are to be identified, reported, and managed. States are now required to notify WHO of all events
that may constitute public health emergencies of international concern in accordance with a set of criteria to assist member states in deciding whether an event is
notifiable to WHO.[57] The criteria are

- Is the public health impact of the event serious?
- Is the event unusual or unexpected?
- Is there a significant risk of international spread?
- Is there a significant risk of international restriction(s) to travel and trade?

Particular diseases are specified either for immediate notification or for assessment against these criteria: smallpox (eradicated, but unfortunately the virus is
still retained in some national laboratories, ostensibly for research and/or defense,
thereby itself constituting an ongoing threat to public health globally), poliomyelitis
due to wild-type poliovirus, SARS, and cases of human influenza caused by a new
subtype. *Case definitions* for each of these four diseases are available from the WHO
IHR website.[58]

Implementation of these regulations faces several challenges, including lack of
capacity in developing countries, the risk of independent action in developed countries, and poor coordination between federal and regional governments in decentralized countries.[59]

The advent of *electronic information* and *communications technologies* is steadily
improving the synergy between individual health practitioners and public health
agencies, linking individuals and agencies around the world. The e-revolution, which
includes systems such as email, interactive websites, tracking systems, social media,
and cell phones, has enabled public health surveillance to operate in virtual "real
time" but has also raised new concerns regarding fear and privacy.[60] Due to varying
levels of complexity and advances in information technology, surveillance systems
now vary from simple data collection from a single source to electronic systems that
receive data from many sources in multiple formats. The number and variety of systems is increasing with advances in electronic data interchange and integration of
data, which will also heighten concerns regarding privacy, data confidentiality, and
systems security.[55]

For example, influenza surveillance today not only includes time-honored data
on hospital admissions and deaths from influenza-pneumonia, but also utilizes sentinel physician panels to assess population susceptibility and active infection trends
and (because this is a zoonotic disease) monitors influenza activity in wildlife and
domestic animals; it is also linked to expanding capacity for vaccine production in

many countries. This is a global collaborative enterprise, coordinated by the World Health Organization, utilizing the full range of information technologies.

Surveillance therefore is a rapidly evolving dimension of the public health enterprise. It is critical to how public health systems navigate and contributes key information for decision making, especially to determine when particular health trends or underlying social-ecological dynamics may require intervention. Surveillance is intimately related to formulating strategies and actions to promote health and combat disease in populations. Examples range from global to local across the health and disease spectrum: coordinated international cooperation to address emerging infectious diseases, risk factor surveillance to guide prevention and control of noncommunicable diseases, and surveillance of groups at increased risk of conditions such as tuberculosis and HIV/AIDS and of institutionalized groups that share particular risks and outcomes (e.g., schools, military, persons in hospitals).

The critical role that surveillance plays in public health interventions may be best appreciated by reference to expectations of what this practice is supposed to accomplish. According to the US Centers for Disease Control and Prevention, this includes[55]

- Guide immediate action for cases of public health importance
- Measure the burden of disease (or other health-related event), including changes in related factors; identify populations at risk and new or emerging concerns
- Monitor trends in the burden of a disease (or other health-related event), including the detection of epidemics (outbreaks) and pandemics
- Guide the planning, implementation, and evaluation of programs to prevent and control disease, injury, or adverse exposure
- Evaluate public policy
- Detect changes in health practices and the effects of these changes
- Prioritize the allocation of health resources
- Describe the clinical course of disease
- Provide a basis for epidemiologic research

Data requirements for surveillance applications must emphasize simplicity, flexibility, timeliness, local operational applicability, and the requirements of legislation. In addition, *all other criteria* that generically apply to health information systems must also be applied to indicators selected for surveillance, but emphasizing its purpose as "information for action." Some important data requirements are now listed:

Simplicity in surveillance systems refers to ease of data collection, entry, retrieval, interpretation, and presentation. It should always be remembered by higher end users that the most important user is working at local level, where most interventions take place; supporting this effort in a timely manner is more important than producing aggregate reports for policy makers, although this is also a desirable surveillance output.

Flexibility refers to the capacity to adapt to modified case definitions, new syndromes, and new data elements. This should be facilitated at the local health authority level, while retaining a common core (minimum data sets) at higher levels (e.g., provincial, national).

The meaning of *timeliness* varies with the condition: for those that spread rapidly (e.g., hours, days, weeks), the allowable time for the whole task from collection, consolidation, analysis, interpretation, and dissemination must be very short for intervention and control to be effective; by contrast, conditions that develop more slowly (e.g., most noncommunicable diseases; NCDs) function with a slower and lower frequency information-to-action cycle. For this reason, the need for active surveillance is greater for infectious diseases and acute toxic agents than for NCDs; NCD surveillance applications have more in common with the data needs of planning and evaluation than for initiating immediate action.

The *sensitivity and specificity* of case definitions for surveillance purposes must include the ability for enhancement, depending on the stage of surveillance. For example, occurrence of either *"rash or fever"* is more sensitive but less specific than *"rash and fever,"* and may be more appropriate to use early in a potential measles epidemic. Adding laboratory confirmation will increase specificity but reduce sensitivity (and timeliness).

Acceptability refers to the need for surveillance to be both effective and as nonobtrusive as possible and non-stigmatizing. The extent to which this may be achieved can vary a lot across jurisdictions and with conditions. For example, HIV/AIDS case reporting is workable in some jurisdictions, less so in others, and even life-threatening in some. Issues of privacy, confidentiality, and security are critical to such surveillance.

Representativeness: as noted earlier, physician and other single-source notification of disease results in relatively incomplete and inaccurate data, and public health agencies must augment this with more purpose-designed surveillance. For some conditions, to await reports of human cases is tantamount to missing both the progression of epidemic activity and the potential for intervention. For example, HIV/AIDS case notification, while useful, is "too little too late," given that transmission is due mainly to sociobehavioral factors; second-generation surveillance combines sociobehavioral data (e.g., from focus groups, KAP surveys) with serological surveys and case reports.

Potential for Integration: The ability to view otherwise different kinds of data within an integrated framework is essential to sound surveillance. A good example is surveillance for West Nile Virus: a virtual "early warning system" that takes into account ecological considerations,[61] integrating data from virus isolation from mosquito traps, virus and serological monitoring of sentinel chickens, similar testing of wild birds, and serological surveys and case monitoring in humans and horses.

Electronic Database Systems: relevant operational requirements include

- Compatible hardware and software
- Standard user interface
- Standard data format and coding
- Quality checks
- Confidentiality and security standards

In some instances, even internally well-integrated systems may still be insufficient, as *surveillance findings must be complemented by investigations* that take place outside the information system. This is where designing surveillance around information technology (IT) requirements alone can get into difficulty, by forgetting that "shoe leather" is equally important. In other words, surveillance cannot be achieved solely by someone sitting in front of a computer screen. Surveillance data have to be integrated by human beings who can recognize when a field investigation is needed, perhaps urgently. By definition therefore the "business requirements" of a public health information system alone and the IT solution do not address the full scope of surveillance. The worst of worlds may arise if IT capacity is all that exists but the skills to interpret and follow up with investigation are missing in action. A competent public health system must deliver these capacities in a seamless manner.

In other words, there is more to surveillance than the data flow itself. *Skills enhancement* is a perennial need in many departments of health around the world, including countries with otherwise well-developed health systems. Recruitment of appropriately trained individuals (e.g., field epidemiologists)[62] and proper application of their skills cannot be taken for granted. For example, in some health ministries, senior managers (often recruited from outside the public health system) may seek *more comprehensive surveillance data* to answer questions that more correctly fall within the domains of health planning or research. This is not always appropriate: while more comprehensive data may have greater potential value, greater also are the costs of collection and risks of noncompletion. The inclusion of extraneous data fields may clutter the surveillance system and render it inefficient.

As noted earlier, surveillance entails important considerations of *privacy and confidentiality*. However, sometimes the call for such protections may reflect obsession with *jurisdictional autonomy* more than either of these principles. In the public interest, *data-sharing agreements* are therefore needed to facilitate legitimate inter-jurisdictional applications. For example, immunization data sharing is universal in New Zealand but not in some Canadian provinces. Impediments to vaccination record sharing between adjacent health areas has the potential to impede prompt and efficient investigation of outbreaks, where poor vaccination coverage or even vaccine failures may be responsible.

Global Surveillance Challenges: It is increasingly clear that, living in a "global village," we cannot escape our common responsibilities, whether these be for the health impacts of climate change or for prevention and control of pandemic diseases. It is long recognized that population mobility and rapidity of travel has facilitated transmission of emerging diseases for which there has been major global concern (e.g., SARS, Avian influenza). However, with the globalization of cultures, many of the forces that have given rise to pandemic chronic disease also apply as readily in one country as to another. This is the nature of the epidemiological transition, especially as countries slowly converge in this respect. Consider the now globalized rural-urban drift, the associated lifestyle risks e.g., sedentary living and nutritional challenges brought about by mass marketing of processed food products; agrarian lifestyles are slowly but steadily receding everywhere.

Given the evolving backdrop, there is a stronger role than ever for bodies such as the World Health Organization, but an even greater need to find ways to reduce the political and logistic barriers to communication and cooperation that separate people around the world from one another. Indeed, there is a critical need for local to global governance structures to ensure consistency in policies and practices, mechanisms for assistance, rules to ensure compliance with globally accepted procedures, and the related need for evidence to support rational decision making. Beyond the revised International Health Regulations, such needs exist across the full range of population and public health from neglected tropical diseases[63] to the global pandemic of noncommunicable diseases and potential new pandemics of infectious diseases, as well as to address their underlying determinants, including all forms of preventable inequity from local to global.

Appendix A: Concepts and Terms Commonly Used in Demography—A Selection

Mid-Year Population: Estimates of population at July 1 are used as the denominator in calculating rates and ratios for given years (e.g., birth rate, death rate). These estimates are ideally based on a census or inter-census projections (these take recent censuses into account along with relevant survey data). Normally these tasks are carried out by countries themselves e.g., by the US Census Bureau in the United States, or by international agencies (e.g., the United Nations Statistics Division), or by private organizations (e.g., Population Reference Bureau). Efforts are made to take into account the effects of refugee movements, foreign workers, and population shifts due to contemporary political events.

Birth and Death Rate: The annual number of births and deaths per 1000 total population. These are referred to as "crude rates" as they do not take age structure of the population into account. Thus, for example, crude death rates in developed nations with a relatively large proportion of high-mortality older groups are often higher than those of less developed nations with lower life expectancies. Conversely, developing counties may exhibit lower crude rates.

Standardization: A set of techniques used to remove as much as possible the effects of differences in age or other variables when comparing two or more populations, or the same population over two or more time periods. For methods the reader should consult a more specialized text.

Rate of Natural Increase: The birth rate minus the death rate, implying the annual rate of population growth without regard for migration; expressed as a percentage.

Net Migration: The estimated rate of net immigration (immigration minus emigration) per 1000 population for a recent year based upon the official national rate or derived as a residual from estimated birth, death, and population growth rates. Migration rates can vary substantially from year to year for any country as can the definition of an immigrant.

Total Fertility Rate (TFR): The average number of children a woman would have assuming that current age-specific birth rates remain constant throughout her childbearing years (usually considered to be ages 15 to 49).

Total Dependency Ratio: This is a measure of the combined population under age 15 and aged 65 years or older, expressed as a ratio to the population aged 15 to 64 years. However, because the similar ratios could derive from countries with very different age structures, depending on the contributions of younger or older group to the numerator in the calculation, it is often useful to do separate calculations for the *Child Dependency Ratio* and the *Aged Dependency Ratio*.

Life Expectancy at Birth: The average number of years a newborn infant can expect to live under current mortality levels.

Infant Mortality Rate: The annual number of deaths of infants under age 1 per 1000 live births. Rates shown with decimals indicate national statistics reported as completely registered, while those without are estimates from the sources cited above. Rates shown in italics are based upon fewer than 50 annual infant deaths and, as a result, are subject to considerable yearly variability.

Child Mortality Rate: Also known as under-5 mortality, this refers to the death of infants and children under the age of 5, expressed per 1000 live births. The child mortality rate is a leading indicator of the level of child health and overall development in countries. It is also an MDG indicator.

This chapter departs from the tradition of depicting types of disease as virtually independent entities. Instead, we focus on their interdependence, encouraging ways of thinking that may give rise to innovative intervention designs. The chapter explores core concepts, such as natural history of disease, Haddon's matrix, and others, and examines the organizational implications for integrated approaches in crossing organizational and disciplinary boundaries. It recognizes that wherever public health and primary health care intersect, especially at community level, disease prevention and control, health promotion, health protection, clinical prevention, and health services organization must work in synergy, not at cross-purposes. This reflects the evolving recognition of national and global agencies that their initiatives must align with local realities in order to be effective, efficient, and accepted by the communities they are intended to benefit.

6

INTEGRATED APPROACHES TO DISEASE PREVENTION AND CONTROL

WHAT IS DISEASE? As introduced in chapter 2, disease implies any departure from good health or from normal physiological and/or psychological function and therefore also encompasses "disorders." Operationally, it is defined by clinical, pathological, and epidemiological criteria that enable systematic study and application. As discrete entities, diseases and disorders are organized into categories— such as infectious, chronic noninfectious, traumatic, and psychological—then subclassified into specific conditions.

Early beliefs attributing disease to mystical origins were referred to in chapter 1. Empiricism and rationalism grew alongside these beliefs, blooming ultimately in our historically recent scientific era. Even now, elements of mystical beliefs about health and disease pervade all societies, from superstition to formalized healing arts, beliefs, and practices. This is so even as scientific knowledge accumulates. There is a resurgent interest today in traditional health belief systems, for a very good reason: they are still relevant. Recognizing earlier belief systems helps health practitioners contextualize how different people interpret apparently the same (or different) afflictions, understand why some are resistance to adopting approaches offered by the formal health system, and appreciate the continuing role of complementary and alternative practices.

The scientific method itself has given rise to perceptual distortions of cause and effect: constructing and deconstructing, knowledge advances mostly in small increments.

In the early 20th century, diseases were considered mostly in relation to organ systems, reflecting the central importance of anatomy in how physical ailments were understood, and mirroring how ill persons presented to clinicians. But it has long been recognized that many disease processes may simultaneously affect several organs as well as social and behavioral dimensions, due to underlying multi-system and relational processes. In effect, human biology and pathology are intertwined with social ecology in a virtually seamless manner; but when this relationship is disturbed, social and health pathologies emerge, as reflected in the social-ecological model (chapter 4).[1]

An early scientific legacy pertaining to disease concepts is the notion of single dominant causes. Following discovery in 1940 of "the wonder drug" penicillin (Nobel Prize awarded to Britons Alexander Fleming and Ernst Boris Chain and Australian Howard Florey), the notion of disease as mostly "unifactorial" was strengthened and that discovering the analogous remedy, or so called "magic bullet," is the key to controlling them. This earlier term, coined by German scientist Paul Ehrlich (1854–1915), inspired generations of scientists to devise powerful remedies for innumerable conditions from infectious diseases to various cancers. However, "magic bullets" turned out to be rare, while epidemiologists meanwhile steadily revealed that most diseases are substantively influenced by social, behavioral, and environmental conditions of exposure and susceptibility; thus today most diseases are considered multifactorial.

The multifactorial approach is now the preferred scientific way of understanding health and disease and is useful in identifying potential interventions. It also applies to conditions with a genetic predisposition for which it is now recognized that gene-environment interactions are at play, as well as for sociobehavioral disorders and for conditions once thought of in terms of one dominant cause (e.g., motor vehicle injury, toxic exposures). Virtually all processes resulting in disease or disorder interact with personal environments and behaviors that may influence the process at any stage from susceptibility and risk of exposure to clinical outcome. Multifactorial thinking therefore offers a range of avenues for new ideas about prevention and control (e.g., engineering, educational, organizational, and social policy solutions), not only biomedical ones.

A key to understanding many diseases lies in first examining their occurrence in populations so as to identify characteristics of time, place, and person. When we observe disparities such as clustering in particular geographic settings or higher prevalence among people in common circumstances, opportunities arise to explain them, as does a public health obligation to seek to alleviate them. We do this by searching for associated risk factors and underlying determinants, drawing from the public health sciences (chapter 2). In examining disparities in disease occurrence we often uncover underlying social inequalities; other times we find cultural or behavioral patterns;

sometimes there is no obvious explanation: this may require further investigation at the basic science level or embracing the complexity with more integrative analyses.

While disease prevention and control owes much of its historical success (chapter 1) to the conceptual and applied knowledge that continues to flow from epidemiology, as public health moves to address more adequately the full spectrum of chronic diseases, mental and social disorders, and disabilities now dominating the global burden of disease, we must look beyond disaggregated risk factors and determinants to embrace how these interrelate throughout the life course, taking into account cultural and social influences. For example, considerable evidence reveals that biological processes and experiences in early life, including fetal life, affect life-long susceptibility to adult disease processes and outcomes. Viewing health through the life course and applying a social ecology lens may advance our understanding and reveal new ways to prevent disease.[2]

As a public health enterprise, disease prevention and control integrates scientific, organizational, and ethical dimensions. There are challenges here for health systems development, combining science and technology with building organizational capacity to deliver services, and a body of law and regulation in some instances to enforce public health measures. For example, health protection measures (e.g., food hygiene, potable water, and clean air; chapter 7) require legislation in order to be to be enforceable. Equally, preventive technologies (e.g., immunization, cervical cancer screening) must first be mandated and then integrated within a service delivery capacity that must be funded. Sociobehavioral interventions, such as providing a safe injection environment for drug addicts, can run into legal barriers not designed with public health in mind. Relevant to political leadership, underlying determinants may require attention to social policy and legislated programs (e.g., literacy, affordable housing, food security, universal health care).

Overlaps and Interactions Across Disease Groupings

The following definitions of four broad disease groupings are useful in considering how they arise and interrelate: (1) An *injury* refers to unintentional or intentional damage to the body resulting from acute exposure to thermal, mechanical, electrical, or chemical energy or from the absence of such essentials as heat or oxygen.[3] (2) A *communicable disease* (*Syn* infectious disease) is an illness due to a specific microbial agent or its toxic products arising through transmission of that agent or its products from an infected person, animal, or other reservoir to a susceptible host, either directly or indirectly through an intermediate plant or animal host, vector, or the inanimate environment.[4] (3) A *noncommunicable disease* (NCD), simply defined, is a condition that is noninfectious. Most NCDs are highly multifactorial, of long duration, and generally slow progression. (4) *Mental and behavioral disorders* are conditions that manifest by abnormalities of thought, feeling, and/or behavior that result in distress or impairment.[5]

Globally, an earlier predominance of communicable diseases has steadily given way to NCDs, now dominant in all regions except for sub-Saharan Africa (SSA), and even here they are increasing in their share of the disease burden. Disease occurrence everywhere is associated with the correlates of poverty, such as nutritional status, housing, illiteracy, and poor living conditions. And it works both ways: all forms of disease are potentially socially destabilizing, for example: the impact of HIV in SSA on the widespread phenomenon of child-led families; the impact of famine in the Horn of Africa on mass migration; the impact of 9/11 terrorist attacks not only in terms of casualties but also on the global security environment and psychosocial health of millions around the world.

At community level, numerous conditions are found simultaneously such that we can no longer justify the traditional practice of approaching disease categories as if they exist in separate silos, with exclusive underlying determinants and no overlap or interaction. There is a need to integrate patient care and disease prevention and control strategies with community health promotion initiatives. For example, the World Health Organization's Department of Mental Health and Substance Abuse prevention strategy emphasizes the importance of nutrition, housing, access to education, economic security, and strengthening community networks.[6] As these conditions also heavily influence the occurrence of many other diseases, it is clear that a broadly based strategic approach to improving human conditions is required, and indeed this thinking lies behind the Millennium Development Goals (MDGs, chapter 5). An analogous principle applies to individuals: for example, the elderly often develop complex multiple disorders such that the tradition of focusing on one disease at a time is outmoded. While the same is true for other groups (e.g., adolescents) whose needs also should not be approached piecemeal, as countries age demographically it has become increasingly clear that the health system must offer more coordinated responses, and deliver integrated care for a wider spectrum of conditions.

An increasing disease burden is also arising from interactions across disease categories. Of course, that infection may lead to chronic conditions is not a new idea. Half a century ago it was discovered that paralytic poliomyelitis (a motor neuron disease once the primary domain of neurologists) was due to an enterovirus infection and that rheumatic heart disease was due to disordered immune response to Group A streptococcus throat infection; these discoveries subsequently led to interventions by vaccination and antibiotic prophylaxis, respectively. Similarly, we now know that several cancers (e.g., Burkitt's lymphomas, hepatocellular carcinoma, cervical cancer,

Kaposi's sarcoma, and some oral cancers) arise from infections. Taking the reverse sequence, people with chronic obstructive pulmonary disease (COPD), which is strongly associated with smoking, are at risk of death from bacterial pneumonia, especially if infected with influenza. A key measure in managing COPD therefore is to ensure annual influenza immunization, and antibiotics may be needed to treat secondary bacterial infections. Similarly, diabetes predisposes to infections that can exacerbate hyperglycemia; quality care therefore is not only a matter of metabolic control and reducing risk factors for severity (e.g., hypertension, smoking), but also attending to ongoing risks of infection.

These realities are evident also in developing countries: as progress is made in combating immunodeficiency disorders, chronicity, and complications associated with longevity arise. For example, increasing numbers of people with HIV infection are becoming at risk of chronic conditions resulting (indirectly) from life-long antiretroviral treatment (e.g., diabetes, heart disease, and stroke).[7] Similarly, the malnutrition that accompanies widespread infectious diarrhea due to unclean water contributes in pregnant women to intrauterine growth retardation, culminating, decades later in higher risk of chronic diseases in the offspring.[8] A case can be made that intervening on contaminated water to prevent gastroenteritis in children is therefore also an important strategy in reducing the future burdens from chronic NCDs.

The case for integrated programs notwithstanding, some highly specific disease control initiatives remain justifiable. Beyond the eradication of smallpox (chapter 2), other initiatives realistically aim for this level of success: Guinea worm, poliomyelitis, iodine deficiency disorders, and others. However, public health has learned that success in "vertical initiatives" should not come at the expense of developing capacity in primary health care: as an integrating strategy to ensure access to health for all people, and which (if properly developed) can enhance the prospect of success in disease prevention and control initiatives. This is why global initiatives such as GAVI (Global Alliance for Vaccines and Immunization) now support health systems strengthening (HSS), and why HSS is valued by the Global Fund for AIDS, tuberculosis, and malaria. In other words, highly specific initiatives need not be at the expense of broader program development.

Creating Useful Public Health Interventions

The first challenge here is *problem definition*. Once a health situation is defined as a public health problem, we can investigate its underlying causes and move toward intervention strategies. In the disease control context, the process is influenced by how disease is conceptualized. For example, in addition to medically defined conditions such as infection, cancer, and heart disease; issues such as violence, drug addiction, adolescent pregnancy, and problem gambling are also legitimate targets for public health action.

It is important to recognize that the International Classification of Diseases (ICD), introduced in chapter 1, was originally designed with clinical, pathological, and administrative applications in mind. This legacy significantly influences how a disease entity may be viewed for other purposes such as health promotion, self-management, rehabilitation, and even prevention. Although public health science evolved from the ICD foundation, strict adherence to it in the past sometimes impeded the flexibility needed to address prevention and control in a more innovative manner, such as through addressing its underlying risk factors and determinants or by creating new cross-cutting organizational entities more able to respond with an integrated approach to several diseases that share similar causes, settings, or interrelated outcomes.

To take lung cancer for example, the diagnosis is highly accurate but too late to be of value to most persons who develop it. However, because over 90% of lung cancer is due to tobacco smoking, and because this exposure increases the risk of virtually all other forms of cancer as well as circulatory and pulmonary diseases, for preventive purposes, an etiological classification (even an informal one) is more useful. Since smoking is a powerful influence on this array of outcomes, the elements for prevention purposes of greatest importance are behavioral and environmental, not clinical nor pathological. Therefore, instead of thinking and acting in terms of "lung disease" (anatomical location) or "cancer" (a pathological process), it is more useful from a prevention perspective to consider the broader etiological label: "diseases of smokers." Addressing this broader issue through a comprehensive tobacco control strategy is much more cost-effective than medical treatment of specific disease outcomes after the fact.

The art and science of classification continue to evolve: a supplementary classification of Impairments, Disabilities and Handicaps to the 9th Revision of ICD led to widespread adoption of the now free-standing *International Classification of Functioning, Disability and Health* (ICF).[9] Briefly stated, *impairment* refers to a physical or mental defect of function or structure in a body system or organ that usually leads to a disability and sometimes to a handicap. *Disability* refers to reduced capacity of a person to perform usual functions, usually the result of impairment, such as limited mobility or intellectual capability. *Handicap* refers to reduced capacity to perform designated tasks or fulfill expected occupational or social roles and functions because of impairment, disability, inadequate training for the task or role, or other circumstances. This development, a classification focused primarily on functions and roles, enables us to address more effectively the entities of impairment, disability and handicap in their own right. These may now be taken as either outcomes or as starting points for intervention at individual or population level, legitimate targets for public health interventions (e.g., their inclusion in the Healthy People 2020 strategy of the USA).[10] Their recognition as entities worthy of assessment may also lead to incorporating them into studies of other diseases and conditions and as modifiers in efforts to reduce related disease burdens.

To take another development, with the emergence of effective vaccines for a range of infectious conditions (e.g., measles, pneumonia, hepatitis B, rotavirus), it has become more operationally useful to refer to these collectively as "vaccine preventable diseases." In other words, it is the intervention technology, not the diagnostic label or pathologic process that is the more useful defining characteristic, at least with regard to primary prevention. Further, as it is now accepted that hepatitis B may lead to hepatocellular carcinoma and that human papilloma viruses are the underlying cause of most cervical cancers (and increasingly oral cancers), *ergo* some cancers may now be included within vaccine preventable diseases for which prevention starts within a childhood immunization program. Thus, with advances in science, technology, and the reorganization of service delivery, aspects of cancer and infectious disease are converging within a new field called "vaccinology": compartmentalizing infectious disease and cancer is thereby obsolescent, although not yet actually obsolete.

So what does this mean for creating useful intervention categories? Philosopher Marshall McLuhan (1911–1980), originator of the idea that "the medium is the message," was concerned that we tend to focus so much on the obvious that "we largely miss the structural changes in our affairs that are introduced subtly or over long periods of time. Whenever we create a new innovation many of its properties are fairly obvious to us. We generally know what it will nominally do, or at least what it is intended to do, and what it might replace. We often know its advantages and disadvantages. But it is also often the case that, after a long period of time and experience with the new innovation, we look backward and realize that there were some effects of which we were entirely unaware at the outset." [11] Applying this to public health, we must remain open to new ways of seeing and doing things, especially in how we approach health situation analysis (chapter 5) and public health interventions, including integrated disease prevention and control.

Epidemiological Transition Theory: Double Burdens and Unfinished Agendas

Epidemiological transition theory (chapter 5) refers to the demographic transitions attributable to declining mortality (particularly early in life) and fertility rates, which are the main contributors to the demographic aging of societies and consequent shifts in variables that produce disease patterns.[12] This process was experienced slowly by Western industrialized societies over three centuries, accompanying improved literacy, hygiene, nutrition, and sanitation; medical interventions played a late role. The "classical" model of Western Europe and North America revealed declining infant mortality, increased life expectancy (LE), and aging populations, with a gradual shift in predominance from infectious diseases (IDs) to NCDs and injuries. Less developed countries are undergoing faster transitions, the timing and pace of fertility decline varying with socioeconomic, medical, technological, and political settings.[13]

Numerous transition variants have been proposed to characterize observed changes in different world regions, but to review each is beyond our scope. However, one of these, an *intermediate transitional variant* (Figure 6-1),[14] is relatively widespread throughout the developing world, where many countries are coping with a double burden of disease: this refers to a growing NCD burden, superimposed on an "unfinished agenda" of IDs.

This dynamic pattern is attributed mainly to improvements in water and sanitation, food safety, adequate housing, together with disease control measures (e.g., immunization, insecticides, antibiotics) and organized health care, as well as to rural-urban population drift. The population drift is associated with dramatic changes in nutrition (the "nutrition transition" introduced in chapter 5) and other lifestyle variables, especially

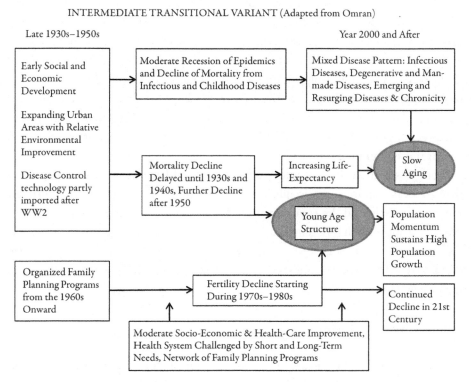

FIGURE 6-1 Epidemiological transition conceptual framework.

physical activity, transforming health and disease patterns. The increasing prevalence of overweight or obesity, due to a shift from traditional diets to diets high in sugars, fats, processed foods, and meats, along with sedentary living, is driving increasing rates of cardiovascular and metabolic disorders (e.g., diabetes), especially in lower income groups. This trend is compounded by globalized mercantile forces, such as aggressive marketing by tobacco companies in countries lacking adequate health protection policies, offsetting global gains in tobacco control, with a consequent surge of associated preventable diseases in middle and low income countries. By 2020, NCDs will account for 70% of deaths in developing regions, and injuries will rival IDs in priority.

Notwithstanding that NCDs are now the leading cause of mortality globally, "new infectious diseases" continue to be recognized while others, once thought controlled, are reemerging as global challenges. Within the past four decades, the following have been recognized (among others): HIV/AIDS, Legionnaire's disease, Ebola virus, toxic shock syndrome, Lyme disease, hepatitis C, hantavirus, bovine spongiform encephalopathy (BSE), avian influenza, and severe acute respiratory syndrome (SARS). Meanwhile, diseases such as dengue fever and West Nile Virus are expanding geographically, even as "old infectious diseases" are far from solved: respiratory infections and gastroenteritis still dominate child deaths globally, while tuberculosis and malaria remain important causes of morbidity and mortality in SSA and parts of Asia. The same underlying forces that are influencing the growth of NCDs also drive these changes, although the pathways to disease may differ: demographic shifts leading to urbanization with poverty, overcrowding, and other behavior-associated changes (e.g., injection drug use, unsafe sexual practices), and the inaccessibility of health services, especially primary health care, for large numbers of people. To these we can add other factors conducive to a resurgence of some IDs: changes in climate (chapter 8), globalized travel and trade, and increasing numbers of persons with compromised immune systems.

From this complexity has emerged the One Health Concept: a strategic vision that advocates more interdisciplinary collaboration on all aspects of health for humans, animals, and the environment.[15] The synergy that could emerge from this ecological approach has potential to advance health in the 21st century by accelerating health science research, expanding the knowledge base, enhancing public health efficacy, as well as medical education and clinical care, thereby to benefit present and future generations.[16]

Natural History of Disease

The "natural history of disease" is a core concept of disease prevention and control, and is an invaluable practical framework for public health problem analysis and identifying intervention opportunities. We now explore this concept and its applications.

The meaning of "disease" varies with perceptions and social context. Those directly affected experience it as "illness." Informal care givers (families, friends, others), become aware at an early stage. Self-care and mutual support may be sufficient to get through the process and may also be critical, depending on the extent to which the formal health system offers access. Clinical practitioners become aware when someone presents with symptoms and/or signs: those in primary care see more of the early process, whereas specialists encounter later stages of more severe disease, when symptoms, signs and test results are more advanced. How a disease is labeled across cultures also varies, emphasis being given to what it means to the observers in their settings and based on their roles. For example, a patient may experience adjustments required for daily living, the impact of the disease on responsibilities, family, or employment; a diagnostician may recognize opportunities for treatment or referral; other observers apply values such as social support or even stigmatization (a negative value), while public health professionals may emphasize the implications for prevention, control, or public policy.

The term *natural history of disease* refers to the way in which disease evolves and progresses. Most diseases pass through several stages: susceptibility, pathological onset, presymptomatic, clinical, then resolution. The process may be modifiable by intervention, such as prevention, treatment, and rehabilitation, as well as by self-care and social adjustments. Depending on disease type and severity, the process may involve a range of outcomes from full recovery to death, with intermediate outcomes such as impairment, disability, or handicap. With variations, the model in Figure 6-2 applies to all diseases.

This model illustrates how, with passage of time (shown in Figure 6-2 by the thick line moving from left to right), a healthy person may enter a subclinical process that in turn may cross a threshold to become recognized as clinical disease, and how it may emerge from this stage at any level from death to partial or complete recovery. While a full discussion of pathophysiological mechanisms exceeds the scope of this chapter, this dynamic sequence holds for virtually all types of conditions: for infectious diseases, the transition from subclinical to clinical disease reflects the incubation period (time interval between invasion by an infectious agent and onset of symptoms or signs of the disease), while for cancer (for example) it is the latent period or time interval between exposure and manifestations (a complex multistep process whereby initial cell changes may become irreversible and there is progression to detectable neoplasia). For the individual who crosses the clinical threshold to become "sick," treatment becomes the priority. However, of central importance to

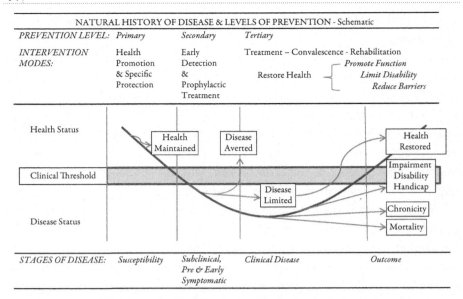

FIGURE 6-2 Natural history of disease and levels of prevention—schematic.

public health interventions are the depictions of "level of prevention" and "modes of intervention" shown in the upper parts of the diagram, and as discussed next.

Levels of Prevention

Prevention refers to actions aimed at eradicating, eliminating, or minimizing the impact of disease and disability, or if none of these is feasible, slowing its progress and reducing associated disability as well as social impacts.[17] This concept is usefully subclassified into levels: primary, secondary, and tertiary prevention. A fourth level, called primordial prevention, was later added. In epidemiological terms, primordial prevention aspires to establish and maintain conditions that minimize hazards to health, primary prevention aims to reduce disease incidence, secondary prevention aims to reduce disease prevalence by shortening its duration, and tertiary prevention aims to reduce the number and/or impact of complications.

While public health practitioners are often strong advocates of health promotion and primary prevention, they also understand that even with complete application of these measures, numerous people will still enter the disease process and progress through it in stages that offer subsequent opportunities for preventive actions. To address prevention only at the level of health promotion and primary prevention is therefore inadequate (necessary but not sufficient) as a policy framework for public health. For a fully formed response to human needs, it is important to incorporate within such a framework the full spectrum of disease prevention and control. A sound grasp of these concepts is essential to all professionals in public health; it also forms a basis for appreciating the efforts of others across the prevention spectrum. We now explore these levels of prevention, starting with primary prevention as the most immediate form and leaving primordial prevention to last due to its alignment with some (not all) health promotion measures. Because some knowledge of epidemiological measures of disease frequency is necessary, we supply selected definitions in Box 6-1.

PRIMARY PREVENTION

Primary prevention is directed toward reducing disease incidence by intervening on known modifiable risk factors or other preventive measures that influence the likelihood of a disease outcome. Reducing incidence by primary prevention usually leads to commensurate reductions in rates of related complications and mortality. Those reductions, when achieved mostly by primary prevention, may be termed an "incidence effect," keeping in mind that there will be a time lag between reductions in the incidence of particular diseases and changes in the rates for subsequent outcomes. Variations in incidence and incidence effects are usually detected by disease surveillance (chapter 5). An excellent example of incidence effects is mass vaccination against rubella: this leads not only to a major reduction in the incidence of this viral disease, but also to a secondary reduction in congenital rubella syndrome (the core rationale for rubella vaccination).

BOX 6-1

MEASURES OF FREQUENCY COMMONLY USED IN DISEASE
PREVENTION & CONTROL

Incidence Rate: The rate at which new events occur in a population. The numerator is the number of new events that occur in a defined period; the denominator is the population at risk of experiencing the event during this period.

Attack Rate: The cumulative incidence rate observed over a period during an epidemic.

Secondary Attack Rate: The number of cases of an infection that occur among contacts within the incubation period following exposure to a primary case in relation to the total number of contacts; a measure of infectivity.

Prevalence Rate: The number of individuals with a disease at a particular time (or during a particular period) divided by the population at risk. The prevalence is a function of both disease incidence and duration.

Case Fatality Rate (CFR): The proportion of cases of a specified condition which are fatal within a specified time; it is a measure of disease severity.

Primary prevention initiatives in public health vary with the priority needs of particular populations. These include protection of health by personal and communal efforts (e.g., smoking cessation); contraceptive counseling; enhancing nutrition generally and by specific nutrition supplementation in pregnancy and fortification of staples with key elements, minerals, or vitamins without which deficiency conditions may arise (see Iodine deficiency Case Study); eliminating environmental risks such as contaminants in air, food, and drinking water; and immunization against childhood infectious diseases.

Few interventions are more cost-effective than childhood immunization against common infectious diseases. All nations accept this as a public health priority, and these programs are usually publicly financed. National schedules are revised periodically depending on need and circumstances of the particular country. For illustration, Figure 6-3 shows the recommended immunization schedule for 2011 for persons aged 0 through 6 years in the United States. Alternative schedules are promoted for other age and risk categories.

Responsibility for primary prevention is shared among primary care practitioners and frontline public health staff working with individuals at risk or through agencies working with communities at risk. This effort is supported by *regulatory agencies* at national and global levels that set standards for air, water, and food quality (see chapter 7) and offer specialized functions relating to radiation protection, other hazardous products and wastes, and the regulation of vaccines, drugs, and devices. Primary prevention also applies to hazards in the workplace, their removal, reduction, or amelioration such as by *industrial hygiene* (e.g., air exchange, temperature control, ventilation, protective clothing and equipment, and best practices), thereby performing a central role within the discipline of occupational health. It also applies in the home, in terms of safe handling of food, building standards, child safety measures, and so on. At times of threat from epidemic disease, community exposure to toxic chemicals, or other emergencies, primary prevention also requires timely decisions that lead to prompt practical measures.

A CASE STUDY OF PRIMARY PREVENTION—IODINE DEFICIENCY DISORDERS

Iodine deficiency is historically associated with goiter (thyroid enlargement associated with metabolic dysfunction, iodine being a constituent of thyroid hormones) and cretinism (a form of nutritional dwarfism with arrested mental development). How the link between goiter and iodine deficiency became recognized was reviewed in chapter 1. But it was not until the 1960s that epidemiological studies of the fetus during pregnancy revealed various levels of iodine deficiency as a major cause of commensurately varying degrees of impaired brain development, and that correcting this deficiency before pregnancy would prevent this damage. Other studies revealed 130

Vaccine ▼ Age ▶	Birth	1 month	2 months	4 months	6 months	12 months	15 months	18 months	19–23 months	2–3 years	4–6 years
Hepatitis B[1]	HepB	HepB			HepB						
Rotavirus[2]			RV	RV	RV[2]						
Diphtheria, Tetanus, Pertussis[3]			DTaP	DTaP	DTaP	see footnote[3]	DTaP	DTaP			DTaP
Haemophilus influenzae type b[4]			Hib	Hib	Hib[4]	Hib	Hib				
Pneumococcal[5]			PCV	PCV	PCV	PCV	PCV			PPSV	
Inactivated Poliovirus[6]			IPV	IPV	IPV	IPV	IPV				IPV
Influenza[7]					Influenza (Yearly)						
Measles, Mumps, Rubella[8]						MMR	MMR		see footnote[8]		MMR
Varicella[9]						Varicella	Varicella		see footnote[9]		Varicella
Hepatitis A[10]						HepA (2 doses)	HepA (2 doses)	HepA (2 doses)		HepA Series	
Meningococcal[11]										MCV4	

Range of recommended ages for all children

Range of recommended ages for certain high-risk groups

FIGURE 6-3 Recommended immunization schedule for persons aged 0 through 6 years—United States, 2011[99].

Note: Abbreviations given in each cell correspond with the vaccines listed in the first column.

Source: Centers for Disease Control and Prevention. Recommended immunization schedules for persons aged 0–18 years—United States, 2011. MMWR 2011;60,5. As cited in reference #18.

countries to be affected by iodine deficiency, representing over 2 billion at some risk of brain damage. Associated social and economic impacts included reduced school performance in children and lower productivity in adults, and the World Bank determined that correcting iodine deficiency would result in net economic benefits. The problem became understood as one of human ecology: that is, people living in environments where soil has been leached of iodine due to flooding of river valleys or in hilly and mountainous areas by high rainfall or glaciation. Deficiency in soil leads to deficiency in all forms of plant life, including all cereals grown in the soil. Hence large populations living in subsistence agriculture, as in the great river valleys of Asia, were locked into iodine deficiency disorders (IDD). The IDD "iceberg" (Figure 6-4) illustrates the effects gradient (See Box-6-2 for a general review of the "Iceberg Phenomenon").[18] The correction of iodine deficiency produces a dramatic reversal of the condition of cerebral hypothyroidism (shown in Figure 6-4 as loss of energy due to hypothyroidism) due to restoration of brain thyroid hormone levels. This is a different effect from brain damage during pregnancy, which is not reversible but completely preventable. Iodine deficiency thus became recognized by WHO as the world's most common cause of preventable brain damage, and provided the basis for a program of *global elimination of brain damage caused by iodine deficiency* by the use of iodized salt and cooking oil.[19]

Major progress has been made since the 1990 World Summit for Children meeting at the United Nations, New York, when the goal of iodine deficiency elimination was first adopted. By 2000 substantial progress had been achieved with almost 70% of at risk households having access to iodized salt. This ensured protection of close to 80 million newborns with an estimated saving of over one billion IQ points.[17] However, 41 million were still unprotected, and more work to be done in many nations: the challenge remains a first for mankind—elimination of a major noncommunicable disease.

WHAT INGREDIENTS ENABLED THIS GLOBAL ELIMINATION INITIATIVE?

1. The problem was of *sufficient public health importance* to justify a major resource allocation. The "at risk" population was estimated to be 2.2 billion from 130 countries.

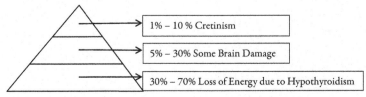

FIGURE 6-4 Nature and magnitude of IDD—the IDD Iceberg[100].

BOX 6-2
ICEBERG PHENOMENON

A common situation where only a relatively small proportion of cases of a given disease, "the tip of the iceberg", comes to the attention of the health care system. The "submerged part" goes undiagnosed and unreported

The proportion of missed cases varies with the disease and its severity, especially during early phases of the natural history when prevention is likely to be most efficacious.

For examples, for Type 2 ("adult onset") diabetes, the submerged portion is about 50% in many western countries; for psychiatric disorders, it may be as high as 75% to 80%; and for hypertension, it may be as high as 90%. Corresponding estimates are generally higher for developing countries.

For some conditions such as HIV/AIDS, and cancer of the cervix, the size of the submerged portion has decreased with improved screening methods (screening is discussed under Secondary Prevention in this chapter).

2. There were effective *preventive measures* suitable for mass application in the form of iodized salt and iodized oil, applicable to both developed and developing countries.
3. There was an *available system for delivery* of iodized salt through the salt industry and for iodized oil through primary health care systems, at minimal cost.
4. There were *practical methods for program monitoring* to ensure that it was effective and sustainable in all settings: checks on salt iodine at factory, retail or household level, and measurements of urine iodine excretion to validate dietary intake.
5. To this core list, we add the critical importance of *effective and sustained leadership* at all levels, not least of which is the continuing role of the International Council for Control of Iodine Deficiency Disorders (ICCIDD), in support of WHO and UNICEF.

In conclusion, Global Elimination of Brain Damage Due to Iodine Deficiency is an inspirational primary prevention initiative, and an authentic global program for human development. It is a model for how the global community can improve public health by working together on evidence based policy and programmatic initiatives.

SECONDARY PREVENTION

This refers to measures available to individuals and communities for early detection and prompt intervention to control disease and minimize disability (e.g., screening programs). Screening is defined as presumptive identification of unrecognized disease or defect by the application of tests, examinations or other procedures that can be applied rapidly. A screening test is not intended to be diagnostic:[17] it sorts out apparently well persons who probably have a disease from those who probably do not. A decision to offer a screening program must be justified in accordance with established decision-making rules that take into account: disease severity and prevalence in a given setting; that the proposed screening test has good performance characteristics (e.g., acceptable error rates and predictive values); feasibility and acceptability of test procedures including cost and resource implications; attributes such as age, sex, family history, and whether risk factors are present; and evidence of intervention effectiveness.[20]

Although much screening activity takes place in physician's offices, similar secondary prevention applications take place in public health settings. For example, in well baby and child health clinics, in addition to routine immunization (primary prevention), children may undergo anthropometry: parents of children not meeting height and weight projections for dates (using standard charts) may then be either counseled (e.g., regarding nutrition and measures to prevent infection) or referred for medical assessment. Clinics focusing on adult health (or "wellness") may screen adults for blood pressure: if found to be consistently elevated, nonpharmacological advice may be offered on how to reduce risk (e.g., physical activity, dietary modification, weight loss, or if such measures are unsuccessful pharmacological intervention may be advised). It is a public health responsibility to promote other effective secondary prevention measures (e.g., cervical cancer screening), usually available from family planning clinics and family physicians.

It is an ethical requirement of screening initiatives that presumptive identification of disease will lead to improved prognosis. This principle is not always respected by advocates of particular screening practices for which the evidence base may be flawed, incomplete, or controversial. In assessing screening initiatives, the "appearance" of improved prognosis can arise as a result of bias (systematic error), the most common forms being: selection bias, lead-time bias, and length bias, each now briefly defined. *Selection bias:* error due to systematic differences in characteristics between those who take part in screening and those who do not; if those differences are associated with a better outcome, the apparent "improvement" may be erroneously attributed to the screening program. *Lead-time bias:* overestimation of survival time, due to the backward shift in the starting point in measuring survival; that is, early diagnosis does not necessarily result in improved prognosis. *Length bias:* selection of disproportionate numbers of long-duration cases in one group (more likely to show up at any point in time, especially if screened) but not in another (unscreened people include persons with all durations).

Screening is a technically complex area of public health decision making, for which adequate validation can be scientifically demanding. Additional reading in epidemiology texts and relevant scientific papers is advisable, especially on topics that are controversial (e.g., breast self-examination[21] and PSA testing for prostate cancer).[22]

There are many good examples of well-validated screening programs, such as for high blood pressure and cervical cancer, already mentioned. A core principle is always that the early identification must lead to improved prognosis: for example, the efficacy of mammography for breast cancer depends on effective treatments once the disease has been identified by the screening process. Another with global impact is illustrated in HIV-endemic areas, where screening for HIV is offered to pregnant women within VCT (voluntary counseling and testing) protocols: if infection is detected and then confirmed by supplementary testing, anti-retroviral (ARV) therapy is offered to the mother. Because mother to child transmission can occur during pregnancy, childbirth, or through breast feeding, additional protocols subsequently apply for the baby from birth;[23] this improves prognosis for both mother and child. In epidemiological terms, a "treatment effect" is expected from secondary prevention: both prevalence and severity (e.g., complications or death) may decline due to this intervention. In some situations there may also be an "incidence effect" (e.g., reduced HIV transmission to babies born to HIV infected mothers as a result of their ARV treatment and reduced risk to their sexual partners). Such effects may be detected at community level by surveillance (chapter 5). In fact, use of ARV drugs in preventing mother-to-child transmission has resulted in virtual elimination of neonatal HIV-1 infection in resource-rich settings.[24] This achievement underlies the "treatment as prevention" movement, which is now highly relevant in all countries.

Treatment effects of public health significance long predate prevention technologies per se. For example, before pneumococcal vaccines were introduced (primary prevention), pneumonia mortality declined due to the impact of antibiotics. Similarly, major declines in tuberculosis mortality were observed in developed countries following introduction of specific antibiotic therapy, well before introduction of TB screening programs (designed to bring people with previously undiagnosed infections into treatment). In some instances, both "incidence and treatment effects" are observed or can be anticipated due to the combined efficacy of both primary and secondary prevention, such as now applies for cervical cancer: primary prevention by vaccination will result in reduced incidence, secondary prevention due to screening interrupts progression of the disease.

Screening activities vary by jurisdictions depending on need and availability of technical and financial resources. Some are routinely offered to entire cohorts of people (e.g., antenatal, early childhood and school entry testing), while others may be offered to persons with particular risks (e.g., for genetic conditions, discussed later in this chapter).

TERTIARY PREVENTION

This consists of measures aimed at mitigating the impact of long-term disease and disability by eliminating or reducing impairment, disability, and handicap; minimizing suffering; and maximizing potential years or useful life. To some clinicians, even some epidemiologists, tertiary prevention "seems a lot like treatment." However, it differs from what many clinicians see as their role, in that it envisions the preventive act not only in terms of achieving a better clinical outcome, but also in terms of the health objectives expressed in the *International Classification of Functioning, Disability and Health* (ICF, as described earlier): restoring function and roles in society. While achieving this larger outcome does require a tertiary prevention vision on the part of clinicians, it requires more than clinical interventions, even beyond related rehabilitation measures (e.g., speech therapy for stroke patients). It also encompasses broader societal measures (e.g., public education to reduce stigma surrounding conditions like HIV, harm reduction measures for addictions, and wheelchair-friendly building designs). Such measures are not "treatment," but they do require public health involvement, including leadership.

PRIMORDIAL PREVENTION

This refers to measures that inhibit the emergence and establishment of environmental, economic, social, and behavioral conditions and cultural patterns known to increase the risk of disease.[25] Primordial prevention therefore is focused on underlying determinants that are amenable to long-range policy shifts and other broad strategic approaches, most of which also fall within the domain of health promotion. Like primary prevention, this prevention mode acts mostly to reduce incidence, but does so through more complex chains of causation such that its impact is generally less immediate and more diffuse. The core rationale of primordial prevention is its link to health disparities (chapters 4 and 5). Using an ecological approach, remedial action involves searching for underlying inequities that give rise to them (including deficits in human rights, literacy, gender equality, opportunity, and so on) and related needs for democratic reform or other social interventions. Of course, not all disparities are rooted in inequities; some are due to aspects of culture, environment, and circumstances, often with historical and geographical origins that need to be understood before being attributed to inequity per se.

Applying Prevention to Public Health Problems: The Haddon Matrix

This is a framework for analyzing injury developed by William Haddon (1926–1985), an early developer of injury epidemiology. Trained both as a physician and an engineer, he was founding head of a Commission that evolved into the US National Highway Traffic Safety Administration. The framework derives from the "epidemiological triad" of host-agent-environment (Figure 6-5); readers will encounter generic discussion of this simple model in virtually all introductory epidemiology textbooks. Originally developed and still applied in the context of infectious diseases, it has other practical applications, including, in addition to injuries: toxic exposure, violence and emergency preparedness.[26]

In the context of injuries, the host is considered the person at risk, the agent a source of energy that causes the injury (e.g., mechanical, thermal, electrical) transmitted through a vehicle (inanimate object) or vector (person or other animal), while the environment refers to the physical and social contexts in which the injury occurred. Enlarging on the last mentioned, physical environment includes characteristics of the setting in which the event takes place (e.g., road, building, playground, sports arena), while social environment refers to the social and legal norms and practices in the culture or society where the event takes place (e.g., alcohol or drug consumption, gun access and control, use of restraints, licensing policies, use of mobile phones while driving).

Consistent with the Natural History Model, these components are examined over three critical periods: (1) leading to the event; (2) the event itself; and (3) directly following the event. From a prevention standpoint, these consecutive phases of an injury process offer opportunities for primary, secondary and tertiary prevention respectively. The pre-injury event phase (primary prevention) is directed toward averting injuries by acting on causes (e.g. protective fences, divided highways, sound building design). The event phase (secondary prevention) offers opportunities to prevent injury or reduce its severity by designing and implementing protective mechanisms (e.g. seatbelts, helmets, faceguards, bulletproof vests). The postinjury

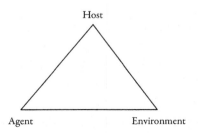

FIGURE 6-5 The epidemiological triad.

phase (tertiary prevention) offers opportunities to reduce injury severity or potential disability by providing adequate care immediately after an event (e.g., application of prompt First Aid or cardio-pulmonary resuscitation [CPR]), and working during convalescence to stabilize, repair, and restore the highest possible level of physical and mental function for the injured person. Using the matrix to analyze injury represents a three-tiered approach to prevention that includes opportunities for behavioral, environmental and policy interventions. The Matrix in Table 6-1 illustrates the context of motor vehicle injuries.

Because all public health interventions have sociopolitical and resource implications choosing intervention options cannot be made simply by extrapolating from such a matrix. Other decision-related criteria include effectiveness, cost, issues of personal freedom, equity, stigmatization, preferences, and feasibility. Taking this into account a three-dimensional version of Haddon's matrix has also been developed.[27] As discussed in chapter 4, to be fully effective requires a participatory approach.

Communicable Diseases

There are an enormous number of communicable diseases, reflecting an even larger number of "causal agents." Although all are "multifactorial," for an infectious disease (ID) to occur a microbial agent is a "necessary cause" without which infection will not take place. Nonetheless, presence of a necessary cause is not always a "sufficient cause," as several other components must come into play, such as: host susceptibility, exposure, cultural and environmental influences. However, it is not usually necessary to identify all components of a sufficient cause to achieve effective prevention or control, because removing even one may impede the causation process. The classic example is how John Snow (chapter 1) curtailed a cholera epidemic in the Soho district of London by breaking off the handle of a street pump that was a common source of contaminated water; this was in 1854—decades before the cholera bacillus was identified as the "necessary cause."

Communicable diseases may be classified by causal agent, clinical presentation or mode of transmission. Two or more characteristics are often used in their description (e.g., cutaneous leishmaniasis; pulmonary anthrax; sandfly fever). Sometimes an occupational descriptor is used, due to historical association with a type of work (e.g., "milkmaid's disease" for listeriosis, "wool-sorters disease" for cutaneous anthrax, and so on). The microbial agents themselves exist within categories: bacteria, viruses, parasites (protozoa, metazoa), fungi, and prions (microscopic protein particles similar to a virus but lacking nucleic acid). As noted earlier, some IDs may lead to chronic conditions (e.g., rheumatic heart disease, Burkitt's lymphoma): these outcomes are

TABLE 6-1

Haddon's matrix applied to motor vehicle injuries (Illustrative—not comprehensive)

Phase	Host	Vehicle or Vector	Physical Environment	Social Environment
Pre-event	Driver eligibility rules; training & driving tests; license categories; vision testing; speeding; alcohol use; cellphones; other risk taking.	Tire & brake maintenance; vehicle inspection; regulation of restraints (airbags, seatbelts, child restraints, roll-bars); obligatory use of headlights; roadside checks.	Safe highway designs (e.g., visibility at intersections, adequate shoulders; road signage; speed limits; traffic advisories; road maintenance).	Cultural norms and personal attitudes regarding speeding, red light running, drunk driving, use of restraints; education & enforcement (e.g, breathalyzer tests).
Event	Human tolerances to crash forces; seatbelt & helmet use & correctly fitting child restraints.	Crash worthiness of vehicle, belts, helmets, & child restraints. NOTE: some jurisdictions approve devices based on national test standards.	Presence of fixed objects near roadways; poorly designed guardrails; unsecured objects within vehicles.	Legislation requiring seatbelt installation and use, child restraints, helmets; enforcement; penalties for noncompliance.
Postevent	Crash victims general health status (age, susceptibility, alcohol, drug use & smoking etc).	Emergency communications; flashing lights; fire-safe fuel tank design; First Aid kit in vehicle; food & water; blankets.	Available, timely, effective emergency care: First Aid training, CPR; prompt transportation to referral services.	Political recognition & public support for timely, effective trauma care & rehabilitation; trained staff available.

classified as noncommunicable even though primary prevention depends on preventing infection.

The next section examines the key principles of communicable disease control, using selected examples. For a full range of IDs of public health importance we recommend the Control of Communicable Diseases Manual,[4] a regularly updated pocketbook that sets out for each disease details on clinical description, geographic distribution, reservoir, transmission modes, incubation periods, communicability, susceptibility, and resistance.

COMMUNICABLE DISEASE CONTROL

This term means the reduction of incidence, prevalence, morbidity, or mortality of a specified disease to a level deemed locally acceptable as a result of deliberate efforts; critically, *control* implies the need for continued intervention to maintain this reduction. It stands in contrast to *elimination* (reduction to zero of the incidence of a specified disease in a defined geographic area as a result of deliberate efforts, continued intervention measures still being required), *eradication* (permanent reduction to zero of the worldwide incidence of infection caused by a specific agent as a result of deliberate efforts, intervention no longer needed), and *extinction* (the specific infectious agent no longer exists in nature or the laboratory).[28]

The success of smallpox eradication (chapter 2) is inspirational for the potential of eradicating other diseases, or at least eliminating them as a public health problem. In fact, elimination and eradication have been an ongoing focus of public health research and development activity for over a century, and many candidates have been considered. However, as a cautionary note, unbridled enthusiasm for eradication is not an appropriate stance for public health: such goals must never be declared without attention to the scientific, technical and logistical challenges to be overcome in launching a sustainable effort; to do otherwise and then to fail could call into question the credibility of the public health profession and its institutions as did the collapse of the malaria eradication program four decades ago.[29] However, despite the failure of early eradication initiatives for malaria, yaws and yellow fever, these experiences did help to improve understanding of the social, biological, political, and economic requirements for effective disease control. Current targets for global eradication, as recognized by the World Health Organization (WHO), include dracunculiasis (Guinea worm disease) and poliomyelitis; WHO-sanctioned elimination targets also exist for neonatal tetanus, leprosy, onchocerciasis (West Africa and the Americas), trachoma, and lymphatic filariasis.[30] Each such initiative requires detailed operational planning and resource allocation: the scientific and logistical conditions required for success are presented in chapter 2.

A key to the control of all communicable diseases is *mode of transmission*. This falls within the following broad categories: direct, indirect, and airborne. *Direct transmission* refers to direct contact such as touching, biting, kissing, or sexual intercourse, or direct projection of droplet spray into the eye, nose, or mouth during sneezing, coughing, spitting, singing, or talking, usually within a distance of 1 meter.[4] Examples of direct contact transmission include sexually transmitted infections and rabies, while direct projection transmits influenza, meningococcal meningitis, and measles among others.

Indirect transmission may occur through a vehicle or an arthropod vector. A *vehicle* is an inanimate object or substance; the microbial agent may or may not multiply or develop in or on it. Examples include water, food, biological products, and articles (e.g., toys, door knobs). Sharing contaminated needles by injection drug users spreads blood-borne diseases (e.g., hepatitis B and C). Contaminated water is responsible for millions of child deaths annually from gastroenteritis in developing countries; contaminated food results in outbreaks in all countries. Arthropod *vectors* also spread disease mechanically (due to contamination of their feet or passage of organisms through their gut); however, by far the more important mode of vector transmission is biological. For example, in malaria (see chapter 2, Figure 2-2) the parasite first develops within the mosquito vector, and its transmission to man via mosquito bites accounts for millions of cases and hundreds of thousands of deaths annually. In fact, many insect vectors are important to human health (Table 6-2); aside from malaria, several give rise to major disease burden (e.g., trachoma, leading infectious cause of blindness globally).[31] Vector-borne diseases are also a key focus for veterinary public health, especially for animals of economic importance. Their effective control requires an integrated ecologically minded approach combining technical solutions with community input, decision making, and action.[32]

Some infectious agents spread by air over long distances. *Airborne spread* requires infectious particles to be small enough for airborne suspension, or contained within liquid (mist) and inhaled (e.g., Legionnaire's disease) (chapter 2). Fungal diseases such as histoplasmosis and coccidiomycosis may also be spread in an airborne manner, often in dusty environments, sometimes by novel means (e.g., inhaling dust while chopping a contaminated tree). Airborne transmission of anthrax and smallpox has been considered to have potential for biological warfare and bioterrorism.

Diseases of vertebrate animals that can spread to humans under natural conditions are called *zoonoses* (Table 6-3), which include some of the most common human diseases (e.g., influenza: new strains often emerge first in pigs, then disseminated by aquatic birds). Many new, emerging and reemerging diseases of humans are caused by pathogens that originate from animals or products of animal origin (e.g., Severe Acute Respiratory Syndrome or SARS, due to a coronavirus originating in civet cats;

TABLE 6-2

Vectors important in disease transmission to humans

Selected Examples

Vector Group	Diseases
Mosquitoes (culicidae)	
• Anopheles	Malaria; lymphatic filariasis
• Culex	Lymphatic filariasis; Japanese encephalitis; West Nile Fever; Western equine encephalitis; Other viral diseases
• Aedes	Yellow Fever; dengue fever; lymphatic filariasis; other viral diseases
• Mansonia	Lymphatic filariasis
Other biting Diptera	
• Tsetse flies (Glossina)	African sleeping sickness
• Blackflies (Simulium)	River blindness (onchocerciasis); Mansonellosis (usually asymptomatic)
• Sandflies (Phlebotomus, Lutzomyia)	Leishmaniasis; sandfly fever
• Horseflies (Tabanidae)	Loiasis, tularaemia
• Biting midges (Ceratopogonidae)	Mansonellosis (usually asymptomatic)
Triatomine Bugs	Chagas disease
Ectoparasites	
• Bedbugs	Not considered vectors of disease, a biting nuisance that can cause allergic reactions and dermatitis.
• Fleas	Plague; flea borne typhus (murine typhus); also a biting nuisance that can cause allergic reactions and dermatitis.
• Lice	Typhus fever; relapsing fever' trench fever. Also cause severe irritation and dermatitis (body, head, pubic forms).
• Ticks	Lyme disease; Tick-borne relapsing fever, Rocky Mountain Spotted fever; Q fever; tularemia; Colorado tick fever; Crimean-Congo hemorrhagic fever; other hemorrhagic diseases and encephalitides.
• Mites	Scrub typhus; scabies; also severe irritation and dermatitis

(continued)

TABLE 6-2 (Continued)

Vector Group	Diseases
Scavengers in Human Settlements	
• Cockroaches	Play a role as carriers of enteric diseases (e.g., diarrhea; dysentery; typhoid fever; cholera).
• Houseflies	Associated with spread of enteric, eye (including trachoma,), skin and skin infections.
Cyclops	Intermediate host of Guinea worm disease (dracunculiasis).
Freshwater snails	Intermediate host of trematode larvae, Schistosomiasis (bilharzia); also foodborne fluke infections affecting the liver (e.g., Chinese liver fluke), lungs and intestines.

see chapter 3 for a Case Study of ethical difficulties encountered in controlling a SARS epidemic involving human to human transmission). Given the wide distribution of animal species, effective surveillance, prevention and control of zoonotic diseases pose a significant challenge.[33]

Finally, having examined modes of transmission one by one, it is important to note that some IDs may spread in several ways, depending on circumstances. For example, direct person to person transmission often accounts for some cases in outbreaks of food or waterborne origins (e.g., *Salmonella* gastroenteritis, hepatitis A). HIV may be contracted directly by unprotected sex, through perinatal transmission (mother to child), and indirectly by sharing contaminated needles. Brucellosis may be contracted directly by exposure to infected animal tissues, indirectly through vehicles such as unpasteurized dairy products, and via airborne exposure to aerosolized blood in abattoirs.[34] Rabies is usually contracted from the bite of an infected animal, but may also be contracted by inhaling bat saliva aerosols in caves. Knowledge of this type is not theoretical; it is obtained from epidemiological field investigations[35] (for two examples see legionellosis and foodborne disease Case Studies, chapters 2 and 7, respectively).

EPIDEMIC THEORY AND PRACTICAL IMPLICATIONS

The literature on the causation of epidemics that spread from person to person, why they propagate or die out, is substantial. A core principle holds that the course of

TABLE 6-3

Zoonoses—organisms and selected vertebrate species Selected Examples

Category of Organism	Organism	Associated Vertebrate Species
Viral		
• Pandemic Influenza	Influenza A subtypes H1N1,H2N2,H3N3	Swine, ducks, chicken, quail; seabirds
• Severe Acute Respiratory Syndrome (SARS)	Coronavirus	Palm civets (other wild bush species under investigation)
• Rabies	Rabies virus	Wild carnivores (e.g., skunks, raccoons, foxes); bats; domestic animals: dogs, cats ferrets, livestock (e.g., cattle).
Bacterial		
• Anthrax	Bacillus anthracis	Herbivores (domestic and wild)
• Brucellosis	Brucella abortis; B mellitensus; B suis; B canis	Cattle, swine, goats sheep; also wild ungulates (e.g., bison, elk, deer); occasionally dogs, coyotes
• Leptospirosis	Leptospires	Feral rodents (e.g. rats); swine, cattle, dogs, raccoons; reptiles and amphibians.
• Plague	Yersinia pestis	Wild rodents (esp. ground squirrels), lagomorphs (rabbits, hares), wild carnivores, domestic cats
• Psittacosis	Chlamydia psittaci	Mostly parrots, but also poultry, pigeons, canaries and seabirds.
• Tularemia	Francisella tularensis	Rabbits, hares, voles, beavers, muskrats, other rodents

(continued)

TABLE 6-3 (Continued)

Category of Organism	Organism	Associated Vertebrate Species
• Salmonellosis (nontyphoidal)	Salmonella enterica (numerous serovars)	Poultry, swine, cattle, and a wide range of pet species
Parasitic		
• Cystercosis and Taeniasis	Taenia saginata, Taenia solium	Cattle, swine.
• Clonorchiasis (i), Opisthorciasis (ii), Metorchiasis (iii)	i Clonorchis sinensis (Chinese liver fluke); ii Opisthorcis felinus (Europe and Asia); iii Metorchis conjunctus (N. America)	i Cats, dogs, swine, rats, freshwater fish, ii Cats, dogs, swine, rats, freshwater fish, iii Freshwater fish, sled dogs, other mammals
• Echonococcosis (Hydatid disease)	Echinococcus granulosis	Dogs and other canids; also domestic herbivores and others
• Toxoplasmosis	Toxoplasma gondii	Cats; also sheep, goats, rats, swine, cattle, poultry, other.
• Trichinellosis	Trichinella spiralis and related designations	Domestic mammals: swine, dogs, cats, horses, rats; wild species: fox, bear, boar, hyena, jackal, lion, leopard; marine mammals in the Arctic.
Prionic		
• Variant Creutzfeldt-Jakob disease (vCJD)—a.k.a. "Mad Cow Disease"	A prion (a filterable, self-replicating agent)	Cattle

an epidemic depends on the frequency of contact between infectious and susceptible individuals. For example, the success of smallpox eradication (chapter 2) can be explained on this basis: maintaining the "reproductive rate of infection" below one ($R_0 < 1$), using surveillance to detect transmission chains and ring vaccination to intercept them.[36] Conversely, a rate of one ($R_0 = 1$) implies sustained propagation; greater than one ($R_0 > 1$) and the epidemic will grow.[37]

Persons harboring infectious organisms can transmit them at various stages: some are most infectious during the *incubation period* (interval between infection and onset of symptoms during which the agent multiplies and initial host responses develop). Persons with active disease are mostly infectious, and some remain infectious after the host is apparently well again: this is known as the convalescent carrier (e.g., typhoid carriers). Some become asymptomatic carriers with potential to infect others (e.g., TB, many STDs).

Exposure and incubation are associated with the phase of susceptibility (Figure 6-2). Where effective treatment exists (e.g., tuberculosis), treatment during incubation may curtail infection thereby averting both disease and transmission, an important secondary public health gain. Such treatment may be "presumptive" and if started before exposure takes place is called "chemoprophylaxis." For most viral diseases, there is no effective therapy (e.g., measles), for which reason primary prevention by immunization is the key.

Inapparent infections (subclinical cases and carriers) are the most likely to propagate, and therefore are most significant in the spread of IDs. This reality underlies such public health practices as quarantine and contact-tracing. Conversely, the more serious the clinical disease, it is more likely that the person affected will be confined to bed or home, and precautions taken to limit transmission to others. This reality underlies infection control practices such as hand-washing, enteric and respiratory precautions, and isolation.

Quarantine refers to restriction of activities of well persons (or animals) who have been, or are assumed to have been, exposed to a case of communicable disease during its period of communicability (i.e., contacts); the purpose is to prevent disease transmission during the incubation period, should infection occur. The clinical distinction between *isolation* and quarantine is that isolation applies to persons already sick, whereas quarantine is usually applied to apparently healthy contacts. This has legal and ethical implications (see chapter 3) if apparently healthy persons must submit to restrictions on their freedom of movement: for this reason "absolute quarantine" is rarely practiced today. Instead, forms of *modified quarantine* are more common, such as restriction from normal school or work environments. More common is *personal surveillance*: close supervision of contacts so as to permit prompt recognition of infection or illness without necessarily restricting movement. Such alternative procedures are more feasible today due to new communication technologies (e.g., mobile phones).

Contact-tracing is a public health procedure used in the control of certain communicable diseases (e.g., tuberculosis, STDs, meningococcal disease), whereby diligent efforts are made to locate and treat persons who have had close or intimate contact with a known case. This term is also applied to seeking persons who have been exposed to epidemic conditions (e.g., foodborne disease outbreaks).

The term *herd immunity* refers to the resistance of a population to invasion and spread of an infectious agent, either from prior exposure (natural immunity) or by vaccination, or both, and is a function of the proportion of susceptibles and the probability that those who are susceptible will encounter a source of infection. For example, unvaccinated individuals derive benefit from living in a well-vaccinated population.[38] Herd immunity thresholds have been estimated mathematically to reflect the proportion of the population at risk that must be immunized in order to reduce propagation, ultimately to zero. However, thresholds vary with disease, and also with other factors such as population mobility, age structure, nutrition levels, concomitant diseases (especially immune system disorders), and extent to which clustering of susceptibles may occur within population subgroups. Ultimately, even in well-vaccinated populations, susceptibles may cluster and accumulate over time; later reintroduction of the infectious agent can result in outbreaks, often at older average ages than may originally occur.[39] Because much of this is unpredictable in the long term, operationally it is more important not simply to aim at a vaccination coverage level that may suppress transmission, but at a higher level that will protect against these longer-term shifts. Ideally this means virtually 100% vaccination, and in some instances additional rounds of immunization may be required.

DEVELOPING METHODS OF COMMUNICABLE DISEASE CONTROL

Considering mode of transmission is central to identifying opportunities for prevention and control: breaking the transmission cycle requires developing practical measures that are likely to work for the disease condition in a particular setting. Some measures are well proven standards, such as guidelines for the control of nosocomial (hospital-acquired) infections, or may be developed from the findings of specific investigations. Table 6-4 lists generic approaches to particular communicable disease categories; all are consistent with the concepts presented, and are operationally proven.

Another core principle of communicable disease control, introduced earlier (Figure 6-5) is the *epidemiological triad*. An alternate representation of the triad is now shown in Figure 6-6, disease being depicted as an outcome of interaction involving host, agent and environment. Prevention and control may be directed to one or more of these elements, at individual or community level. It is also useful once again to note the alignment with Haddon's Matrix principles: pre-event, event, and postevent phases can be usefully considered as consistent with the levels of prevention: primary, secondary, and tertiary.

At the level of *host*, most fundamental is to promote resistance through measures such as nutrition, protective clothing, and immunization. Where justified, preexposure treatment can prevent infection (e.g., ARV treatment of HIV-infected pregnant

TABLE 6-4

Common measures used in breaking the transmission cycle

Respiratory Infectious Diseases
- Reduce potential for direct contact
- Isolate if serious infection
- Chemoprophylaxis
- Face masks
- Immunization against selected pathogens (e.g., pneumococcal disease)
- Contact Tracing, Personal Surveillance, Modified Quarantine (e.g., school exclusion)

Enteric Infectious Diseases
- Sanitary Measures
- Food hygiene
- Personal hygiene
- Contact insect pests (e.g. scavengers)
- Immunization against selected pathogens (e.g., rotavirus infection)
- Contact Tracing, Personal Surveillance, Modified Quarantine (e.g., school exclusion)

Sexually Transmitted Diseases
- Responsible Sex Practices
- Avoid unprotected sex; Use Condoms
- Promote evidence based safer sex practices
- Prompt diagnosis and treatment of STD; chemoprophylaxis
- Contact Tracing, Personal Surveillance

Vectorborne Diseases
- Ecological control of breeding sites
- Prevent vector access (e.g. bednets)
- Selective use of insecticides
- Integrated vector control

Zoonoses
Similar specific measures (as apply to the above categories) also apply to animals.
    Control of transmission from animal to man needs to focus on that aspect of the
    transmission cycle.

Mixed Modes of Transmission
Multiple measures maybe applicable for conditions that reveal multiple transmission
    modes

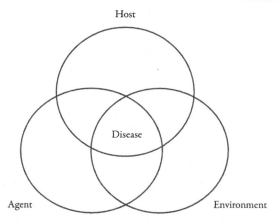

FIGURE 6-6 The epidemiological triad as applied to disease.

women to reduce transmission to their offspring).[25] Prophylactic antibiotics are also given to persons with high risk occupational exposures (e.g., mouth-to-mouth resuscitation, needle-stick injuries, contaminated aerosols). Antimicrobial treatment following infection may render cases and carriers noninfectious: prevention by reducing onward transmission.

Thus, *facilitating timely diagnosis and treatment can be part of a public health strategy.* The context of international travel illustrates this: persons traveling to malaria-endemic areas may take anti-malarial drugs before arriving, during their stay, and for several weeks after leaving so as to protect themselves. If the area to which they return is malaria-receptive, this regimen also prevents introduction of the parasite to that area. Similarly, persons infected with tuberculosis (e.g., skin test conversion following exposure) can receive six months of treatment to prevent development of clinical disease, thereby preserving their own health and reducing the likelihood of becoming an infective carrier. (Note: It is clearly in the public interest that such services are normally provided without charge, especially for persons in high risk groups, e.g., international refugees.)

Regarding the *agent*, although the focus again is to reduce exposure, this is done through measures such as ensuring safe water and food by preventing contamination and spoilage (see chapter 7). In the context of vector control, an agent-oriented measure would be to disable or kill the insect by applying insecticides. In settings such as hospitals, where host measures such as personal protections and precautions are applicable, agent-oriented measures, such as instrument sterilization, are also emphasized.

Addressing the *environment* itself offers many avenues for communicable disease control. For examples, drinking water safety achieved by filtration and chlorination; food kept hot or cold (not warm) to prevent multiplication of organisms that cause food spoilage as well as disease; good housekeeping to reduce exposure to pathogens (and toxic agents); reducing mosquito breeding sites, especially those close to human habitation; enhancing air quality in buildings and industrial settings (air conditioner maintenance, ventilation) to protect against both infectious and toxic agents; sound environmental management on farms to protect animals, people and the environment. Barrier techniques such as masks can reduce respiratory transmission. Preventing overcrowding (e.g., homeless shelters, dormitories, military barracks) can reduce droplet transmission. Proper management of waste (sewage, animal and food residue) averts cross contamination and promotes environmental quality.

It should by now be clear that there are many instances where all components of the triad are addressed. For example, protection against mosquito-borne pathogens (e.g., malaria, dengue) may be achieved through insecticide-treated bednets plus daytime protective clothing and use of repellants. These measures combine personal protection with an insecticide active against the agent, but more fundamental still is to keep domestic and worksite spaces free of containers that may serve as breeding sites (an environmental measure). In health care institutions, infection control rules combine personal with environmental actions. In the food industry, protective clothing (e.g., gloves, gowns, goggles) protects both worker *and process* from contamination (the latter is an environmental measure). In chapter 7, we explore airborne, foodborne, and waterborne diseases and their control in further depth. In all instances, disease surveillance, and monitoring and evaluation of control procedures, are highly relevant to effective control (chapter 5).

Often communicable disease control measures are *legally mandated* and resources committed to ensure that standards are upheld, by professionally qualified inspectors. For example, regulations under public health legislation commonly govern drinking water safety, food control, waste management, and aspects of the building code. Other policy measures address roles and responsibilities of the individual and society ranging from use of aprons and hairnets in food preparation to immunization and chemoprophylaxis. Virtually all such mandated measures benefit recipients and also prevent the transmission of communicable diseases to others. In some jurisdictions, immunization is required as a condition for school entry. Similarly, some forms of quarantine and personal surveillance are designed to prevent transmission as already discussed.

Sociocultural environments affect virtually all disease occurrence. Consider the situation of colonized minorities (chapter 4): due largely to systematic discrimination by colonial societies, virtually all forms of morbidity from alcoholism, to diabetes, to gastroenteritis are more frequent than in the general population. For example, an investigation into drinking water supply systems on First Nations (aboriginal) lands in Canada revealed 24% to pose a high risk to water quality and safety and therefore to human health; the bacteriological monitoring frequency was only 29% of that recommended nationally.[40] Corrective measures are now being taken by the Canadian government, as First Nations health protection falls mainly within federal jurisdiction. Comparable situations have confronted others who have suffered sociocultural deprivation (e.g., endemic roundworm infection in a peri-urban minority community in Canada).[41] No nation is free of such scenarios.

Purely medical approaches fail in such situations: one must tackle root causes, but this is easier said than done. To take an example from Africa, bringing the HIV pandemic under control is complex:[42] aside from risk behaviors (which apply in all global settings, e.g., unprotected sex with multiple partners), other determinants are active: complex cultural and social factors, human rights and status of women, and comorbidities (e.g., tuberculosis, malaria). Weakness in health management systems is part of the public health challenge: bottlenecks in distribution and utilization of funds and in procurement and supply of preventive and therapeutic goods. The *social-ecological model* (chapter 4), as further developed below (Figure 6-7), offers an analytical framework through which strategies may be designed, implemented and assessed: to ensure that preventive actions are reinforced at all levels from individual to family, community and society at large.

The model's essence is that individual behavior is determined largely by the external social environment. Barriers to healthy behaviors are often shared across

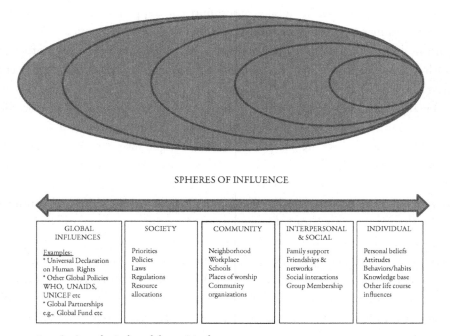

SPHERES OF INFLUENCE

GLOBAL INFLUENCES	SOCIETY	COMMUNITY	INTERPERSONAL & SOCIAL	INDIVIDUAL
Examples: * Universal Declaration on Human Rights * Other Global Policies WHO, UNAIDS, UNICEF etc * Global Partnerships e.g., Global Fund etc	Priorities Policies Laws Regulations Resource allocations	Neighborhood Workplace Schools Places of worship Community organizations	Family support Friendships & networks Social interactions Group Membership	Personal beliefs Attitudes Behaviors/habits Knowledge base Other life course influences

FIGURE 6-7 Socioecological model—revisited.

a community, even society as a whole; as these are lowered or removed, behavior change becomes more achievable and sustainable. The optimal approach may be to combine efforts at all levels: individual, interpersonal, organizational, community, and public policy. In the disease prevention and control context, this model does not replace operational tools such as the natural history model, modes of transmission, or Haddon's matrix; however, it does help to facilitate multilevel approaches to these challenges.

NUTRITION AND IMMUNITY

Returning to natural history (Figure 6-2), individuals may transition from susceptibility, through disease, toward recovery (or not). During this process, interactions involving nutrition, immunity and infection take place: host susceptibility varies with all three factors, each amenable to action. By acting on both nutrition and immunity we reduce the likelihood of infection and improve individual and population outcomes.[43] This strategy is critically important in situations of deprivation, such as settings where acute respiratory infection and gastroenteritis are leading causes of child death: in these situations, underlying malnutrition heightens the risk of infection, and renders children more susceptible to severe outcomes (discussed in chapter 7). Nutrition supplementation helps to rectify this situation, by attending to both general and specific nutrition requirements (e.g., protein and caloric intake, micronutrient supplementation). Similarly, breast-feeding promotes protection against infant deaths, while specific immunizations not only prevent specific conditions, but also reinforce the ability to cope with other infections as well, thus enhancing the prospects of normal growth and development.

Finally (right side of Figure 6-2) if a person survives a communicable disease, specific immunity usually develops to protect against future occurrence if reexposure occurs. However, there are exceptions, such as dengue fever (further discussed in chapter 9), for which primary infection may set up a complex immune response that can result in more serious disease on exposure to other serotypes.[44] Another exception is influenza A virus, which undergoes periodic antigenic shifts and continual drifts, thereby trending ahead of human immunity, ensuring its own survival.

To conclude this section, it is important to note that so many different types of infectious conditions exist, some with enormous antigenic variety, as well as occasional emergence of new ones (e.g., HIV, SARS), that the potential for individual exposure to previously unencountered pathogens is ever-present. Communicable disease control will remain a major public health challenge: for as far as the mind can foresee, "an unfinished agenda."

Noncommunicable Diseases

For almost two decades, noncommunicable diseases (NCDs) have been the leading category of morbidity and mortality worldwide, the only exception being Sub-Saharan Africa, although here too, the NCD burden is increasing. As already noted, these trends reflect epidemiological transitions (Figure 6-1). Following our natural history model (Figure 6-2), NCDs may result in death, various levels of dysfunction, or healthy resolution depending on the natural course and/or effectiveness of intervention.

Typically, after disease manifestations develop, most persons with NCDs will experience varying degrees of functional impairment, related economic adjustments, and altered quality of life. Generally, NCDs arise from prolonged exposure to environmental and social determinants and risk factors strongly influenced by behavior; underlying this, genetic susceptibility plays a role. Many common NCDs (e.g., diabetes, hypertension, heart disease, cancers) strongly reflect multifactorial etiology. However, although simply defined as a condition that is noninfectious, some (as earlier discussed) are initiated by acute infectious processes (e.g., numerous forms of cancer, rheumatic fever, many postinfectious neuropathies). In this sense, there is no hard boundary between IDs and NCDs: not all diseases classified as NCDs are necessarily noncommunicable, although most are.

Comparing unlike conditions (whether IDs or NCDs), especially for purposes of priority ranking and resource allocation, is challenging. Direct measures such as disease incidence, prevalence and mortality, do not adequately reflect the comparative disease *burdens* across settings (different places, persons and time periods). For this purpose a "burden of disease" measure was developed by the World Health Organization. Referred to as the DALY (disability-adjusted life years), one DALY represents the loss of the equivalent of one year of full health. DALYs combine the following components: YLL (years of life lost due to deaths in a given year), and YLD (equivalent healthy years of life lost through living in states of less than full health for cases of disease and injury incident in a given year). Using DALYs, it is possible to compare the burdens of diseases that cause early death but little disability (e.g., drowning or measles) to those that do not cause death but do cause disability (e.g., cataract causing blindness). Globally, 60% of DALYs are due to premature mortality; disability accounts for the remaining 40%.

Using this measure, NCDs now cause almost half the disease burden in low and middle-income countries. The top 10 causes of disease burden globally in 2004 are listed in Table 6-5, which shows number of DALYs for common conditions and the percentage distribution for the world as a whole, and for three country groups classified by gross national income.[45] The table reveals how disease burdens are

TABLE 6-5

Leading causes of disability-adjusted life years (DALYs) all ages 2004: World and countries by income group

WORLD	Millions	%
1 Lower respiratory infections	94.5	6.2
2 Diarrhoeal diseases	72.8	4.8
3 Unipolar depressive disorders	65.5	4.3
4 Ischaemic heart disease	62.6	4.1
5 HIV/AIDS	58.5	3.8
6 Cerebrovascular disease	46.6	3.1
7 Prematurity and low birth weight	44.3	2.9
8 Birth asphyxia and birth trauma	41.7	2.7
9 Road traffic accidents	41.2	2.7
10 Neonatal infections and other*	40.4	2.7

MIDDLE INCOME COUNTRIES	Millions	%
1 Unipolar depressive disorders	29.0	5.1
2 Ischaemic heart disease	28.9	5.0
3 Cerebrovascular disease	27.5	4.8
4 Road traffic accidents	21.4	3.7
5 Lower respiratory infections	16.3	2.8
6 COPD	16.1	2.8
7 HIV/AIDS	15.0	2.6
8 Alcohol use disorders	14.9	2.6
9 Refractive errors	13.7 13.1	2.4
10 Diarrhoeal diseases	3.1	2.3

LOW INCOME COUNTRIES	Millions	%
1 Lower respiratory infections	76.9	9.3
2 Diarrhoeal diseases	59.2	7.2
3 HIV/AIDS	42.9	5.2
4 Malaria 32.8 4.0	32.8	4.0
5 Prematurity and low birth weight	32.1	3.9
6 Neonatal infections and other*	31.4	3.8
7 Birth asphyxia and birth trauma	29.8	3.6
8 Unipolar depressive disorders	26.5	3.2
9 Ischaemic heart disease	26.0	3.1
10 Tuberculosis	22.4	2.7

HIGH INCOME COUNTRIES	Millions	%
1 Unipolar depressive disorders	10.0	8.2
2 Ischaemic heart disease	7.7	6.3
3 Cerebrovascular disease	4.8	3.9
4 Alzheimer and other dementias	4.4	3.6
5 Alcohol use disorders	4.2	3.4
6 Hearing loss, adult onset	4.2	3.4
7 COPD	3.7	3.0
8 Diabetes mellitus	3.6	3.0
9 Trachea, bronchus, lung cancers	3.6	3.0
10 Road traffic accidents	3.1	2.6

* About 20% of DALYs shown in this category are due to other noninfectious causes arising in the perinatal period apart from prematurity, low birth weight, birth trauma and asphyxia.

Source: Adapted from Table 13 In: Global Burden of Disease Report 2004, as cited in reference #48, and reproduced with permission from the World Health Organization.

being experienced differently across these groups, reflecting varying stages of epidemiological transition. For example, in low income countries, the challenges of unequally distributed ecologically and environmentally determined disease burdens (e.g., for respiratory infections, malaria, diarrheal diseases) remain prominent, even as ischemic heart disease is now in the top ten. For middle income countries, neuropsychiatric and circulatory conditions are now leading, while the longer-standing dominance of chronic NCDs in high income countries is readily apparent.

DEVELOPING NCD INTERVENTION OPTIONS

The key to prevention and control of NCDs is understanding the *causal pathways*. Using multifactorial frameworks, epidemiologists have identified various *risk factors* for specific NCDs, which predict the likelihood of their development. These fall within two categories: modifiable and nonmodifiable, a distinction that partly depends on the state of knowledge. While full examination of the science behind risk factors exceeds our scope, it is important to recognize that the strength of a risk factor, its prevalence, and extent to which it is modifiable are important keys to NCD prevention and control.

Another core principle, arising from the seminal work of Geoffrey Rose (1926–1993) on "Sick individuals and sick populations," is that *a large number of people at small risk may give rise to more cases of disease than a small number at high risk.*[46] Referred to as the "Rose Theorem," this is also called the "prevention paradox": *a preventive measure that brings large benefits to the community may offer little to most participating persons.* For example, to reduce the lung cancer death rate, many people must refrain from or cease smoking, while only some who have been exposed to tobacco smoke will die prematurely from this disease. Similarly, to prevent one death from a motor vehicle accident, many hundreds of people must wear seatbelts. Applying this principle to cardiovascular disease (CVD) disease in east Asia, estimates suggest that a reduction of just 3% in average blood pressure (as might be achieved by sustained reductions in dietary sodium or caloric intake) would be expected to reduce the incidence of disease (largely among clinically defined nonhypertensive persons) almost as much as would be hypertensive therapy targeted to all hypertensive persons in the population.[47]

By contrast, the traditional approach to prevention is focused mostly on individuals with higher levels of a risk factor, who may present with symptoms or signs of related ill-health, or be detected through a case-finding effort while visiting a physician's office or other screening venue. While this "high-risk strategy" is generally in the best interests of those individuals, it will miss a much larger number of people at lower risk. Given the "Rose theorem": a public health approach will therefore

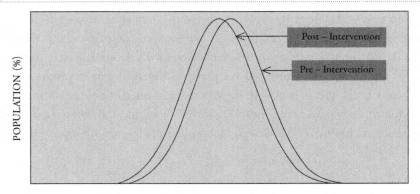

POPULATION MEAN BLOOD PRESSURE (systolic or diastolic mm Hg)

FIGURE 6-8 Effects of a population-based intervention strategy on distribution of blood pressure—schematic.

consider a "population strategy" of attempting (by nonpharmacological means) to shift risk factor distributions so as to prevent disease burden at the population level (Figure 6-8). This approach underlies much of the success of integrated disease prevention and control initiatives (discussed further later in the chapter) and forms much of the evidence base for related health promotion, especially those determinants and risks that are primarily behavioral in origin.

Causal Factors: Determinants and Risk Factors

Addressing NCDs from a public health perspective thus emphasizes the occurrence of common exposures and diseases that affect society as a whole. Broadly speaking, while NCD risk factors are mostly genetic or behavioral, social and environmental determinants are fundamentally important: these operate mostly indirectly at societal level and are considered "distal" from the perspective of individuals—to act on them depends more on social change, even legislation. At population level, a high prevalence of either class of *causal factors* (determinants or risk factors) will place communities at increased NCD risk. This said, it is the "proximal" risk factors that offer the more immediate prospects of improving individual outcomes, mainly through behavioral or clinical interventions.

In the context of our natural history model (Figure 6-2), determinants and risk factors, and the links and interactions among them, act most critically during the period of susceptibility. It is "risk factors" that mostly drive the molecular, structural, and physiological damage that takes place virtually undetected during the period of susceptibility; this is why the dominance of NCDs in the global burden of disease is often referred to as "the silent pandemic" (by the time damage is done to the individual, the optimal opportunity to intervene has passed). At the level of persons, after sufficient time has elapsed, functional impairment may emerge, followed by symptoms and signs of disease. The same influences may continue to act (especially without intervention) throughout the disease course: however, intervention even when disease is apparent, can improve outcomes, mostly through secondary and tertiary prevention modalities.

Nonmodifiable Causes

In terms of overall population health impact, the most powerful risk factors for NCD occurrence are age, sex and genetic traits. The mechanism of aging is assumed to be cumulative, long-term exposure to factors that alter function and structure, including DNA; apparent differences in rates of aging may reflect variations in this process. Regarding the influence of sex, particular risks are associated with being female or male, many genetically determined (e.g., from pregnancy-related to sex-linked disorders), while others are influenced more by associated gender roles (e.g., anxiety and depression, some occupational diseases). Regarding the role of genetics, some genotypes are potentially beneficial, having evolved as protection against particular risks (e.g., sickle cell trait, which confers a selective advantage in malarious environments even as it places homozygous persons at risk of sickle cell disease).[48] Indigenous circumpolar peoples have basal metabolic rates higher than people of temperate zones, hypothesized to be a genetic adaptation to colder climates.[49] With exceptions, genetic susceptibility for disease does not imply that it will occur. In most instances, genes interact with personal behaviors and environmental exposures to modify the probability of disease development: just because a condition is genetic in origin does not mean that we can do nothing to influence its natural history.

To the contrary, many age, sex and genetically linked conditions are amenable to risk reduction by modifying behavior or environment. This may entail early identification, risk modification and focused health education, especially in childhood, adolescence and early adulthood. For most NCDs, improving personal behavior and reducing exposures are important universal primary prevention strategies that are applicable at several levels: from health promotion for society as a whole (e.g., healthy public policies) to clinical prevention. One must caution, however, that disease processes that take years, even decades, to develop usually require much time and resources to reduce their impact. Further, addressing only susceptibility through health promotion or primary prevention will not be sufficient for everyone: a fully developed and humane public health strategy must also address progression among those who develop disease. In other words, a balanced approach will also consider secondary and tertiary prevention.

Genetic Disorders

Medical genetics as a discipline is about half a century old; a definition with potential for public health application is: "the science of human biological variation as it relates to health and disease." This field is transforming into "genomic medicine" calling attention to the genome as the source of life's continuity and variety, and the origin of health and disease in molecular and genetic terms. It has potential to account for all aspects of disease expression, and pathogenic processes.[50] In 2003 the Human Genome Project (HGP) released a complete map of the genome;[51] new genetic markers for disease susceptibility have since been identified and begun to clarify host-genome-environment interactions (Figure 6-9).

Discovery of a genetic susceptibility provides potential for alerting individuals at increased risk. However, despite this promise, *the ethical basis for genetic screening programs has not changed, nor should it*: these may only be considered when formal criteria are met, such as: the natural history of the disorder is understood, screening test characteristics have been determined (sensitivity, specificity, reliability), disorder prevalence and test predictive values can be estimated for settings where it may be applied, effective intervention is available and relevant (sometimes lifelong) follow up is feasible. In particular, an acceptable measure must be available that will improve the outcome (e.g., instruction to avoid an exposure; counseling to help with family decisions). Where such conditions are not met, problems arise, such as: unnecessary testing conducted for little or no benefit to the subject, and that have significant resource implications.[48] Ethical aspects of medical and public health genetics are explored further in chapter 3.

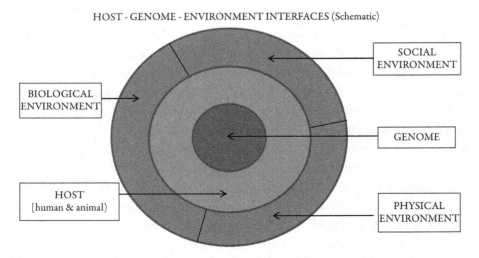

HOST - GENOME - ENVIRONMENT INTERFACES (Schematic)

FIGURE 6-9 Host–genome–environment interfaces (schematic).

Consistent with formal criteria and ethical principles, intervention based on genetic screening for severe, often life-threatening conditions has long been practiced. Testing of newborns for selected conditions is widely available in many nations (Table 6-6).

Consider now genetic conditions that manifest mostly as adult-onset disease, for example, familial hypercholesterolemia. This disorder arises from a single abnormal gene that results in blood cholesterol levels up to four times above normal. However, this does not mean that such persons are not amenable to environmental (including dietary and lifestyle) interventions, but it does mean that—to be effective in light of current knowledge—the intervention must be individualized and medically aggressive.[52]

TABLE 6-6

Newborn screening programs for serious genetic disorders commonly available in some or all US states (examples only)

Disorder	Outcome If Left Untreated	Treatment
Phenylketonuria	Mental retardation, seizures	Diet restricting phenylalanine
Congenital hypothyroidism	Growth failure, mental retardation	Oral levothyroxine
Sickle cell disease	Anemia; "sickle cell crises"	Prophylactic antibiotics
Galactosemia	Liver, renal and brain damage; high infant mortality	Galactose free diet
Maple syrup urine disease	Brain damage	Diet restricting intake of branched-chain fatty acids
Congenital adrenal hyperplasia	"Addison's disease"; impaired genital and sexual development	Glucocorticoids; mineralocorticoids; salt
Cystic fibrosis	Frequent lung infections, growth retardation, infertility	Improved nutrition; management of pulmonary symptoms
ACADD—Acyl CoA medium chain dehydrogenase deficiency	Lethargy, hypoglycemia, liver and brain damage	Avoidance of fasting; aggressive medical management during illness

Genomic research has the potential to identify more *single gene abnormalities* such as this, and thereby move clinical and public health prevention further away from traditional "one-size-fits-all" approaches. It may well advance the evidence base for public health concerns such as obesity, particular infections, and susceptibility to toxic exposures.[53] This said, despite speculation regarding the potential for genetic engineering solutions to such human disease, so far no current preventive strategy uses such an approach.

As a result of the HGP, our ability to identify more genetic links with disease raises the possibility of interventions at many ages. For example, the (American) Society of Gynecologic Oncologists Education Committee recently stated (partial quote):

Women with germline mutations in the cancer susceptibility genes, BRCA1 or BRCA2, associated with Hereditary Breast/Ovarian Cancer syndrome, have up to an 85% lifetime risk of breast cancer and up to a 46% lifetime risk ovarian cancer. Similarly, women with mutations in the DNA mismatch repair genes, MLH1, MSH2 or MSH6, associated with the Lynch/Hereditary Non-Polyposis Colorectal Cancer (HNPCC) syndrome, have up to a 40–60% lifetime risk of both endometrial and colorectal cancer as well as a 9–12% lifetime risk of ovarian cancer. Genetic risk assessment enables physicians to provide individualized evaluation of the likelihood of having one of these gynecologic cancer predisposition syndromes, as well the opportunity to provide tailored screening and prevention strategies such as surveillance, chemoprevention, and prophylactic surgery that may reduce the morbidity and mortality associated with these syndromes. Hereditary cancer risk assessment is a process that includes assessment of risk, education and counseling conducted by a provider with expertise in cancer genetics, and may include genetic testing after appropriate consent is obtained.[54]

This statement illustrates the emerging guidance on identifying individuals who may benefit from hereditary cancer risk assessment, and emphasizes that options are available to help a person manage their risk. As new knowledge emerges from the HGP, we must stay alert to how applications evolve, including policy developments and implications.

Although these are early days, the "genomics revolution" may have adverse potential to divert attention and resources away from more cost-effective community solutions to human health challenges that focus on external influences such as environment, social structure, lifestyle, and public policy. This said, we must also recognize that we are also on a threshold where viewing "genes as determinants" of health is no longer just a theoretical construct: as we move forward it may gain practical and favorable application.

Genomic medicine is expected to transcend the current boundaries of medical genetics. Its leaders assert that it will be applicable for the health of the many or all, not just the few.[55] Given current inequities in health systems, and the underlying influence of social determinants, how this actually plays out requires vigilance. The future may depend on the extent to which such principles as equity and universality are upheld. The hope that genomic research will lead to better recognition of environmental diseases and identification of individual susceptibility, in addition to more personalized medical care, is also stimulating the development of a new field within public health called Public Health Genomics. Ethical aspects of this discussion are further reviewed in chapter 3.

Modifiable Causes

The underlying premise here is that modifiable causes can be addressed either through risk factors or underlying determinants, ideally both. The classical risk factor approach in public health is to conduct a baseline survey so as to map risk factor prevalence thereby revealing related disease risks for communities or particular groups. Interventions can then be designed to reduce risk factor prevalence, while outcomes can be tracked using surveillance systems (chapter 5). However, one may also impact development of risk factors by modifying the underlying social and environmental conditions that influence behaviors, for example through health public policies and promoting health literacy. Conceptually, the risk factor approach is likely to deliver a more immediate intervention effect, i.e., morbidity and mortality may be averted or forestalled more promptly. By contrast, the determinants approach may take longer but offers the prospect of more sustainable improvements. The two approaches are different but complementary: an optimal strategy may be to combine them so that they are mutually supportive and potentially synergistic; these ideas are further developed in the next section.

INTEGRATED APPROACHES

The North Karelia Project is an integrated NCD prevention and control initiative that started as a demonstration project, then scaled up to a nationwide intervention.[56] As a Case Study in chapter 4, we noted its emulation throughout the CINDI-CARMEN network of projects active in numerous countries in Europe and the Americas. Here we examine some of the operational features that made this integrated model a success.

Launched in 1972, within two decades the incidence of ischemic heart disease was more than halved in both sexes in this Finnish province;[57] 80% of this was attributable to reduced tobacco use, hypertension and blood lipids. Intersectoral policy initiatives were combined with community action, medical intervention and public-private partnerships. The main behavioral change was dietary: the local diet was high in salt and fats, and a combination of education and industry cooperation effectively reduced the use of butter on bread from almost 90% to 10%, associated with a rise in use of soft margarine and butter-vegetable oil mixtures. Traditional butter use for cooking and baking was largely replaced by oils and margarines, and whole milk replaced by low-fat and skimmed milk. The initiative extended in the late 1970s to Finland as a whole, stimulating declines in smoking, serum cholesterol and blood pressure.[58] After 25 years, cardiovascular disease declined 73%, lung cancer 71% and total mortality 49%.[59] While this demonstrates the use of epidemiological evidence for outcome evaluation, North Karelia also pioneered process evaluation: documenting *how* it was done—not the norm during the 1970s.[60,61]

Nonetheless, the global landscape of NCD prevention and control remains dominated not by such integrated approaches, but by disease-specific interventions. For every example of integrated interventions, there have been dozens of stand-alone initiatives focusing on single disease entities. Consensus has emerged that the collective impact on clinical prevention and health promotion might have been greater over the decades had more coordinated approaches been applied to both health policy frameworks and disease prevention initiatives. After all, the core prevention message for many of these entities is similar, especially with regard to three risk factors (tobacco use, poor diet, and physical inactivity) that contribute to four conditions (heart disease, type 2 diabetes, lung disease, and cancers) that together account for the majority of deaths globally.[62]

The Call for More Integrated Approaches: A United Nations Declaration on the Prevention and Control of Non-Communicable Diseases was issued in 2011.[63] This sets out the global challenge and its socioeconomic and developmental impacts; it calls for what is described as "a whole of government and whole of society" effort to reduce risk factors and create health promoting environments; to strengthen national policies and health systems. It calls for international cooperation, collaborative partnerships, new efforts in research & development, monitoring & evaluation, and requires UN follow up.

This UN declaration builds upon the "Global Status Report on Non-communicable Diseases 2010,"[64] the first worldwide report on the state of NCDs, ways to map them, reduce risk factors, and strengthen health care for people affected by them. The report found that NCDs (including CVDs, lung diseases, cancer, and diabetes) were responsible for 36 million deaths in 2008 (63% of all deaths worldwide). Every year, hypertension causes 7.5 million deaths, tobacco causes 6 million deaths, lack of physical activity causes 3.2 million deaths, and overweight and obesity causes 2.8 million deaths. Three priority areas for action were advocated: surveillance, prevention, and health care. *"Best buys"* applicable to all countries were highlighted: public smoking bans, enforcing bans on tobacco and alcohol advertising and sponsorship, raising taxes on these products, reducing salt in foods, replacing trans-fat with polyunsaturated fat in foods, and promoting public awareness about nutrition and physical activity.

SCALING UP INTERVENTIONS

As discussed in scaling up community interventions (chapter 4), before one can aspire to integrated approaches, whether for NCD or other disease control initiatives, the components to be integrated must be conceptualized and developed. Disease-specific approaches are the building blocks for this. Once the conceptual approach to a type of disease is worked out, taking into account operational requirements, a decision can be made as to whether the initiative should "stand-alone" or whether it could be effectively delivered in an integrated manner within a broader disease prevention and control initiative, or within a health promotion framework, or both.

To illustrate how initiatives focused on one set of conditions may interrelate with others, we now consider diabetes and arthritis as case studies.

CASE STUDY: APPLYING INTEGRATED PREVENTION
PRINCIPLES TO TYPE 2 DIABETES

The modern pandemic of Type 2 diabetes emerged as a result of global trends in its underlying risk factors, driven by broad social determinants, as portrayed in Figure 6-10. In individuals who develop the condition, it arises due to a confluence of polygenetic, behavioral, environmental, and metabolic (including intrauterine) influences, resulting in reduced insulin secretion and diminished insulin sensitivity. If left to run its course, diabetes results in premature morbidity and mortality; globally it is also a leading cause of blindness and nontraumatic limb amputation. Over 300 million people worldwide have diabetes now, projected to rise to 500 million within a generation. Globally, a high proportion of people with diabetes go unrecognized and receive no prevention or treatment. Millions face stigma and discrimination that can create barriers to services, employment, and normal social interactions in many societies; it is both cause and a product of social inequity, in terms of both health and social consequences.[65]

Turning now to diabetes prevention, the three main levels are addressed in Table 6-7. This also lists broader health promotion measures that serve as a societal framework to facilitate preventive actions, as well as having independent merit.

Primary prevention, through promotion of healthy living and optimizing maternal nutrition, diet and physical activity (to prevent overweight—a powerful risk factor

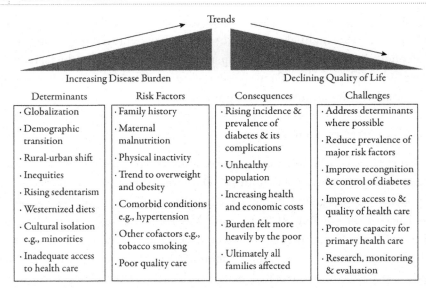

FIGURE 6-10 Pandemic Type 2 Diabetes-Determinants, Risk Factors, Consequences and Challenges.

for diabetes), is now scientifically well-established.[66] Being aware of one's family history is useful, as diabetes tends to run in families (reflecting both genetic and environmental influences). We now know that secondary prevention is ideally focused at the biochemical level (it applies mostly to apparently healthy people) rather than at the time of clinical presentation (often too late due to the onset of complications, which implies that the disease process is advanced); it involves detection of glucose abnormalities (e.g., elevated fasting glucose or impaired glucose tolerance) followed by diabetes education and monitoring; management of hypertension and smoking cessation are equally important. If diabetes develops, home-based self-monitoring of blood glucose (SMBG) using a glucometer (glucose meter) is becoming recognized as a critical skill in maintaining metabolic control, and illustrates the principle of self-care—maintaining the independence of the person affected. This may be augmented by periodic monitoring of glycosylated hemoglobin (HbA1c), facilitated by a health care provider: the A1c test measures the amount of glucose in red blood cells, and reflects an average of glucose control over a period of 2–3 months. Tertiary prevention implies early detection and treatment of complications, by screening for retinopathy, cardiovascular and peripheral vascular disease and neuropathy (especially signs of "diabetic foot").

While some of the foregoing falls within the spectrum of "clinical prevention," to achieve impact at the level of population health requires *public health involvement*: promoting professional, patient and public education on diabetes, smoking

TABLE 6-7

Illustrating diabetes (type 2) health promotion, primary, secondary, and tertiary prevention

Health Promotion	Primary Prevention	Secondary Prevention	Tertiary Prevention
Healthy public policy	Promotion of healthy living	Access to affordable health care	Access to affordable health care
Transportation policy	Physical activity (e.g., cycling, walking)	Early detection of glucose intolerance	Early detection of complications
Food pricing & labeling,	Healthy nutrition	Patient education	Patient education
Healthy workplaces	Avoidance of overweight/ obesity	Primary prevention in secondary context (e.g., weight control)	Primary prevention in tertiary context (e.g., quit smoking)
Improving public knowledge	Awareness of family history	Self-monitoring of metabolic control	
Creative use of public media	Optimal maternal nutrition	Blood pressure control	Community care systems

prevention and cessation programs, facilitating screening initiatives, and supporting self-care and community care systems free of stigma for people affected by this condition. Because good outcomes depend on metabolic control (facilitated by SMBG and HbA1c monitoring) and removal or management of risk such as smoking and hypertension, a quality of care monitoring system offers major advantages.[67] To ensure that this is put in place is arguably a public health responsibility: not necessarily to do it, but to facilitate its development and use, especially as it may be adapted for other NCD prevention and control applications.

Finally, there is *a powerful take-away message* about diabetes that resonates with the call for more integrated programming: what works for type 2 diabetes prevention also works for other common NCDs and for community health generally. Conversely, integrated public health approaches to NCD health promotion and disease prevention will benefit people at risk for diabetes. For readers wishing to delve deeper into diabetes, from public health and program development perspectives, references are cited.[68, 69, 70] There is also discussion of the role of international cooperation in integrated diabetes program development in chapter 8 (see Public Health Goals and Objectives at Societal Level).

CASE STUDY: ARTHRITIS—AN INTEGRATED
APPROACH TO PREVENTION AND CONTROL

A complex health problem, arthritis is a diverse set of conditions, each with comparable clinical and social impacts. In 2003, the US Centers for Disease Control and Prevention (CDC) launched a national arthritis action plan that included the following elements:[71]

Primary Prevention: Being overweight is associated with increased risk for arthritis in general. In particular, weight loss reduces risk for osteoarthritis of the knee. Physical activity not only helps prevent obesity but also maintains joint health and reduces risk for premature death, heart disease, and diabetes. Proper warm-up routines, strengthening exercises, and use of protective equipment during activity can prevent traumatic injuries that may result in arthritis. Occupational injury prevention programs, especially those that reduce repetitive joint stresses, also reduce the risk.

Secondary Prevention: Early diagnosis and appropriate management of arthritis can be beneficial, especially for people with inflammatory arthritis. Early use of disease modifying drugs (e.g., methotrexate for rheumatoid arthritis) can profoundly affect the course of some forms by reducing joint destruction and improving long-term outcomes. Some drugs can prevent exacerbations (e.g., drugs to control uric acid levels help prevent attacks of gout; anti-inflammatory medications can help relieve pain and improve function).

Tertiary Prevention: Although joint replacement surgery is highly effective for reducing pain and improving functionality, several nonsurgical strategies can reduce pain and disability, increase a person's sense of control, and improve quality of life. The key strategies are *physical activity*, *weight control*, and *self-management education programs*.

CDCs purpose in developing this plan was to catalyze a public health response to a nation's leading cause of disability, thereby complementing medical interventions to address arthritis at the individual level. Considering these measures within an integrated health promotion framework is useful: for example, promoting *physical activity*, *weight control*, and *self-management education programs* should also result in cardiovascular and other benefits, thus delivering the broader value of an integrated approach. However, in the context of arthritis, both primary *and* tertiary prevention must be addressed. For example, many existing health promotion efforts emphasize healthy people (to keep them that way), but the question relevant to a national arthritis strategy is whether they also cater to the needs of people suffering arthritis or convalescing from related clinical interventions. As CDC points out: People with arthritis are often more vulnerable to stress, depression, anger, and anxiety because of pain, loss of functional ability, and fewer social contacts. Because of joint pain, they may also be less physically active, placing them at higher risk for obesity, heart disease, diabetes, and high blood pressure. A fully developed strategy must therefore address these impacts as well as facilitate secondary prevention, including access to medical care and community support.

Chronic Care Management Models

Having just reviewed integrated approaches to the prevention of type 2 diabetes and arthritis, it is timely to consider the chronic disease management models that have been evolving in concert with the trend toward integrated approaches. The most widely cited chronic care model (CCM) describes chronic care broadly as "prevention and diagnosis, management, and palliation of chronic disease."[72] Based on a systematic review of chronic care interventions the model responds to calls for continuous, coordinated integrated systems of health service delivery. Key elements include the following:[73]

- Personnel and processes to support proactive care, including planned care and care coordination and scheduling or coordination of visits and follow-up
- Decision support for providers, including disease management guidelines and protocols
- Information systems to ensure access to timely and relevant information
- Support for patient empowerment and self-management
- Community resources to inform and support patients
- System support for chronic illness care among providers integrated into care networks

Enhancements have been made to the CCM in various settings so as to more adequately incorporate elements of health promotion and community health not fully recognized in the original model.[74] Such adaptations are clearly in the interest of proactive patients, families, communities, and providers.[75]

Prevention and Control of Mental and Behavioral Disorders

What are mental and behavioral disorders? As defined earlier, these manifest by abnormalities of thought, feeling and/or behavior that result in distress or impairment, and may have relational and social consequences. Collectively they are a leading cause of ill-health globally. Some are heavily influenced by cultural and religious norms especially with regard to perceptions of deviance. Others are defined on the basis of harm to others, regardless of the affected individual's perception of distress. Most are accompanied by varying degrees of stigma resulting in discrimination. Many mental and behavioral disorders have physical components or consequences to self or others: depression can result in suicide; injection drug use conveys a high risk of contracting blood-borne diseases and is associated with nutritional deficiencies; fetal alcohol spectrum disorder, due to alcohol abuse during pregnancy, is characterized by growth and mental retardation, cranial and facial malformations, and cardiac defects.

Concepts of mental health and illness have varied across time and cultures; approaches to definition, classification, assessment and intervention continue to evolve. There is ongoing debate regarding how best to approach particular disorders from the perspectives of individual and public health. As evidence emerges from research into their nature and from the evaluation of interventions, such issues will steadily become clarified.

According to the US National Institute of Mental Health (NIMH), over the past 15 years, discoveries in genetics, neuroscience, and behavioral science largely account for the gains in knowledge that have helped to understand the complexities of mental illnesses and behavioral disorders.[76] This includes such aspects as cognition, emotion, social interaction, learning, motivation, and perception. The underlying complexity continues to be revealed from studies of genes, proteins, cells, systems and circuits, and builds on increasing understanding of the neurochemistry of the brain and advancements in pharmacological sciences that have led to the introduction of several affordable drugs for some mental illnesses (e.g., treatment of depression and prevention of relapses).

Once again, the natural history model (Figure 6-2) offers a valuable framework for analysis in the context of mental and behavioral disorders: in fact, the U.S. Institute of Medicine (IOM), in 1994, put forward an intervention framework based on the public health distinctions between primary, secondary and tertiary prevention.[77] In 2004, the World Health Organization (WHO) embodied these principles within its policy approach to intervention initiatives.[78] Mental disorder prevention, thus defined, aims at "reducing incidence, prevalence, recurrence of mental disorders, the time spent with symptoms, or the risk condition for a mental illness, preventing or delaying recurrences and also decreasing the impact of illness in the affected person, their families and the society."

To appreciate the full scope of mental and behavioral disorders, we need to recognize the conceptual boundaries, gaps, overlaps and continuities that exist across physical and mental health and illness, and between disease prevention and health promotion.

Interrelationships between biological processes and pathologies that result in behavioral signs and symptoms have long been recognized in conditions such as epilepsy, cerebral palsy, and traumatic brain injury. Each of these readily fits the natural history model (Figure 6-2), as do some secondary forms of Parkinsonism. Conditions such as multiple sclerosis exhibit both neurological and behavioral outcomes, while bipolar disorders and schizophrenia are less well understood. Such conditions continue to attract research into neurological and biochemical pathways, as well as social and behavioral research.

It is important to keep an open mind as new scientific evidence emerges: there can be surprises, including the potential to virtually eliminate some conditions, but there can also be downsides to some of the upsides. To take pellagra as an historic example (chapter 1), a disease often characterized by psychotic depression, research revealed it to be a nutritional disorder (thiamine deficiency) of the poor. Now eliminated in most parts of the world, the pellagra story reveals the value of both primary prevention (nutritional intervention) and of health promotion (poverty alleviation).[79] Psychotherapeutic drugs also relieve much human suffering, and have dramatically improved the prognosis for patients with severe mental illness. But drugs have side effects and not all patients can be helped. Also, while they allow large numbers of people to be discharged from hospital, all too often they return to communities poorly prepared to provide continuing care.[80]

To take another early example of the potential for misunderstanding the biological basis of some mental disorders, King George III of the United Kingdom suffered from insomnia, headaches, visual problems, restlessness, delirium, convulsions, and stupor as well other more physical manifestations of illness. His confused thought processes are considered by some to have contributed to the American Revolution (1775–1783). From 1811 until his death in 1820 the royal patient became progressively insane and blind. He was nursed in isolation, and kept in straight-jackets behind bars in the privacy of Windsor Castle. We now know that that he suffered from the treatable genetic disease porphyria. A steady progression of 20th century research reveals that there are at least eight types of porphyria, each with different clinical manifestation, and each determined by deficiency of a different enzyme, usually inherited. This stream of research led to porphyria being classified as an "inborn error of metabolism" and not primarily a mental disorder. Although there is no cure for porphyria, treatment is available for each type of the disease.

Turning now to the distinction between mental health and mental disorder, and the differing roles of health promotion and prevention, this relates mostly to differences between their targeted outcomes. Together, they may be described as overlapping and interrelated components of *a unified concept of mental health*.[80] Mental health promotion aims to promote psychological well-being, competence and resilience, by creating supportive living conditions and environments. By contrast, mental disorder prevention targets the reduction of manifestations of mental disorders. It recognizes and uses health promotion strategies as one means of achieving these goals. In a complementary way, mental health promotion when aiming to enhance mental health in the community may also have the secondary outcome of decreasing the incidence of mental disorders or their sequelae. Strategically, prevention and promotion may be combined so as to produce complementary outcomes. In addition to interventions at individual or group level, achieving optimal outcomes in mental disorder prevention requires supportive health promoting actions across domains such as human rights, literacy, environment, housing, social support, employment, poverty reduction and justice, achieving broader benefits.

Even recognizing the synergy between approaches, there remains divergence of opinion regarding the applicability of the disease prevention paradigm to a number of sociobehavioral conditions, at least to the extent that it draws from the "medical model." This is portrayed as viewing disability as a deficiency or abnormality: being disabled is negative, disability resides in the individual, the remedy for disability-related problems is cure or normalization, and the agent of remedy is the professional.[81] A juxtaposed "sociopolitical model" holds that disability is a difference: being disabled is neutral, it derives from the interaction between the individual and society; the agent of remedy is the individual, or advocate, or anyone who affects arrangements between the individual and society.[82]

Both depictions, though helpful in challenging the *status quo*, are oversimplifications that tend to ignore both individual realities and the continuing evolution of evidence. In the meantime, the public health approach is flexible enough to utilize several models based on evidence of what actually works. Public health at its best is eclectic, neither ideological nor dogmatic. It may call upon a full range of biomedical and behavioral sciences, such that to juxtapose the two as if competing rather than complementary overlooks the core goal: to determine the best mix of interventions that will help individuals, reduce the disease burden on society, and promote health.

MENTAL AND BEHAVIORAL DISORDERS AS A PUBLIC HEALTH PRIORITY

Almost half a billion people suffer from these disorders worldwide; one in four persons will develop one or more during their lifetime. In 1996, neuropsychiatric conditions accounted for 13% of DALYs lost due to all diseases and injuries in the world and were projected to increase to 15% by 2020.[83] In 2002 estimates, four of the ten leading causes of YLD globally were due to neuropsychiatric disorders.[84] In addition to common conditions such as anxiety and depression, and less common but generally more serious psychotic conditions, the category includes sociobehavioral disorders such as alcoholism, drug abuse, problem gambling and various forms of violence. Mental disorders are often associated with stigma and human rights violations: affected individuals and their families suffer intense and pervasive discrimination. In part, these phenomena are consequences of a general perception that no effective preventive or treatment modalities exist against these disorders; this inaccurate perception is often reflected in the unsupportive policy making that forms part of the historical legacy of mental and behavioral disorders. Most of them also increase the risk of physical illnesses.

Much more even than for physical health, resources for prevention and treatment of mental disorders, and for mental health promotion, are unevenly distributed worldwide. Global initiatives are desperately needed to reduce this gap and to help low income nations to develop prevention knowledge, expertise, policies and interventions that are responsive to their needs, culture, conditions and opportunities. Conditions such as child abuse, violence, war, discrimination, poverty and lack of access to education all contribute to mental ill-health and the development of mental disorders. Policy actions that improve the protection of human rights represent a powerful preventive strategy.

Disorders with multiple determinants call for integrated approaches: Social, biological and neurological sciences have revealed much about the role of risk and protective factors in the developmental pathways to mental disorders and poor mental health. Numerous factors and interactions have been identified across the life-course: because many are modifiable they offer potential targets for prevention and promotion measures. Their interrelatedness with physical illnesses and social problems point to a need for integrated policies and programs, targeting clusters of related problems, common determinants, and populations at multiple risk. To make optimal use of limited resources, priority should be given to programs and policies based on evidence of effectiveness.

In adopting the prevention model, the World Health Organization's Department of Mental Health and Substance Abuse,[80] emphasizes primary prevention and adopts strategies from health promotion (e.g., improving nutrition, housing access to education, economic security and strengthening community networks), as well as from the field of human development (e.g., early child development, the family context, the workplace, and mentally healthy aging). Specific strategies have been developed to help deal with conditions such as aggression and violence, depression and anxiety, eating disorders and psychotic conditions. In the arena of addictions, WHO puts forward strategies aimed at reducing harm from addictive substances and the physical and behavioral correlates.

MENTAL AND BEHAVIORAL CASE STUDY #1—PROBLEM GAMBLING

To illustrate the phenomenon of seemingly competing models for mental and behavioral disorders, consider problem gambling (social definition), also known as pathological gambling (medical definition):

Problem gambling: The Canadian Problem Gambling Index (CPGI) is used to screen for problem gamblers in the general population (in Canada and in several other countries). It defines problem gambling as "gambling behavior that creates negative consequences for the gambler, others in his or her social network, or the community"[85]. Consequences can be severe: bankruptcy, job loss, marital breakdown, suicide. Scores are used to classify persons across a spectrum: from *at risk gambling* to *severe problem gambling*.

Pathological Gambling: The American Psychiatric Association's Diagnostic and Statistical Manual (DSM IV) defines this clinical term as an *impulse control disorder*. Ten criteria are used to guide diagnoses, ranging from "repeated unsuccessful efforts to control, cut back, or stop gambling" to committing "illegal acts such as forgery, fraud, theft or embezzlement to finance gambling." These criteria represent three dimensions: damage or disruption, loss of control, and dependence.

Most public health practitioners tend to use the term "problem gambling" because it places emphasis on behavioral and social impacts and is often used in population surveys of gambling prevalence. However, most also would agree that these two terms describe virtually the same condition, the DSM term focusing more on the individual and the CPGI severe problem gambling category being more applicable to populations.

Gambling disorders affect 0.2–5.3% of adults worldwide, although measurement and prevalence varies according to screening methods used, and availability and accessibility of gambling opportunities.[86] While aspects of these sociobehavioral disorders are amenable to some approaches derived from the "medical model," other approaches are better aligned with social intervention. For example, individual treatments have been favorably evaluated (e.g., cognitive behavioral and pharmacological interventions). Regarding the social model, family therapy and support from Gamblers Anonymous (while promising) are less supported by evidence. However, overriding such contrasts, gambling disorders are highly comorbid with other mental health and substance use disorders: one must therefore consider the needs of the whole person, with attention to both medical and social models; research is needed into both underlying causes and intervention efficacy.

Taking a human ecology approach, while various genes confer susceptibility to gambling, environmental influences facilitate gambling behavior disorders among susceptible persons. These include accessibility and type of establishment, size and number of prizes, proximity to alcohol, and social considerations. Early negative childhood experiences, such as abuse and trauma, seem to be higher in frequency among individuals with gambling disorders than among social gamblers, with severity of maltreatment associated with severity of gambling problems and earlier age of gambling onset. That childhood exposure to gambling may affect behavior later in life is suggested by reports of associations between gambling problems and parental gambling. Studies of aboriginal populations reveal a higher risk of problem gambling. The recent introduction of more rapid online and interactive games is likely to lead to an increase in the prevalence of problem gambling.[87]

When one takes into account the associated issues of organized crime, the addictive social and economic impacts of gambling on people who can least afford it, and the corrosive effects on responsible government, problem gambling is surely a "sociopolitical" problem that goes well beyond the medical model and even beyond the usual limits of public health. However, as a public health problem, the challenge still must be met: the key avenues for prevention are public education regarding its risks, measures to address the harm it is causing (harm reduction for the individual and the family), and policy advocacy to control and perhaps even to shut down some kinds of gambling.

MENTAL AND BEHAVIORAL CASE STUDY #2—DRUG ADDICTION

A public health approach to drug addiction offers positive alternatives to responding to this disorder primarily as a matter of law enforcement as many nations do. That superior outcomes can be achieved is illustrated by "Insite." Operating since 2003, Insite is North America's first legal supervised site for injection drug use (IDU). Located in a disadvantaged area of Vancouver, Canada, Insite's front line team includes nurses, counselors, mental health workers and peer support personnel. About half the clients are marginalized: homeless or living in shelters or have mental health issues. Many are older, have used drugs for many years and have compromised their health. The operation has booths where clients inject pre-obtained illicit drugs under supervision. While it does not supply drugs, it supplies clean equipment (syringes, cookers, filters, water, and tourniquets). If an overdose occurs, a nurse-led team intervenes immediately: despite 1418 overdoses at InSite between 2004 and 2010, there has never been a fatality.

Insite represents a "harm-reduction" model: striving to decrease adverse health, social and economic consequences of drug use without requiring abstinence from drug use. This embodies primary and secondary prevention: reducing the incidence of infections through safe injection, and reducing HIV and TB transmission by facilitating highly active antiretroviral therapy (HAART) for HIV infected persons. Clients develop trust with health and social workers in a safe place where they may inject drugs under supervision and access addiction counseling and treatment, other diagnosis and treatment services, housing and community support. The Ministry of Health provides funding, while Vancouver's public health agency operates InSite in collaboration with community organizations. Insite promotes continuity of care for people with addiction, mental illness and HIV/AIDS: clients ready to access withdrawal management are accommodated at Onsite, a partner program where counselors, nursing and medical staff help people stabilize and plan their next steps. People then move to transitional support for further stabilization and connection to community services, treatment programs and housing.

Supported by the Urban Health Research Initiative of the British Columbia Centre for Excellence in HIV/AIDS, an initial evaluation (2003–6) revealed that the facility attracted IDUs who were hard to reach through conventional programs, coinciding with a reduction of public injection drug use and publicly discarded syringes, suggesting that the facility has also enhanced public order.[88] Among clientele, Insite reduced the rate of syringe sharing, a practice identified as a primary mode of HIV transmission. Clients were more likely to enter into addiction treatment and Insite was not associated with an increase in levels of drug related crime in the area where it is located. There is evidence of reduced overdose mortality after the opening of Insite: fatal overdoses within 500 meters of Insite decreased by 35% after the facility opened compared to a decrease of 9% in the rest of Vancouver.[89] A study of user perspectives revealed that, of 1082 clients surveyed, 809 (75%) said that they injected more safely as a result of Insite.[90] When asked to list barriers, participants most commonly reported travel time, limited operating hours, and waiting time, reflecting the demand for its services. In-depth interviews have revealed that Insite has provided women temporary refuge from street-based drug scene violence.[91] By learning how to inject themselves safely, women gain more control over the circumstances of their drug use. This, in turn, reduces their risk of becoming infected with HIV or hepatitis C. Study details, available online, should be useful to other cities considering supervised injecting facilities, and to governments regulating their use.[92]

In conclusion, the purpose of supervised injection facilities is to reduce harms associated with injection drug use, one of the four pillars of a comprehensive drug strategy (the others being prevention, treatment and enforcement). This said, the way forward is complex for any society that pits the perceived interests of "law and order" against public health. Insite's legal status in Canada reflects this dichotomy, as it has been subjected to legal challenges by a conservative federal government, even while supported by a liberal provincial government and the Vancouver Police Force who observed first hand its effectiveness. Its commitment to research and evaluation built an evidence base that eventually served as an effective counterpoint to political opposition based on ideology. On September 30, 2011, the Supreme Court of Canada ordered the federal Minister of Health to grant an exemption to

Vancouver's supervised injection facility in accordance with the Controlled Drugs and Substances Act. It is relevant to note that several European countries have similar facilities in major urban centers, as does Australia. By ruling that addiction-related drug use is a health issue and not simply a criminal justice issue, the Supreme Court decision upheld Canada's constitutional rights to life, liberty and security of the person and the role of public health interventions of this nature.

Integrating Disease Prevention and Control through the Life-Course

Consistent with integrated thinking, it is timely to consider again how people live their lives, rather than disease categories as such. For example, in the NCD context, focusing only on risk factors in a given generation, while potentially successful in reducing disease burdens, runs the risk of younger generations being exposed to similar influences. In the ID context, the heavy international donor focus on disease-specific initiatives has undermined the development of primary health care in some settings.[93] For example, globally supported vaccination initiatives have come at the opportunity cost of displacing locally framed priorities. Often also, gains in disease control through categorical approaches have been achieved mostly in mainstream populations, with much less success in socioculturally disadvantaged hard-to-reach groups, and others experiencing barriers to their health that remain unaddressed. These deficiencies in global disease control initiatives are only recently being recognized by donor agencies, and efforts finally being made to correct them by allocating a greater portion of their funding to health systems strengthening and encouraging countries to build this into their proposals.

In light of these observations also a shift has emerged over the past decade in favor of studying the occurrence of health and disease throughout the life-course, especially for vulnerable populations.[94] *Life-course epidemiology* has been defined as the study of long-term effects of physical or social exposures during gestation, childhood, adolescence, and throughout adult life on developmental health and disease risk.[95] The benefit of this perspective is that it expands conventional models of disease risk by recognizing that psychosocial as well as physiological factors occurring throughout an individual's life can affect diverse outcomes. The perspective allows one to see disease as an integral part of an individual's life and argues that disease prevention and control must be intimately integrated into normal daily life, and sustained to benefit the health of communities.[96] Thus, strategies that address risk factors must not do so in a vacuum: they must take into account underlying economic, gender, political, behavioral and environmental factors that foster these risks within all age groups and across generations. This recognition also is consistent with the "whole of government and whole of society approach" (now advocated by WHO for the global approach to NCDs, as noted above).

The life-course approach applies to a wide spectrum of conditions. For example, Figure 6-11 illustrates how nutrition impacts health throughout life, from mental development to risk of chronic disease. This reinforces the premise that susceptibilities and conditions that take years to emerge, with overt manifestations occurring in middle to late adult life, offer potential for early identification and risk modification during pregnancy, in early and later phases of childhood, adolescence, and early adulthood. Similarly, ID risks may be addressed well before they take their toll: by public health and preventive measures appropriate to age, sex and circumstances.

In relation to the life-course approach, integrated programming is highly relevant. For example, in primary health care, scheduling childhood immunization provides an opportunity for contraceptive education of parents, and cervical cancer screening of mothers. Offering these services together is a cost-effective way to prevent unintended pregnancies among many women, and contributes to a healthier population. If well organized, integrated health services have the potential to result in net savings and benefits for both society and individuals. For example, integrated services save people time, enabling them to be more active in the workforce, improve household income, and to invest more in their own, and their children's health, education, and well-being.[97]

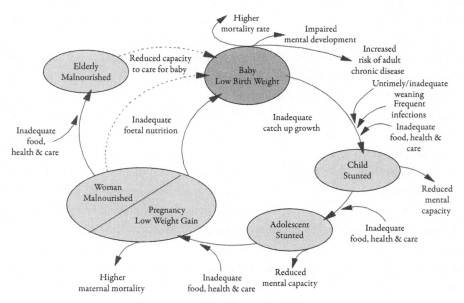

FIGURE 6-11 Nutrition and health throughout the lifecourse[101].

Acknowledgment: Reproduced from Figure 1.1 in reference #101 with permission from the United Nations System Standing Committee on Nutrition (UNSCN).

A Global Perspective on Integrated Health Services

The World Health Organization defines integrated service delivery as "the organization and management of health services so that people get the care they need, when they need it, in ways that are user friendly, achieve the desired results and provide value for money."[98] In the context of public health, Figure 6-12 depicts this principle in relation to disease prevention and control services, contrasting the "vertical" (discrete) approach of individual programs doing their own policy planning and implementation, monitoring and evaluation, with the alternative possibility of pooling common capacities to serve the interests of several programs. While individual programs may retain their own dedicated leadership, the challenge is to develop and utilize these capacities within a shared support framework so as to achieve synergy across goals and objectives, to avoid duplication of valuable resources and expertise, thereby to become mutually supportive and more effective at community level, and potentially at other levels. While integrated approaches also call for greater commitment to interprogrammatic coordination than exists in many public health organizations even today, improved coordination at virtually all levels is a justifiable investment to achieve more effective and efficient public health systems.

The following lessons on how to promote integrated programs are adapted from WHO:

1. Supporting integrated services does not mean that everything has to be integrated into one package, or necessarily delivered in one place. It does mean arranging services so that they are mutually supportive and easy for users to navigate. This in turn means providers have management support systems

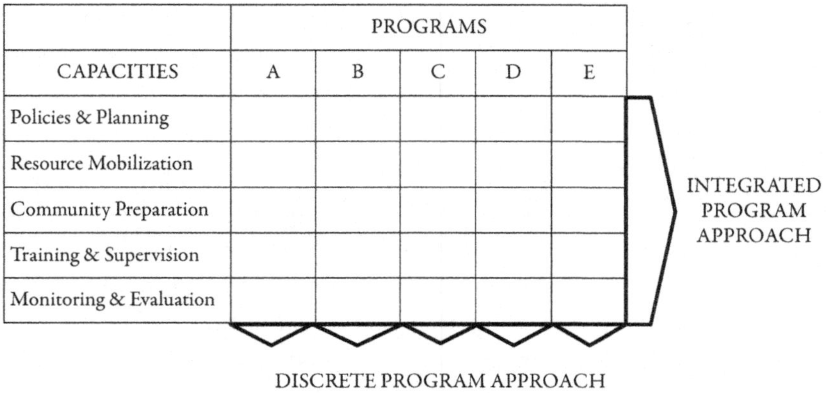

	PROGRAMS				
CAPACITIES	A	B	C	D	E
Policies & Planning					
Resource Mobilization					
Community Preparation					
Training & Supervision					
Monitoring & Evaluation					

INTEGRATED PROGRAM APPROACH

DISCRETE PROGRAM APPROACH

FIGURE 6-12 Integrated versus discrete approaches to disease prevention and control programs—a schematic contrast.

(e.g., for medicines or financial management) that help make this happen, and also make the best use of resources.

There are also arguments in favor of some discrete or "single-issue" programs:

- As a short-term measure in fragile states
- For the control of some epidemics and the management of some emergencies
- So that appropriate services can be provided for specific client groups such as commercial sex workers, drug addicts or prisoners

2. Integration isn't a cure for inadequate resources. While it may provide some savings, integrating new activities into an existing system can't continue indefinitely without the system as a whole being better resourced. For example, a public health workforce cannot be expected to add to their workload without expanding the overall workforce at some point. As *Quality* can also be affected by integration it needs to be monitored.

3. Evolving public health programs in favor of integrated services involves a mix of political, technical and administrative action. People are asked to change the way they work, including control over resources. Incentives may need to be altered. Powerful interests (e.g., specific disease lobbies, donor driven priorities) may have to be actively managed. For related discussion see chapter 8.

Conclusion

Integrated approaches to disease prevention and control, as portrayed in this chapter, are becoming recognized as a paradigm that can work well for both health systems and the people they serve, especially at community level. However, in advocating a transition to more integrated approaches, resistance will be encountered and legitimate concerns need to be addressed, especially to reassure "single disease" champions more familiar with traditional stand-alone initiatives. In this respect, unique and important aspects of particular conditions must receive the priority they deserve, and not lost in the process; in some instances stand-alone programs will remain justifiable. Success in transforming separately organized programs into a more integrated model requires vision and guidance from leadership and management levels, as well as a training strategy that will instill new knowledge, skills and attitudes to front-line staff. This process should be guided by evidence, and a commitment to monitoring and evaluation.

You can survive for 3 minutes without air. After 3 days, you need water or you'll perish. You can make it 3 weeks without food. The purpose of this chapter is to discuss the relationships between human health and access to clean air, a safe drinking water supply, sanitation, food security, food safety, and nutrition. The relationship linking water, food and human health rests on complex connections between the water requirements of crops and animals used for human consumption and the human needs for water to survive. Human health and survival is inextricably linked with the provision of air, water, and food and the protection of these basic determinants of life from pollution and contamination.

7

AIR, WATER, AND FOOD

THE BASIC ELEMENTS of life—air, water and food—are generally considered as part of the discipline of environmental health within public health programs. Our inclusion of the nutritional aspects of food expands on most discussions of environmental health that deal with food safety but not nutrition. All three elements involve a dynamic tension between the need for economic and resource development and the need to maintain the health of populations. Virtually all forms of economic development entail health, social, and environmental impacts. The precautionary principle, as discussed in chapter 3 and explored further in chapter 9, applies to many issues raised in this chapter as well. There is a related need to balance concerns about environmental degradation with the need for economic growth and expanding markets, which are also critical to human development. How a society chooses to balance the competing issues involved in health protection and disease prevention and economic growth and development is likely to be influenced by cultural and political values. Economic policies that require polluting industries to pay for the cost of environmental degradation is one approach to ensuring the costs of development include environmental health and restorative costs as well. The complex issue of global warming is addressed in greater detail in chapter 9.

In the United States, recognition that certain populations have been inordinately affected by environmental contamination led the Environmental Protection Agency to establish in 1992 a program on environmental justice.[1] *Environmental justice* is defined by the program as: fair treatment and meaningful involvement of all people regardless of race, color, national origin, or income with respect to the development, implementation, and enforcement of environmental laws, regulations, and policies. International agreements have addressed a wide range of issues concerning management of hazardous chemicals from production to disposal; among these is the 1998 Aarhus Convention on Access to Information, Public Participation in Decision Making, and Access to Justice in Environmental Matters (signed by some 40 European and East Asian countries).[2] Other international treaties have targeted more specific environmental topics such as the Kyoto Protocol (1997) to reduce greenhouse gas emissions so as to mitigate global warming.[3]

Air

Air pollution due to human activity is referred to as *anthropogenic*, and dates from the first use of fire.[4] Indirect human impact includes animal causes such as overgrazing, which contributes to desertification and dust storms, and the overproduction of cattle, which emit methane (a greenhouse gas) in "super-natural" abundance. Meanwhile, the widespread clearing and burning of vast forests to expand land use for agriculture affect the natural balance between oxygen, nitrogen, and carbon dioxide and have reduced the variety of biological species either through toxicity or by removal of delicate ecosystems. Not least, the industrialization of the past two centuries, with its exponential increase in airborne emissions, both outdoor and indoor, has compounded the threat to our ecosystem and the public health. While much of the immediate impact is local, there are also longer-term effects due to long-range dissemination of pollutants by air currents, and their eventual deposition and accumulation around the world, such that all species of arctic wildlife are now affected by toxins that had their origins thousands of miles away.[5]

As far as human health is concerned, poor air quality leads to greater prevalence of a number of illnesses. Air quality can be a community issue for neighborhoods located downwind from refineries or near busy highways or can result from global activities such as from major bush fires, volcanic ash, or radioactive drift from a nuclear power plant meltdown. Personal exposure to poor air also occurs in the context of work and home environments, including indirect exposure to tobacco use by others. Anthropogenic sources thus are the major ongoing underlying cause, which we clearly can and should do something about: the major global sources include fossil fuel emissions (for energy production and industrial processing) and uncontrolled burning in the forestry and agricultural industries.

The World Health Organization estimates that approximately 3.3 million deaths occur each year due to air pollution; a figure that represents about 5% of deaths from all causes that occur annually in the world.[6] Of these premature deaths, indoor air pollution is estimated to cause approximately 2 million, mostly in developing countries, almost half of which are due to pneumonia in children under 5 years of age. Urban outdoor air pollution is estimated to cause 1.3 million deaths. For each death, many others are made ill from asthma, chronic bronchitis, circulatory disorders, and other conditions. Those living in middle-income countries disproportionately experience this burden.

The health impacts of air pollution offer a classic example of the "iceberg phenomenon" (See chapter 6 Box 6-2 for a review of this concept).[7] A simple illustration is shown below as a pyramid (Figure 7-1). Mortality, hospital admissions, and visits to health care providers are shown at the apex or "tip of the iceberg," which includes people least able to withstand the effects of toxic air, often due to underlying conditions that render them more susceptible or circumstances that result in them being more exposed. In some development settings (see relevant discussions in chapters 8 and 9) people suffer from severe cardio-respiratory morbidity and mortality in the face of air pollution disasters without access to formal health care. Toward the pyramid's base is an increasing mass of people with lower severity disease, disorder, and dysfunction that does not come to the immediate attention of health care systems. Many take steps to cope, such as to reduce activity or seek cleaner air, whereas others may self-medicate for symptoms.

Our understanding of the health effects of most air contaminants depends largely on the sciences of toxicology and epidemiology, the former having contributed many theoretical constructs about biological responses to toxic exposures, and the latter most of the human health information. These disciplines also inform decisions and actions to prevent or regulate exposures. As applied to environmental health,

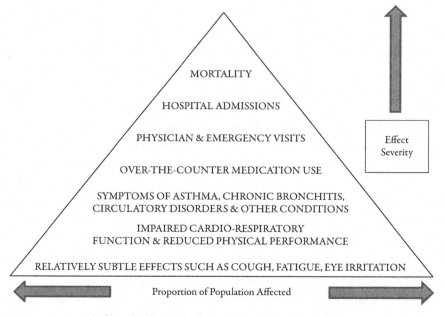

FIGURE 7-1 Pyramid of health effects—the "air pollution iceberg."

they are concerned primarily with harmful effects of substances encountered in our water, food, or air (e.g., outdoor air pollution) or in the often more intense exposures of occupational, residential, or vocational settings (e.g., indoor pollution).

The respective roles of epidemiology and toxicology in elucidating environmental health derive from their inherent strengths and limitations: data mostly from experimental studies in animals is the purview of toxicology and, using those data, findings are extrapolated to people using specified assumptions and mathematical methods. The advantage of this is that human exposure need not have occurred, and that exposure-response relationships are modeled over much shorter periods than usually apply to human populations. Toxicology also employs cell culture studies, where human or animal cells may be used (e.g., genotoxicity tests). In contrast, epidemiology examines human populations for whom exposure has already taken place or is currently occurring, and the findings then applied to that setting or extrapolated to other situations. Simply put, toxicology asks *Could this happen?* while epidemiology answers the questions, after the fact, *Did it happen? Or is it happening?* In practice, the two sciences are complementary.[8]

Toxicology studies generally utilize experimental designs, in which small numbers of animals (or cell culture systems) are randomized into exposure and non-exposure groups, using exposure levels much higher than normal for humans, so that a *result* is obtained that may then be extrapolated to humans.[9] This extrapolation rests on two major assumptions: (1) that very high doses given to small numbers of animals over short time periods can be used to model the effects of low doses to larger numbers over longer periods; and (2) that what can be observed in animal species (e.g., dogs, rats, rabbits) can be applied to humans. Many substances shown to be harmful in such animal studies are assumed thereby to be harmful to people. How reasonable this is depends on considerations such as *species specificity* of a given effect, and whether *thresholds* may exist for lower dose effects.

There are many examples of toxic effects in particular species that do not occur in people, just as there are effects in people that have not been seen in animals. In interpreting animal studies, especially in terms of applicability to humans, one therefore must examine exposure levels, route(s) of administration, absorption, metabolism, translocation, storage, and excretion of the chemical or its metabolites. To assess how plausible it is to extrapolate the findings to humans requires reference to *toxicodynamic* studies: if an experimental animal has metabolic pathways similar to those of people, the likelihood of similar health effects increases, while dissimilar toxicodynamics decreases the likelihood. In practice, this process errs on the side of caution (i.e., if in doubt, assume that extrapolation is justified).

Given the function of the lungs to provide the body with life-sustaining oxygen and to enable the release of carbon dioxide, it makes little logical sense to impede these functions by inhaling substances that could damage these functions, such as tobacco smoke, industrial toxins or ambient air pollutants. Scientific observations from such occupations such as coal mining, confirm that dust inhalation can shorten people's lives and impede quality of life through ill-health. In fact, much of occupational health as a discipline closely allied to public health emerged from such studies into diseases due to dust exposures (known as pneumoconioses) as well as other respiratory hazards in the workplace. Starting with the observations of John Evelyn (chapter 1), air pollution also has been extensively studied in relation to respiratory and (to a lesser extent) circulatory diseases. It is now also known that an array of other (non-cardio-respiratory) adverse outcomes is also associated with poor air quality, and that relevant exposures may be indoors and outdoors.

To illustrate the diversity of air contaminants, Table 7-1 illustrates them, listing their sources and health effects. "Criteria pollutants" are the focus of air pollution monitoring and control efforts, as these are thought to have the greatest impact on cardio-respiratory health; however, non-criteria pollutants also result in many other important outcomes.

Detailed discussions of the direct health effects of tobacco, lead and ozone-depleting chlorofluorocarbons are provided in case studies included in chapter 2. The impact of greenhouse gas emissions on global climate change is discussed in chapter 9.

Water

Humans need water for drinking, cooking and bathing. For communities to thrive, water is needed for agriculture and for manufacturing. Water is also used in many communities as a mode of transportation and as a source of energy. A complex relationship exists between water and sanitation and hygiene knowledge and practices and the role they play in alleviating poverty, promoting human health, advancing educational opportunities, and reducing gender inequity. The United Nations Millennium Development Goals (chapter 5) include two global water targets: by 2015 halve the proportion of people without safe drinking water and halve the proportion of people lacking adequate sanitation.[10]

Over a billion people in developing countries lack access to safe water, and 2.4 billion lack access to adequate sanitation. In rural areas without distribution technology, fetching and carrying water, often performed by women and children, reduces the time available for other subsistence activities. In urban slums from Lima to Karachi, the poor suffer from exploitation by tanker "mafias" delivering water at

TABLE 7-1

Common air contaminants, sources and health effects

Contaminant	Sources	Health Effects
A. Criteria Pollutants-Outdoor Air Quality		
Particulates (fine, coarse inorganic)	Combustion of fossil fuels: vehicle exhaust, wood burning, agricultural burning, forest fires. Emissions from smelters, pulp and paper plants, beehive burners, incinerators. Road dust, volcanic emissions.	*Cardio-respiratory effects*: increased risk of angina and heart attacks, development of atherosclerosis, aggravation of chronic lung disease, risk of pneumonia. Increased health care visits. *Asthmatics*: increased symptoms and reduced pulmonary function, increased emergency visits, hospital admissions and family physician visits. *Cancer*: increased risk of lung cancer
Sulphur dioxide	Coal and oil fired power plants, pulp mills, petrochemical refineries	*Respiratory*: Aggravation of asthma, increased chronic bronchitis.
Carbon monoxide	Vehicle exhaust, wood stoves, tobacco smoke.	*Cardiac*: myocardial ischemia, cerebral impairment, increased hospitalization. *Other*: decreased birth weight.
Nitrogen dioxide	Motor vehicle exhausts, other internal combustion engines, marine vessels, industrial processes. Indoors: unvented gas appliances—stoves, ovens, heaters; ice resurfacers.	*Cardio-respiratory*: aggravation of asthma, chronic bronchiolitis, increased respiratory infections?

Ozone	Photochemical reactions involving nitrogen oxides and VOCs (see below).	*Respiratory*: aggravation of asthma, increased school absence for respiratory disease, hospital admissions, decreased lung function (acute and chronic) decreased lung development, increased mortality.

B. Non-Criteria Pollutants-Outdoor Air Quality
(illustrative selection; note that some also occur indoors)

Lead	Lead smelters. Lead-based paint, lead pipe solder, pipes, toys and cooking utensils.	*Neuro-behavioural*: impaired cognitive development, learning disabilities. *Blood disorders*: interferes with heme synthesis. *Cardio-respiratory*: contributes to hypertension and chronic renal disease.
Benzene	Automotive exhausts; evaporation of gasoline. Tobacco smoke.	*Cancer*: cancers of blood and lymphatic systems (e.g., leukemia). *Neurotoxicity and blood disorders*: at higher concentrations.
Dioxins, furans and polychlorinated biphenyls (PCBs)	Emissions from pesticide plants, incineration of plastics; electrical transformers; dust from waste dumps, herbicides.	*Skin lesions*: burns and chloracne *Breast milk*: chemicals excreted and ingested by infants. *Reproductive effects*: disruption in hormonal balance. *Metabolic*: liver enzyme changes *Cancer*: soft tissue sarcomas, N-H lymphoma; but evidence is controversial.

(*continued*)

TABLE 7-1 (Continued)

Contaminant	Sources	Health Effects
Pesticides	Forestry and agricultural spraying; domestic applications indoors and outdoors. Aerial drift (off-target) of spray operations.	*Neurobehavioral disorders*: headaches, dizziness, twitching, tremors, muscle weakness, parasthesias, balance disturbances, slurred speech, paralysis. *Hypersensitivity reactions*: skin rashes. *Cancer*: mutagenicity carcinogenicity, and teratogenicity *Immune system impacts*: suppresses both humoral and cell-mediated immunity
Hydrogen sulphide	Gas wells; pulp mills; vegetation decay; sewage; geothermal emissions.	*Olfactory*: bad odor ("sewage gas," "rotten egg gas"). *Eyes*: irritation *Central Nervous System*: (high levels) CNS depression, respiratory paralysis.
Pollens and Spores	Seasonal plants	*Respiratory*: allergic responses in susceptible persons; may be expressed as rhinitis (runny nose), eye irritation, and/or asthma.
C. Selected Indoor Air Pollutants (illustrative selection; note that some also occur outdoors)		
Environmental Tobacco Smoke and other Combustion by-products	Smoking cigarettes, cigars and/or pipes; woodstoves, for heating or cooking, if poorly exhausted and when ventilation is inadequate	*Circulatory effects*: increased risk of angina, heart attacks, stroke *Respiratory effects*: aggravation of chronic lung disease, risk of pneumonia, increased risk of lung cancer; increases in the prevalence of asthma; in asthmatics: increased symptoms and reduced lung function, increased health care visits and hospital admissions.

Agent	Sources	Effects
Volatile Organic Compounds (VOCs) (e.g., benzene, formaldehyde)	Gasoline vapors, diesel exhaust, consumer products: paints, carpets, furnishings; chemical industries, compressed construction materials; many natural sources also.	*Variable Effects* depend on the chemical (e.g., see above: benzene; formaldehyde associated with upper airway and eye irritation, and after many years occupational exposure risk of nasopharyngeal cancer); mucous membrane irritation; neurobehavioral effects. [Note: public health significance of this class of chemicals not fully assessed].
Toluene	evaporation from gasoline, vehicle exhaust emissions, solvents; glue sniffing	*Neurobehavioral*: headaches, dizziness, twitching, tremors, muscle weakness, parasthesias, balance disturbances, slurred speech, paralysis.
Asbestos	Released from renovation and demolition of buildings containing asbestos, and removal of insulation.	*Respiratory*: asbestosis, chronic bronchitis, lung cancer, mesothelioma (pleural and peritoneal), gastric cancers; interacts with tobaccos to increase risk of chronic bronchitis and lung cancer.
Radon	Released from ground in mines, tunnels and some basements; may infiltrate other house rooms.	*Respiratory*: Elevated risk of lung cancer; increased risk in smokers.
Microbiological agents	Contaminated AC cooling towers; poorly ventilated and damp buildings/houses; dusty/moldy, inadequately cleaned indoor spaces; water damaged indoor surfaces.	*Respiratory*: Pulmonary infection of bacteria may lead to pneumonia (e.g., legionellosis); inhaled molds may also cause pulmonary infection and/or asthma; allergic responses in sensitive individuals. Other toxic effects from released endotoxins in related dust.

prices up to 20 times that paid by those who enjoy a municipal supply; poor households spend up to 40% of their income on water.[11] In some developing countries the ability to develop water supply systems is inhibited by costs, by civil unrest, and by lack of infrastructure. The abuse of water security as an instrument of conflict has increased exponentially: of 30 such events over a recent 20 year period, half were military actions targeting water supplies, resulting in widespread water-borne diseases, affecting mainly infants and children; this form of biological warfare is not recognized under the Biological Weapons Convention (1972).[12]

Humans have historically manipulated natural bodies of water, located underground aquifers by digging or drilling wells, and captured rainwater for drinking and for crops and livestock. Altering the flow of water in rivers, for such economic purposes as power generation and irrigation, has increased problems with flooding for people living along river banks and in low-lying areas; it has sometimes resulted in silting and salination, ultimately obstructing irrigation schemes and reducing water quality. Flooding can be a part of a natural cycle of soil replenishment, but it can also adversely affect food production and increase contamination from chemicals used by humans (pesticides, chemicals used in manufacturing, petroleum products). One concern with climate change is the potential for changing water levels in low lying areas resulting in an increased number of flooding events, as already experienced in some settings such as Bangladesh and the Tokelau islands in the Pacific, resulting in both internal and external migration pressures. Elsewhere there is concern that climate change is impacting arid areas through aggravating drought conditions. These related issues are further discussed in chapter 9.

Water systems have become increasingly complex throughout history and have provided harbor for pathogens, heavy metals and chemicals that cause human disease. Microbial pathogens in water are globally ubiquitous and include bacteria, viruses, protozoa, and other organisms.[13] As discussed in chapter 6, transmission may occur due to ingestion of contaminated water by humans or animals, often associated with inadequate food and beverage preparation and poor personal hygiene (e.g., insufficient hand-washing, face-washing, and bathing), while some diseases are associated with insect vectors and parasites that contaminate or propagate in and around water. Prevention and control approaches (chapter 6) are primarily based on interrupting modes of transmission, among which the provision of potable water is preeminent for waterborne diseases. Other diseases and adverse health conditions are associated with contamination of water by heavy metals and chemicals: direct effects may be incurred by ingesting toxins in water, while indirectly toxic effects may occur are a result of ingesting fish or wildlife that have consumed from a contaminated source.[14] Chemical pollutants of concern to water quality and health may come from natural or man-made sources; they are increasingly the focus of monitoring studies in many parts of the world, such as by the International Joint Commission under the *1909 Boundary Waters Treaty* (United States and Canada).[15]

In order to control the diseases associated with waterborne pathogens, people developed treatment approaches that have resulted in the introduction of the disinfection byproducts that are themselves associated with new disease risks including cancers and adverse reproductive outcomes.[16, 17, 18, 19] Disinfection byproducts are formed when chemicals used in a water treatment react with bromide or decaying vegetation present in water being treated; different disinfectants produce different types and/or amounts of by-products including the following: trihalomethanes, haloacetic acids, bromate, and chlorite.[10]

The primary goals of water resource management, water supply systems, and sanitation networks are to provide for sustainable use of water resources and to reduce water-related diseases. Given the ongoing need to prevent waterborne epidemics due to microbial pathogens (see later section), the efficacy and safety of treatment technologies in themselves has also become a continuing focus for research and policy development. Augmenting supply methods such as diverting water from natural sources, digging or drilling wells, rainwater catchment, recycling, reclamation, and desalination, efforts are also under way to improve drinking water safety through improved filtering, on-site disinfection, and other developing technologies including lower cost alternatives.

Waterborne Diseases

Waterborne diseases are caused by pathogenic microbes that can be directly transmitted to humans through water. Often the transmission of pathogenic organisms is the result of poor systems of sanitation. Most waterborne diseases cause gastroenteritis: 88% of diarrhea cases worldwide are linked to unsafe water, inadequate sanitation or insufficient hygiene.[20] Most vulnerable are children, who suffer over 3 million deaths annually from diseases due to lack of water, dirty water, and inadequate sanitation.

Cholera is a classic example of a gastrointestinal disease caused by a gram-negative bacterium *Vibrio cholerae*, which first became pandemic in 1817 when it spread from India to Europe then to the rest of the world. The world is currently considered to be experiencing its seventh pandemic; it is believed that the first six cholera pandemics were caused by the classical biotype, but the new El Tor biotype has subsequently spread globally and replaced the classical biotype in the current pandemic.[21] Where cholera is endemic, disasters such as widespread flooding can cause epidemics affecting people who are displaced from their homes, living in crowded and unsanitary conditions. For example, an earthquake in Haiti in January 2010 displaced a large portion of the population. Living in temporary camps under unsanitary conditions with limited water for drinking and for washing, an unprecedented epidemic of cholera occurred. As of December 3, 2011 a total of 91,770 cases of cholera were reported; 43,243 (47.1%) patients had been hospitalized, and 2,071 (2.3%) had died. Cholera had not been documented in Haiti for over a decade at the time of the outbreak.[22] So even in areas where the disease in uncommon, the displacement of a large number of people can result in reintroduction of a disease that is not usually seen in an area, and can be the result of efforts to provide aid to communities affected by a disaster.

However, in most situations where water and sanitation infrastructures are compromised, the disease burden tends to come from an array of enteric pathogens other than cholera (which actually accounts only for a small percentage of global gastroenteritis morbidity and mortality). This stands to reason because it is the same endemic organisms that are normally present in a community that get out of control when disaster strikes.

While effective primary prevention of gastroenteritis requires prudent attention to the quality of drinking water quality, for many people in developing countries this is not feasible due to the realities of their immediate circumstances, and in any event is often too late (epidemic diarrhea can establish itself very quickly). This is why oral rehydration to replace fluid and electrolyte loss (a form of secondary prevention—see chapter 6 therapy—(ORT)) is so important to promote as a core local health practice in developing countries. Since its development and widespread introduction in Bangladesh about 4 decades ago, ORT has saved millions of lives around the world. This said, ORT for diarrhea reaches only about half of those in need. Also, without water for washing, both skin and serious eye infections can become epidemic (see AMREF case study chapter 4).

Only universal provision of hygiene education, potable water and sanitation can virtually eliminate water-borne diseases in the long term. While high-income countries can generally afford to install comprehensive water and sanitation infrastructures, in many parts of the world simple low cost technologies are necessary, such as the use of chlorine drops in dedicated water containers, filter systems locally acquired (e.g., sand, clothe, or boiling, which can be unsustainable); rainwater catchment is an important source for many and can be made safe, while solar technologies are being developed in some settings. The development of safe local water supply systems, properly managed and regularly tested by trained individuals, is a major development thrust in many parts of the world; interventions to improve hygiene education and practices show promise.[23]

Vector or Insect-borne Diseases

Water plays a critical role in the spread of insect-borne diseases because many insects, such as mosquitoes, breed around water. Poorly designed irrigation and water systems and poor water disposal and storage may contribute to vector-borne diseases (chapter 6) including malaria (chapter 2), dengue fever, and leishmaniasis.[24] Flooding can directly impact the number and dispersal of breeding sites of mosquitoes and other insects, thereby creating new environments for disease; often compounding the health impacts of disasters.[25] Concerns about climate change and the changing geographic distribution of vectors of human disease have been expressed;[26] we return to this in chapter 9.

The World Health Organization has promoted integrated vector management, an approach that builds upon the link between health and the environment. Integrated vector management (introduced in chapter 6) stresses the importance of understanding the local vector ecology and local patterns of disease transmission before choosing the vector control methods. Strategies include environmental management to reduce breeding grounds through improved design, improved operation of water resources development projects, and use of biological controls such as bacterial larvicides and larvivorous fish to reduce the need for chemicals. Chemical methods of vector control are used when other measures are ineffective or not cost-effective. Chemical measures are designed to reduce disease transmission by interrupting the lifespan of vectors and include indoor residual sprays, space spraying, use of chemical larvicides and adulticides. Personal protection and preventive strategies combine environmental management and chemical tools such as insecticide-treated nets. Insecticide-treated nets have been effective in reducing child and infant mortality in malaria-endemic countries.

Health Impact Assessment (HIA) of new infrastructure development in water resources, irrigation and agriculture is recommended to help identify potential impacts such as vector-borne disease and to assist in developing effective policies.[27,28] HIAs involve working with a range of decision makers and community groups to assist in determining the potential health effects before a policy, program, or project is implemented.

Chemical Contaminants

A number of chemicals associated with manufacturing, mining, and agriculture and other industries have been shown to contaminate surface and groundwater, causing human exposures and disease such as arsenic, atrazine, cadmium, lead, mercury, nitrates, and radon. There are concerns as well with regard to potential contamination as a result of oil and gas exploration and extraction, especially the newly widespread practice of hydraulic fracturing of rock structures. From the pharmaceutical industry there is concern about the impacts of drugs such as antibiotics and hormones when they reach watercourses.

Studies using ecosystem approaches have identified sources, transmission, and health effects that link water contamination by toxic materials to the contamination of fish consumed as a dietary mainstay in the Amazon and in the Great Lakes.[29] An ecosystems approach to the potentially contentious debate regarding nutritious food (fish) and toxics allows for an approach that takes into account ecological, social, cultural, and dietary influences; the aim is to maximize benefits for all while minimizing risks. This approach is especially relevant for vulnerable populations, for example indigenous peoples with traditional fishing rights, who may be most affected by policies prohibiting fishing in contaminated waters.

The widespread use of the herbicide atrazine has raised concerns with regard to its potential for adverse health consequences, but there is considerable disagreement about whether humans are affected or not. Studies have identified atrazine in groundwater in the Midwest of the United States and the search for human health effects linked to atrazine exposure continues in cancer, preterm delivery and endocrine disruption[30]. Atrazine is widely used to control weeds and while animal studies have suggested serious health effects, studies among humans have been less definitive.[31] However, the persistence of atrazine in groundwater is of concern.[32] The use of atrazine to control noxious weeds has allowed farmers to increase crop yields, further it is the most heavily used pesticide in the United States and perhaps worldwide.[26] Further there have been studies reporting endocrine disruption in frogs leading to feminization of male frogs both in laboratory studies and in the wild.[33, 34] Seven countries in the European Union (EU) have banned atrazine: France, Sweden, Denmark, Finland, Germany, Austria and Italy. These countries have a policy of banning pesticides that occur in drinking water at levels higher than o.1 parts per billion. EU countries that have not banned atrazine include the United Kingdom, Ireland, Belgium, and Luxemburg. Australia has conducted safety reviews of atrazine and has not banned use. In the United States, the Environmental Protection Agency has been conducting a review of evidence that has accumulated since 2003.[35]

Other Water Contaminants and Injuries

Other diseases in humans associated with water have been attributed to algal blooms and fungi (e.g., ringworm). Drowning is also a water related hazard for people.

Worldwide, an estimated 400,000 people die each year from drowning.[36] A majority of drowning occur in open bodies of water (oceans, lakes, ponds, and rivers). Uniform guidelines have been developed for management of recreational waters; these include adult supervision of children, legal blood alcohol levels during water recreational activities, swimming lessons, and use of lifejackets.

Food

Food is discussed from the following perspectives: food production and distribution systems, food security, food safety, and nutrition including conditions resulting from too little or too much nutrition. The first of the Millennium Development Goals (chapter 5) is to halve the proportion of people in extreme poverty and hunger by the year 2015.[37]

The food system is an ideal area to draw on the ecosystem approach to health as there is a complex interaction between the dynamics involved in food production, food culture, international trade policies, and human health. Figure 7-2 provides a schematic diagram for the complex array of factors that constitute the agro-ecosystem.

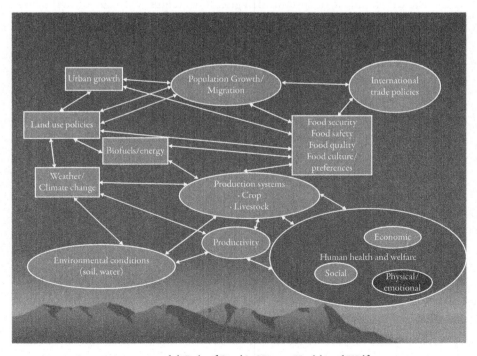

FIGURE 7-2 Agro-ecosystem model. Role of Food in Human Health and Welfare.

The quality and quantity of food are important determinants of human and community health. Contamination of food by pathogenic organisms, toxic chemicals, or other adulterating substances can cause diseases in humans. The absence or deficiency of essential ingredients such as vitamins or minerals can also result in human diseases (see the Iodine Case Study in chapter 6). Nutritional needs of pregnant women, infants, and growing children are of special concern, and increasingly overeating has become a global concern with ever increasing numbers of overweight and obese people.

Food Production

The food production system includes the growing, harvesting, transporting, processing, packaging, storage, distribution, and sales of food. With urbanization and mechanization in agriculture, separation between the production and consumption of food has increased. Food grown in distant parts of the world has become common in grocery stores and markets in many communities. This industrialization of the food distribution system and global distribution of food has led to increased demands for food inspection worldwide. There has also been a call for increased attention to the influence this separation has on human health and on the environment. The development of sustainable agriculture requires an agricultural system that can meet demands for food, fiber, and fuel at a socially acceptable economic and environmental cost.

Current advocates for changes in the food production and distribution system are calling for an agro-ecosystem approach that incorporates an understanding of the role of food in human health, animal well-being, the economics of food production and costs to the environment of distribution systems, and the ecological conditions that are involved not only in the production of food but also influenced by agricultural activity. Agricultural food systems are needed that are economically viable, meet society's need for safe and nutritious food while conserving natural resources and the environment.

Food Safety

Many types of foodborne microbial exposures result in illnesses (Table 7-2); just as for communicable diseases generally, responsible pathogens include bacteria, viruses, parasites, and prions. Most bacterial and viral foodborne diseases have rapid onset (incubation periods measured in hours or days), for example, salmonellosis (a common bacterial disease in many countries) and Norwalk virus disease (the leading viral cause of gastroenteritis globally). Parasitic foodborne diseases have typically

TABLE 7-2

General features of foodborne illnesses and exposures

Type	Features
Parasitic infections	Variable symptoms: enteritis, anemia, pneumonia, skin sores, cysts
	Variable incubation periods
	Transmission through fecal-oral route, undercooking meat and fish
Infections (bacterial, viral)	Vomiting, nausea, diarrhea
	Systemic symptoms (e.g., fever)
	Variable incubation periods and duration
	Transmissible to others
Transmissible spongiform encephalopathies (TSEs) or Prion diseases	Degenerative fatal brain disease
	Transmissible through consumption of cattle ill from bovine spongiform encephalopathy (BSE)
	Transmissible through invasive medical interventions
Bacterial toxins Staphylococcal enterotoxin	Explosive onset after short incubation period
	Vomiting predominates
	Few or no systemic symptoms
	Not transmissible
Botulism	Slow onset
	Neurotoxic symptoms
	Not transmissible
Plant, food poisons	Short incubation
	Dramatic symptoms, usually gastrointestinal
Chemical contamination	Variable incubation-minutes, days, years
	Widespread systemic effects
	Chronic conditions including neurological conditions, birth defects, cancer

longer incubations, usually weeks following exposure (e.g., ascariasis), while much longer incubation periods are observed for transmissible spongiform encephalopathies (TSEs), such as variant Creutzfeldt-Jakob Disease (vCJD): these take decades to become apparent. Bacterial food poisoning differs from other forms of bacterial foodborne illness in that these result from a toxic by-product or metabolite of a micro-organism that has contaminated food (e.g., botulism and staphylococcal enterotoxic gastroenteritis). Other relevant discussion of some of these conditions is found in chapter 6, where we also recommend the Control of Communicable Diseases Manual[38] for more detailed information on distribution, reservoir, modes of transmission, incubation periods, periods of communicability, susceptibility and resistance, as well as methods of prevention and control.

Chemicals can also contaminate the food chain, and mercury is a classic example. Well known as an environmental pollutant for half a century and as an occupational hazard for hundreds of years,[39] community health concerns arise today mainly when fish and wildlife from contaminated ecosystems are consumed by humans. The most well-documented outbreaks of severe methyl-mercury poisoning are from Minamata Bay, Japan in 1956 (industrial release of methyl-mercury) and in Iraq in 1971 (wheat treated with a methyl-mercury fungicide). In each instance, hundreds of people died, and thousands were affected, many with permanent damage. With milder levels of mercury poisoning, adults complain of reductions in motor skills and dulled senses of touch, taste, and sight. However, fetal and early childhood exposures pose the greatest risk.[40]

Chemical food poisoning received recent attention due to contamination of milk products with melamine in China (see Box 7-1). Contamination of food with chemicals can be unintentional or intentional. It can also occur from utensils or containers if the chemical is toxic or if it interacts with the food being stored or prepared.

BOX 7-1

CHEMICAL CONTAMINATION OF MILK PRODUCTS IN CHINA, 2008

An estimated 300,000 children were sickened and six died as a result of consuming dairy products laced with the industrial chemical melamine. The industrial chemical was added to thousands of tons of watered-down milk to deceive inspectors testing for protein content and increase profits in one of the most high-profile contamination issues in recent years. Tens of thousands of Chinese children sickened by melamine-tainted milk showed signs of kidney damage months afterward—with the potential for long-term harm a serious concern, said new research.

The manufacturer, Sanlu, part-owned by New Zealand's Fonterra Cooperative, recalled all of its powdered milk products in China's north-west province of Gansu. However, twenty-two brands of milk powder were quickly identified as containing melamine. Allegedly, someone in the supply chain, a milk supplier or manufacturer, was adding melamine to the milk formula to artificially increase the apparent protein levels. Formula milk had not until this outbreak been tested for melamine, because regulators did not suspect this ingredient might be added.

An example of chemical contamination from containers is the bisphenol A (BPA), an industrial chemical used to strengthen and harden plastic and used in many consumer products, including reusable water bottles and baby bottles.[41] BPA is also found in epoxy resin protective linings on the inside of metal food and beverage cans. Canada is the first country in the world to take action on BPA.[42] In the United States, several counties, Chicago, and Minnesota have prohibited BPAs in beverage containers used for children under 3 years of age.[43] Connecticut has banned BPA in reusable food and beverage containers and in plastic containers, jars or cans that contain infant formula or baby food.[44] Recent legislative activity on BPA has taken place in Oregon, Washington, Wisconsin, and Vermont.[45]

Poisonous plants or animals are sometimes eaten in the mistaken belief that they are edible. Travelers, immigrants and others not familiar with local hazards may be at particularly high risk of consuming poisonous plants and animals.

A detailed foodborne illness is presented in Box 7-2.

BOX 7-2

CONTAMINATION OF PROCESSED FOOD: PEANUT BUTTER AND PEANUT BUTTER PASTE

In November, 2008, an epidemiologic investigation by the Centers for Disease Control and Prevention was initiated due to an increasing number of cases of *Salmonella* serotype *typhimurium*.[79] By January 28, 2009, 529 people from 43 states in the United States and one person in Canada were reported to have been infected with the outbreak strain. Of these, 116 cases were hospitalized and the *Salmonella* may have contributed to 8 deaths. Case control studies indicated significant associations between consumption of peanut butter and specific brands of prepackaged peanut butter crackers with no association reported with national brands of peanut butter sold in stores. The Minnesota Department of Health conducted detailed investigations of patients infected with the outbreak strain, as did many state health departments where there were cases. In December 2008, a number of patients were identified who lived or ate in one of three institutions. The investigation found that the institution had a common food distributor in North Dakota but the only food common to all three was King Nut creamy peanut butter. An open container of King Nut peanut butter was found to contain the outbreak strain of *Salmonella*.

During January, 2009, other states reported similar laboratory results from samples of King Nut peanut butter. All versions of King Nut peanut butter were produced by Peanut Corporation of America at a single facility in Blakely, Georgia. Early in January, the Food and Drug Administration began an investigation of the Peanut Company of America in Blakely, Georgia. King Nut peanut butter was distributed in bulk packaging to institutions, food service industries, and private food label companies but not

(continued)

BOX 7-2 (Continued)

directly marketed to consumers or distributed in grocery stores. A number of patients did not eat peanut butter in institutions but did eat other peanut containing products. The Blakely facility also produced peanut paste and other peanut products that were sold to food companies for use as an ingredient and widely distributed throughout the United States and in at least 23 other countries and non-US territories. Control measures included the voluntary suspension of production at the Blakely plant by the Peanut Company of America on January 9, 2009. On January 10, 2009, King Nut Company issued a voluntary recall of specific lot numbers of peanut butter. On January 16, 2009, Peanut Company of America announced a voluntary recall of all peanut butter and peanut paste produced at the Blakely facility since July 1, 2008 and expanded the recall to include all the same products processed since January 1, 2007. In January, the Food and Drug Administration also began an investigation of a Peanut Company of America facility in Plainview, Texas.[80] By February, 2009 the outbreak strain was confirmed in peanut meal from the Peanut Company of America facility in Plainview, Texas.

This outbreak led to one of the largest product recalls in the nation's history, with more than 2,000 products recalled as of February, 2009. This example provides a perspective regarding the complexity of determining the source of contamination in the current food system where a single facility has such a wide distribution system and the wide array of peanut containing processed foods made the outbreak investigation to track the epidemiological pattern of disease of extreme value in identifying the source.

SANITARY CONTROL OF MILK

Milk and milk products are susceptible to contamination with pathogenic micro-organisms. Pathogenic organisms may be shed even by healthy cows, goats, and sheep. Contamination can come directly from the cow or can be introduced by dairy workers. Raw milk may contain many pathogens including but not limited to *Mycobacterium tuberculosis, Mycobacterium bovus, enterotoxigenic Staphylococcus aureus, Campylobacter jejuni, Salmonella* species, *E. coli, Listeria monocytogenes, Brucella* species, *Coxiella Burnetti,* and *Yersenia enterocolitica.*[46]

Pasteurization is a process developed to kill harmful bacteria by heating milk to a specific temperature for a specified period. Despite the effectiveness of pasteurization in killing pathogenic bacteria, nonpathogenic bacteria may still be present and can cause milk to spoil, therefore refrigeration is used to prevent spoilage. Other ways to safeguard milk products includes boiling, freeze drying, and condensing. Sweetened condensed milk relies on high sugar concentration to kill pathogens. Pasteurization of milk has been recognized as a public health control measure throughout the world. In Canada, federal and many provincial regulations prohibit the sale of raw milk. However, in many countries the direct sale of unpasteurized milk to consumers is allowed with certain restriction and limitations.

Federal regulation of dairy processing plants requiring milk pasteurization and sanitation has been in existence in the United States for nearly 100 years.[47] As a result of regulations under the US Public Health Service and a variety of state and local regulatory agencies, the incidence of milk-borne illness in the United States has decreased from approximately 25% of reported foodborne illnesses in 1938 to less than 1%. Currently in the United States, federal regulation prohibits the introduction of any unpasteurized milk product in final packaged form intended for human consumption into interstate commerce. Some, but not all, states permit the intra-state sale of raw milk intended for human consumption.

Milk may also contain other contaminants such as pesticides, antibiotic residues, polychlorinated biphenols (PCBs), dioxins, and radioactive trace elements that are not affected by pasteurization or other means of reducing pathogens.

QUALITY CONTROL IN FOOD PRODUCTION, MANUFACTURING, AND PREPARATION

The following section provides a few examples of the relationship between human disease and quality control in food production and in manufacturing/processing (also see Box 7-3).[48]

ANIMAL FEEDING PRACTICES AND DISEASE IN HUMANS

In 1986, bovine spongiform encepalopathy (BSE) was recognized in cattle in the United Kingdom (UK).[49] The leading initial hypothesis about the cause of the outbreak that followed was cross-species transmission of scrapie (a fatal transmissible degenerative disease of sheep) to cattle by feeding meat and bone meal that was contaminated with scrapie-infected sheep parts. In 1988, a ruminant feed ban was instituted that prohibited the practice of using rendered BSE infected carcasses for cattle feed and in 1990, a ban was introduced to remove the known infectious parts of cattle in all animal feed. BSE received worldwide attention because of the impact it had on the farming industry and international trade but also because of strong evidence that indicated transmission to humans causing a variant form of Creutzfedlt-Jakob Disease (vCJD).[49] National surveillance of CJD instituted in the United Kingdom yielded an unusual clustering of 10 young patients with a unique clinical and neuropathic profile, described in 1996. The absence of similar cases in other countries with CJD surveillance systems, their continued occurrence in the UK, and additional laboratory studies have strengthened the causal link between

BOX 7-3
UNITED STATES

Food and Drug Administration

The Reportable Food Registry was established by section 1005 of the Food and Drug Administration Amendments Act of 2007 (Pub. L. 110–85), which amended the Federal Food, Drug, and Cosmetic Act (FD&C Act) by creating a new section 417, Reportable Food Registry [21 U.S.C. 350f], and required FDA to establish an electronic portal by which reports about instances of *reportable food* must be submitted to FDA within 24 hours by *responsible parties* and may be submitted by public health officials. These reports may be *primary*, the initial submission about a *reportable food*, or *subsequent*, a report by either a supplier (upstream) or a recipient (downstream) of a food or food ingredient for which a *primary report* has been submitted.

The RFR covers all human and animal food/feed (including pet food) regulated by FDA except infant formula and dietary supplements. Other mandatory reporting systems exist for problems with infant formula and dietary supplements. Submissions to the Reportable Food electronic portal provide early warning to FDA about potential public health risks from reportable foods and increase the speed with which the agency and its partners at the state and local levels can investigate the reports and take appropriate follow-up action, including ensuring that the reportable foods are removed from commerce when necessary.

The RFR does not receive reports about drugs or other medical products, reports about products under the exclusive jurisdiction of the U.S. Department of Agriculture, or reports from consumers.

vCJD and BSE. As of 2004, there were a total of 151 vCJD cases reported in the UK with three cases (one each from Canada, Ireland, and the USA) reported among people with potential BSE exposure in the UK.[49]

Food Security

The World Food Summit of 1996 defined food security as existing "when all people at all times have access to sufficient, safe, nutritious food to maintain a healthy and active life."[50, 51] In developing countries the combination of malnutrition and food-borne diarrhea is a double burden, furthering inadequate nutritional uptake and increasing the risk of severe illness and death.[52, 53]

The primary link between food security and health is through malnutrition. The World Food Summit goal is to halve the number of malnourished people between 1990–1992 and 2015.[54] Recent food and economic crises have increased food price volatility and resulted in higher food prices, challenging the ability to reach the goal.

In 2007 and 2008 commodity prices skyrocketed and locally grown food became cheaper than imported food, but local producers were unable to keep up with the demand.[50] Table 7-3 presents the prevalence of undernourished people by region in the world with reference to the progress toward the World Food Summit goal; except for favorable progress in developed countries, the trends from 1990 to 2008 are not encouraging.

A majority of working people in most developing countries are employed in agriculture. International agricultural agreements in developing countries support the development of export crops and increase local food insecurity by diverting the farmers who might otherwise be raising crops for local consumption. A group of World Trade Organization (WTO) member states have called for agricultural agreements that allow developing countries to raise tariffs on key products to protect national food security and employment.[54] Also of concern is the role of massive agricultural subsidies in developed countries, which suppress the potential for sustainable agriculture (including export markets) in developing ones, and even outweighing the entire value of all foreign aid.[55] Further problems with trade policies include the exporting of crops at prices below the cost of production. With importation of low cost commodities into developing countries, local farmers were unable to compete and reduced their production.[54]

Currently there are concerns about food-price volatility linked to with wide swings in commodity prices; farmers around the world are having a difficult time planning their crop and livestock production. Between 2005 and 2008, global food prices increased 83%.[56] The Food and Agriculture Organization (FAO) of the United Nations estimated that price increases pushed an additional 40 million people into hunger that year, raising the total number of undernourished people in the world to 963 million compared to 923 million in 2007.[57] The economies most impacted by rising prices are developing countries and within these countries the low-income groups who depend on local markets to access food. These groups spend up to four-fifths of their income on food, such that higher prices undermine the ability of poor households to meet essential food needs. To further complicate the food security situation worldwide, the cost of feed, fuel, fertilizers, and seeds has been equally volatile and increasing. This makes it more difficult for farmers in developing countries and in more developed countries to afford to keep production stable.

Another issue raised by the FAO is that of the gender gap for women working in agriculture.[58] Women comprise an average of 43% of the agricultural labor force in developing countries, ranging from 20% in Latin America to 50% in Eastern Asia and sub-Saharan Africa.[53] At this time in developing countries the agricultural

TABLE 7-3

Prevalence of undernourishment and progress toward the world food summit targets in developing countries

Region	Total population 2006–08 (millions)	Number of People Undernourished				
		1990–92	1995–97	2000–02	2006–08	% change
World	6652.5	848.4	791.5	836.2	850.0	0.2
Developed regions	1231.3	15.3	17.5	15.4	10.6	−30.8
Developing regions	5402.2	833.2	774.0	820.4	839.4	0.8
Least-developed countries[a]	796.7	211.2	249.0	244.7	263.8	24.9
Landlocked developing countries[b]	382.8	90.2	101.6	102.5	98.3	8.9
Small island developing countries[c]	52.2	9.6	10.9	9.7	10.7	11.8

a. Afghanistan, Angola, Bangladesh, Benin, Burkina Faso, Burundi, Cambodia, Central Africa Republic, Chad, Comoros, Democratic Republic of the Congo, Djibouti, Eritrea, Ethiopia, Gambia, Guinea, Guinea Bissau, Haiti, Kiribati, Lao People's Democratic Republic, Lesotho, Liberia, Madagascar, Malawi, Mali, Mauritania, Mozambique, Myanmar, Nepal, Niger, Rwanda, Samoa, Sao Tome and Principe, Senegal, Sierra Leone, Solomon Islands, Somalia, Sudan, United Republic of Tanzania, Timor-Leste, Togo, Uganda, Vanuatu, Yemen, Zambia.

b. Afghanistan, Armenia, Azerbaijan, Bolivia, Botswana, Burkina Faso, Central African Republic, Chad, Ethiopia, Kazakhstan, Kyrgyzstan, Lao People's Democratic Republic, Lesotho, Macedonia, Malawi, Mali, Republic of Moldova, Mongolia, Nepal, Niger, Paraguay, Rwanda, Swaziland, Tajikistan, Turkmenistan, Uganda, Uzbekistan, Zambia, Zimbabwe.

c. Antigua and Barbuda, Bahamas, Barbados, Belize, Cape Verde, Comoros, Cuba, Dominican Republic, Fiji Islands, French Polynesia, Grenada, Guinea Bissau, Guyana, Haiti, Jamaica, Kiribati, Maldives, Mauritius, Netherlands Antilles, New Caledonia, Papua New Guinea, Saint Kitts and Nevus, Saint Lucia, Saint Vincent/Grenadines, Samoa, Sao Tome and Principe, Seychelles, Solomon Islands, Suriname, Timor-Leste, Trinidad and Tobago, Vanuatu.

Source: Modified with permission from the Food and Agricultural Organization of the United Nations (FAO). Adapted from Table, Technical Annex. The State of Food Security in the World. FAO Rome 2009.[54]

sector is underperforming, and one of the key contributors is that women farmers do not have equal access to resources and opportunities they need to be productive. Women control less land than men, they own fewer farm animals, the land they have access to is poorer quality, they use fewer modern inputs (e.g. fertilizers, pest control measures, and mechanical tools), and they have less credit, less education, and less access to extension services.[53] These factors prevent women from adopting new techniques that produce higher yields. FAO reports that yield gaps between men and women averages 20–30%, with most of the difference attributed to resource use.[53] If the yield averages of women were raised to those of men, the estimated increase in agricultural output in developing countries would be between 2.5 and 4%. This would reduce the number of undernourished people in the world between 12–17%, or bring the number of undernourished people down by 100–150 million. Closing the gender gap in agricultural production would also serve to put more resources in the hands of women, strengthen their voice in their homes, which is a proven strategy for enhancing food security, nutrition, education, and the health of children.[53]

Nutrition

Human nutrition is the process by which substances in food are transformed into body tissues and provide energy for the full range of physical and mental activities that make up human life. Essential nutrients include carbohydrates, proteins, fats and oils, vitamins, and minerals.

MALNUTRITION

Malnutrition is the physical condition resulting either from an inadequate supply of nutrients or from a physical inability to absorb or metabolize nutrients. The essential nutritional requirements for a healthy diet include some carbohydrates, proteins, fats or oils, and a variety of vitamins and minerals.

Children who do not have sufficient caloric intake or are nutrient deficient are at higher risk of illness and death. The manifestations of undernourishment among children include stunting (low height for age) and wasting (low weight for height). The prevalence of measurable childhood malnutrition (stunting or wasting) in many developing countries falls within 35 and 40%, and malnutrition is an underlying cause in a large proportion of child deaths (e.g., 60% of deaths under 5 years in Pakistan).[59] Protein-energy malnourished children develop marasmus, which is associated with very low weight, weakness, and susceptibility to infections.[60] Those with diets dominated by protein deficiency develop kwashiorkor: while they may appear to maintain a moderate weight, much of this is due to edema (fluid accumulation), often characterized by a swollen belly. Marasmus and kwashiorkor represent a spectrum of severe childhood malnutrition: children with kwashiorkor also lack sufficient caloric intake. Malnutrition renders the child more susceptible to morbidity and mortality from other causes, especially infectious diseases such as gastroenteritis and acute respiratory infections, as well as impaired cognitive development.

VITAMIN AND MINERAL DEFICIENCIES

Food fortification is an important strategy to fight malnutrition. In 2002, the United Nations General Assembly established the Global Alliance for Improved Nutrition (GAIN).[61] GAIN operates projects to fortify foods including wheat and maize flour, sugar, vegetable oil, milk, soy sauce, and fish sauce. Vitamins and minerals used to fortify foods include Vitamin A, Vitamin D, iron, zinc, folic acid (B9), thiamin (B1), riboflavin (B2), niacin (B3), pyridoxine (B6), and cobalamin (B12).

Next are descriptions of three vitamin and mineral deficiencies of global importance now being addressed by GAIN through food fortification.

Vitamin A is an antioxident essential for eye health found primarily in yellow, green and dark green vegetables.[62] Vitamin A deficiency is one of the most common causes of preventable blindness with an estimated 190 million children and 19 million pregnant women affected globally.[63] In some countries milk, sugars and other commercial foods are fortified with Vitamin A. Vitamin A capsule supplements are also available.

Iodine deficiency is a low dietary supply of iodine. It occurs where the soil has low iodine content as a result of past glaciation or the repeated leaching effects of snow, water and heavy rainfall.[64] Crops grown in this soil, therefore, do not provide adequate amounts of iodine when consumed. Iodine deficiency can result in mild to severe impairments including lethargy, abortions, stillbirths, increased perinatal mortality, goiter, hypothyroidism, mental retardation, impaired mental function, and a type of brain damage called cretinism. Cretinism is the most extreme manifestation of iodine deficiency, but the primary goal in eliminating iodine deficiency are the mental and neurological impairments that lead to poor school performance, reduced intellectual ability and impaired work capacity.[61] The recommended strategy for control is to increase iodine intake through supplementation or food fortification. The history of iodine deficiency research is reviewed in chapter 1; Global Elimination of Brain Damage Due to Iodine Deficiency is presented as a primary prevention Case Study in chapter 6.

Iron deficiency anemia is the most common nutritional disorder worldwide. [65] Iron deficiency is due to a diet that is monotonous, but rich in substances (phytates) inhibiting iron absorption so that dietary iron cannot be utilized by the body.[66] WHO estimates the that this form of anemia is experienced by two billion people worldwide, accounting for approximately 50% of all forms of anemia.[59] Food based approaches are recommended to combat iron deficiency[67] but WHO also recommends strategies that combine iron interventions with other measures where iron deficiency is not the only cause of anemia. For optimal effectiveness, such strategies should be integrated within primary health care systems, programs such as maternal and child health, and initiatives such as IMCI:[68] integrated management of child-hood and adolescent illness.[69] Political support and education of local public health providers as well as an operational surveillance system with reliable, affordable and easy-to use methods for assessing and monitoring anemia prevalence and the effectiveness of interventions are recommended.

OVERNUTRITION

There is a global consensus in public health that many countries in the developed world and an increasing number in the developing world have a nutritional crisis reflected in increased numbers of overweight and obese individuals.[70] These conditions in turn are strongly associated with circulatory diseases, cancer and diabetes. Intermediate markers for these diseases are linked with diet, such as total serum cholesterol, low density lipoproteins, and insulin resistance. Global increases in the incidence and prevalence of obesity have been attributed to the globalization of Western food systems and consumer culture that have increasingly penetrated all world societies. High urbanization rates, technology shifts, and industrialization have imbalanced nutrition toward higher intake of fats, refined sugars, and salt.[63] To become effective in responding to this emerging global pandemic of overweight and obesity, public health professionals must move beyond questions of biology and personal behavior, to study the underlying collective, social, economic, political and cultural determinants so as to be able to influence global values and the role of corporations and politics that have given rise to it.

Dietary guidelines to reduce the hazards associated with poor nutrition balance have been in place in the United States since 1977.[71] These guidelines recommended increases in carbohydrate consumption intake and decreases in fat, saturated fat, cholesterol, and salt. These same recommendations were carried further in dietary guidelines that were issued in 2010.[72] These guidelines included a proscription against low carbohydrate diets and increases in whole grain and fiber and decreases in dietary saturated fat, salt and animal protein.[68] Others have argued that the evidence used for these guidelines was incomplete, sometimes inaccurately represented or interpreted and largely did not reflect limitations or controversies in the science.[68] Of concern is that during the period between 1977 and 2000, energy intake among American men and women shifted in the recommended direction since the 1977 recommendations were issued, with decreased consumption of total and saturated fats and increased consumption of carbohydrates. However, during the same period, the prevalence of overweight and obesity epidemic increased in the country, along with a parallel increase in diabetes.[68]

In contrast to the reductionist approach just described, where the role of single nutrients in diet-disease relationships was emphasized, is an approach focusing on the synergy between foods and food consumption patterns.[73,74] Recently dietary-patterning analyses have been used as an alternative method to traditional single nutrient analysis to assess cumulative effects of the overall diet.[69, 70] This work has not incorporated the broader global perspective beyond the classification of the Western diet (high in fried foods, salty snacks, eggs, and meat) as poor and disease promoting in contrast to an Oriental diet (characterized as high intake of tofu and soy and other sauces) and a prudent diet (high in fruit and vegetables), which are viewed as more health promoting.[69, 70, 75] However, the scientists involved in these studies also acknowledge the economic forces and call for initiatives that favor production, distribution and marketing of healthier foods.[69, 70] Consistent with the principles of health promotion, they call for policies that regulate food advertising and promotion, especially to children while also addressing the need to build or reconstruct the physical environment to be more conducive to physical activity.[76]

Economists have argued that an important explanation with regard to the increased prevalence of obesity and overweight in the United States is in the division of labor in food preparation.[77] In the 1960s, the bulk of food preparation was done by families with them cooking and eating at home.[73] Technological innovations since 1970 include: controlled atmosphere processing allowing food manufacturers to control gaseous environments where food is stored, reducing spoilage, slowing ripening, and lengthening shelf life; food irradiation and hydrogen-peroxide sterilization to kill and stretch wrap to keep out harmful microorganisms; development of flavor-barrier technology to prevent migration of flavor related chemicals from packaging; flavor chemists to design food flavors; and control of temperature and moisture using polyethylene plastics and other materials.[73] Other advances include microwave ovens and improvements in kitchen appliances such as ovens and refrigerators. All of these advances contributed to increased commercial production and preparation of food.

By 1997, only 23% of the cost of food represented input from farmers, the rest came from the retail sector excluding restaurants.[73] The argument then is made that the reductions in time of food preparation by individuals contributed to an increase in food consumption. This is reflected in an increased variety of food consumed, increased frequency of food consumption, a switch to high-calorie-high flavor prepared food and an increase in overall consumption of each individual food item.[73] Basically, the composition of peoples diets have changed, the overall food preparation has shifted from homes to factories and people are consuming more calories for less effort than ever before. In addition, the farmers who produce the raw materials that go into our food receive a lower percentage of the money that we pay for food than in the past and the manufacturers receive a higher percentage of our food costs.[73] Therefore it is in the best interest of the companies to keep the cost of food cheap so we will purchase more. In the United States, government farm subsidies have favored grain and oilseed crops (e.g., corn and soybeans), resulting in low prices for these crops, often below the cost of production. Food companies then purchase these commodities cheaply. Similarly, livestock producers can purchase feed for their animals cheaply, which encourages producing grain-fed livestock over grass-fed meat and dairy. Healthier fruits and vegetables and other specialty crops receive little government support and therefore are more expensive for consumers.[73]

Community gardens, by this or similar names, are one way people in numerous countries have attempted to counter the high cost of fruits and vegetables. For example, the history of community gardens in the United States dates from the early 19th century.[78] As a result of social, environmental, and economic conditions of the 1890s, school gardens and vacant lot cultivation began to address urban congestion, immigration, and economic instability.[74] The populations targeted to benefit were children, immigrants and the poor. During World Wars and the Great Depression, community gardening participation became widespread and the gardens served as a food source to offset gross shortages.[74] Community gardens have come and gone in conjunction with socioeconomic circumstances and in the 1970s with high food prices and a renewed concern about environmental stewardship, they made a comeback. In 2009, the recession led to another increase in interest to reduce family food bills and to provide greater self-sufficiency.[74] Community gardens may provide benefits beyond reducing food costs in terms of fostering intergenerational and interracial relationships in urban neighborhoods, creating jobs, increasing food security, improving diets, and enhancing the physical environment while providing physical activity and experiential learning.[74]

Conclusion

Air, water and food are all essential elements to maintain and promote health and well-being. As science and technology advance there are continuing challenges to understanding the influences these advances have in relation to air, water and food and their positive or negative health effects. Continuing to develop new interventions and evaluate previous assumptions about health is an essential role for public health practitioners.

Because health care itself is a resource for public health, this chapter commences with an introduction to how health systems vary among countries, and some key issues of health sector reform now sweeping the world. It is also important that future public health practitioners, as broadly educated professionals, have an appreciation of how health systems are designed and operate. Our focus then moves to public health as a core component of all health systems: its organizations, structures and functions, including the elements of priority setting, planning, monitoring and evaluation. The chapter closes with a review of the role of public health in emergency and disaster response.

8

PUBLIC HEALTH ORGANIZATION AND FUNCTION IN EVOLVING

HEALTH SYSTEMS

ACCORDING TO THE Universal Declaration of Human Rights (as discussed in chapter 3), essential public health measures and access to medical care are human rights. It does not prescribe *how* these provisions should be delivered, and does not imply that access must be to any type of health care at any cost, nor does it state who should bear the cost. Nonetheless, in virtually all countries, essential health care includes publicly financed public health measures. The actual services included and just how they are financed is determined by each nation, according to its values and its resources.

Political and cultural values heavily influence health systems. In many nations debate revolves around the extent to which health services should be a cost to the state. The debate varies by country, mostly depending on whether particular services are perceived to produce outcomes, not only of value to individuals but to society as a whole.

In the World Bank's view, investing in health through basic health care and public health measures is an investment in a nation's human resource.[1] Nations reap what they sow: those that invest wisely achieve handsome dividends in healthy productive populations.

Comparative Health Systems—An Overview

A *health system* comprises all organizations, institutions and resources whose primary intent is to improve health; the four essential functions are service provision, resource generation, financing and stewardship; the health systems of most countries include public, private and informal sectors.[2] While this view emphasizes the economic, fiscal and political management systems that underpin formally organized health services, the informal sector is also recognized and consists of self-help and care by families and communities, as well as the role of alternative and traditional practitioners.

While it might be thought that the objectives of all formal health systems must be similar, they are very much shaped by a country's traditions and political culture, and by economics and resources (material, human), as well as other social forces, including the significant influence that the health professions themselves exercise. Health systems design and management therefore varies around the world.[3] Furthermore, the political priority accorded to health varies among countries, with wide variations in resource allocation, equity, quality of care, and outcomes. So too within the realm of public health services, commitments vary with regard to the extent to which they are designed to be accessible to everyone at risk in a population, the inclusion of specific preventive services, and the adequacy of measures that address underlying health determinants.

In general, the richer a country, the more organized, structured and technically complex the system of health care. At the other extreme, traditional forms thrive even when some are not safe or effective, primarily because they are culturally acceptable, accessible and locally affordable. The informal health sector embodies complementary and alternative medicine (CAM) practices. Widespread in Europe and North America are naturopathy, homeopathy and chiropractic, along with other traditional practices such as Chinese medicine and acupuncture. In South Asia Ayurveda, Siddha and Unani flourish, while elsewhere other indigenous health practices are found such as African herbalism imbued with spiritualism, and a wide diversity of health beliefs among other indigenous cultures.

Recognizing the reality of underdeveloped formal health systems in most poor countries, the World Health Organization (WHO) promotes a policy of bringing traditional systems into the mainstream, seeking a role for these while strengthening health infrastructures, services, and staff, and improving access to effective drugs and emergency measures.[4] The formal systems of many countries are now facilitating CAM practices based on evidence; for example, the Indian Council of Medical Research promotes research into traditional practices, as does the US National Center for Complementary and Alternative Medicine. For example, randomized trials have established the value of massage therapy in the management of osteoarthritis of the knee,[5] low back pain,[6] and several other forms of symptomatic pain management.

An inescapable fact of both formal and informal health systems around the world is that they are shaped increasingly by economic considerations: funding sources (e.g., tax, insurance, out-of-pocket), degree of integration of financing agents and providers (e.g., single payer systems versus multiple private insurers), ownership of providers (e.g., public, private, nonprofit), and the extent to which the whole population has access to all services, or otherwise the extent to which different groups have different entitlements and providers).[3] The health care system performance of six developed nations on several key parameters, are ranked in Table 8-1 (1 is most favorable, 6 is least favorable).[7] This comparison was carried out by the Commonwealth Fund,[8] a respected private foundation in the US that aims to promote a health care system that achieves better access, improved quality, and greater efficiency, particularly for society's most vulnerable, including low-income people, the uninsured, minority Americans, young children, and elderly adults.

According to some analysts,[9] a nation's health system can be understood at three levels. Level 1 is where the goals and aspirations of a society are formulated, reflecting the dominant cultural, political, and economic forces; change is slow and rare at this level. Institutional and structural design forms level 2. Here again change does not occur often, but when it does it redefines the "rules of the game" in a fundamental way.

TABLE 8-1

Ranking six nations on key performance indicators

Country Rankings

	1.00–2.66
	2.67–4.33
	4.34–6.00

	Australia	Canada	Germany	New Zealand	United Kingdom	United States
Overall Ranking (2007)	3.5	5	2	3.5	1	6
Quality Care	4	6	2.5	2.5	1	5
Right Care	5	6	3	4	2	1
Safe Care	4	5	1	3	2	6
Coordinated Care	3	6	4	2	1	5
Patient-Centered Care	3	6	2	1	4	5
Access	3	5	1	2	4	6
Efficiency	4	5	3	2	1	6
Equity	2	5	4	3	1	6
Healthy Lives	1	3	2	4.5	4.5	6
Health Expenditures per Capita, 2004	$2876*	$3165	$3005*	$2083	$2546	$6102

Source: Commonwealth Fund 2004 International Health Policy Survey, reproduced with permission from The Commonwealth Fund, as published by American College of Physicians, cited in reference #7.

Level 3 is the level of policy application, where systemic and institutional features are operationalized within organizational designs and specific programs. Pertinent questions here include the mix of curative and preventive practices, the amount of choice, incentive structures and the assignment of responsibilities within particular programs. At this level change occurs more frequently but need not imply alterations in the fundamental structural and institutional setting, nor in a society's goals and aspirations.

For example, the so-called "Nordic model" of health care contains consistent level 1 and 2 features across all five countries (Finland, Sweden, Denmark, Norway, and Iceland): tax-based funding, publicly owned and operated hospitals, universal access based on residency, and comprehensive coverage. However, despite these features that reflect comparatively similar values, great variation is found across these countries in the way institutions are designed and how strategies are conceived and implemented.[9]

Greater contrasts are apparent in North America. Starting with Saskatchewan in 1962, all other provinces adopting similar systems within a decade, health care in Canada is guided by the principle of universality (access to a defined range of services for everyone) within provincial systems of single payer public administration, with relatively minimal residual roles for private insurers.[10] By contrast, virtually alone among developed countries, health care in the United States remained dominated by private administration and financing. The high cost of obtaining health insurance for those not included in employer-funded plans has resulted in almost 50 million people lacking coverage: insurers historically being allowed to deny coverage based on preexisting conditions, and caps set on life-time payments regardless of medical need. Dominated by a plethora of competing "for profit" insurance schemes that treat health care as a commodity (listed on stock exchanges), most health care is allocated on the ability to pay. A systematic review of thirty eight studies revealed that Canada's system leads to more favorable outcomes when compared with the US predominantly private for-profit system, at less than 50% of the cost.[11]

However, dramatic changes are now taking place: under new legislation (the Patient Protection and Affordable Care Act of 2010 to be fully phased in by 2020) of the Obama administration, the United States will begin to close the gap on universality and other deficiencies will be addressed. The legislation was upheld by the Supreme Court on June 28, 2012, against challenges by twenty-six states, several individuals and the National Federation of Independent Businesses.[12] Nonetheless, even with this policy shift, the US will remain the only developed nation that depends predominantly on a private insurer, private provider entrepreneurial model. This acknowledged, the US system also contains substantial public sector elements that will continue to grow: Medicare for the elderly (comparable to Canada's universal single payer system where providers are not directly employed by government); a program called Medicaid to address essential health care for low-income families based on eligibility criteria, financed jointly by state and federal governments; Veteran's Affairs health care (a single payer system whose providers are employed by the Department of Veterans Affairs, an approach similar to the British National Health Service, although not applied to persons in active service who are covered by private insurers under "Tricare"—an employer based insurance scheme).

The multitiered US system will continue to be a source of learning due to the varying performance of its diverse components. Issues of effectiveness and efficiency will be intensively studied as it tries to provide quality care for all citizens under the new legislation; there will likely be ongoing political challenges to equity and universality.

An insightful study of low and middle income countries that achieve good health outcomes at modest cost (Bangladesh, Ethiopia, Kyrgyzstan, Tamil Nadu, and Thailand), recently revealed four underlying determinants that drive successful health systems.[13] These are capacity (the key role of individuals and institutions in designing and implementing reforms), continuity (the stability required for reforms to be implemented, and the institutional memory that prevents mistakes from being repeated), catalysts (the ability to make use of windows of opportunity), and contexts (policies relevant and appropriate to circumstances). The study also identified the critical role of access to primary health care (especially antenatal care and skilled birth attendants), and high uptake of critical public health interventions (e.g., immunization, oral rehydration for diarrheal disease, and modern contraception). The importance of sustained political support for health, a skilled health workforce, a high degree of community involvement and health promoting polices that go beyond the health sector, are emphasized.

Relevant to global comparisons is the WHO landmark study, in 2000, of health systems performance in almost 200 countries. WHO's assessment was based on five indicators: overall population health; health inequalities within the population; overall health system responsiveness (combining patient satisfaction and how well the system acts); distribution of responsiveness (how well people of varying economic status find they are served by the health system); and the distribution of the health system's financial burden within the population (who pays the costs). While there is a need to repeat this type of international study, the findings were instructive; for example, France was found (on these criteria) to provide the best overall health care followed by Italy, Spain, Oman, Austria, and Japan. The United Kingdom ranked 18th, Canada 31st, and the United States 37th (with the most expensive system in the world). Australia's performance (sociodemographically similar to Canada but with more private sector involvement) was ranked 32nd.[14] Most

European countries ranked higher than Canada, Australia and the United States. Such international ranking exercises are almost always controversial both methodologically and politically.

This brief review of comparative health systems illustrates how nations can learn from one another's experiences. This said, common features across all countries include

- A local to national hierarchy of responsibility that reflects roles and relationships
- Elements ranging from preventive to diagnostic, treatment and curative services
- Referral systems that link across levels to more specialized levels of intervention
- Local systems that tend to reflect the needs of individuals and communities, and that generally fall within state/provincial or national guidelines
- State/provincial or national guidelines that may not be sufficient for all needs
- Roles and services at state/provincial and federal levels that are usually more specialized and defined in legislation, and more involved in setting policies and standards
- Formal systems that are complemented by community organizations and private sector activities (see chapter 4)
- Health service structures and functions that are influenced by political considerations and therefore always subject to change
- A substantial component of self-help and support from families, and a legacy of traditional and complementary health practices

Health Sector Reform

For over two decades, efforts to achieve health sector reform have swept around the world, as countries strive to meet essential health needs at costs that are affordable. A complex process, such efforts must be guided by a nation's economic, cultural and political realities, while addressing such operational issues as planning, financing, management, organizational structure, gender equity, leadership, systems research, and priority setting to achieve effective resource utilization.[15] In countries where the health sector suffers from insufficient or imbalanced allocations of public funding, the private sector often dominates the provision of health services. The challenge therefore, in countries as disparate as Pakistan and the United States, is to rationalize the private sector's role, even while its participation may remain essential.

In virtually all countries, "reform" is driven more by fiscal than health priorities, largely due to rising costs and competition for resources. A common challenge is to resolve cost and efficiency concerns while simultaneously improving population health. Part of the solution in most settings may be found within primary health care, especially through promoting prevention and self-management. While health may be improved indirectly by investing in other sectors (e.g., education), optimal results require investment in the health sector itself. Lack of investment by many developing countries, especially in Africa, contributes to a "brain drain" that diminishes national capacities while subsidizing the health systems of developed nations, some of whom actively recruit this talent (e.g., technologists, nurses, doctors). Health human resources, discussed more fully at the end of this chapter and in chapter 9 also, is a key area for international development assistance.

Lack of knowledge is a barrier to how to prevent or care for illnesses and how best to access the health care system. It is commonly found that high literacy among women is associated with better overall health literacy; however, it is equally well demonstrated that this is not likely without high general literacy including science literacy.[16] Over-reliance on health professionals in itself can be a cause for escalating health care costs. Incentives for self-education or self-discipline, and ways of improving this situation have been advocated, including school-based health education, health information packages, promoting the internet and the media as public information tools, translation of materials into minority languages, and extending education to rural communities through mobile facilities, thereby to increase the accessibility of self-care resources.[10] In examining issues surrounding self-care generally, there is increasingly recognition that people must be enabled to take more responsibility for their health—a core principle of the Ottawa Charter on Health Promotion (1986), discussed in chapter 4.[17]

Many health systems fail to address priority needs with equity (universality, accessibility, affordability), especially for groups lacking power or recognition.[10] However, public debate about health care tends to focus instead on costly items that preoccupy institutional administrators and politicians, often overlooking "upstream" fundamentals that preserve health: healthy environments and workplaces, primary prevention (e.g., nutrition education, immunization, ante-natal care, physical activity, smoking prevention, and social policies that affect literacy, employment, crime, public safety, housing quality, and community well-being). It may reflect basic human nature that societies are preoccupied with acute care issues, which are crisis-prone and often glamorized, all but ignoring the upstream factors and even important downstream ones (e.g., long-term care, home care), whose availability determines the speed with which acute care patients may move on to more appropriate levels of care for their convalescence. Almost everywhere it is necessary to reexamine what services should be core or essential, to evaluate what is needed and effective, and to consider the needs of vulnerable groups.

Role of the Private Sector

The role of the private sector and perceptions of *public-private partnership* (or P3, as introduced in chapter 4) vary across countries. In the context of health systems reform, the term *privatization* means different things to different people, and can be both politically and emotionally laden. For example, in countries strongly committed to public financing and administration of health services, such as Canada, P3s are often viewed as a threat, with potential to undermine universal health care and resulting in a two-tier system with regard to access and quality. In others, such as the United States, whose system may be described as multitiered, government involvement is seen by many as a political threat, while in many European countries and Japan, a mixed system is considered sensible. In many developing countries, in light of massive under-funding of public sector health care, there would be virtually no health care at all for the majority of people without the private sector (in all forms). This said, in virtually all settings the issue of how much public or private mix is desirable is politically charged, which can impede rational debate. As we explore this issue, our intent is to recognize that, regardless of the form private sector involvement may take, government has a responsibility to ensure that the system as a whole delivers essential public health measures and access to effective health care for all.

For about three decades, conditions for financial assistance from the International Monetary Fund (IMF) and the World Bank forced developing country governments to reduce their responsibility for providing health services.[15] Economic development was promoted as separate from, and more important than, health development, even though both are closely linked. IMF conditions provoked privatization of health services, and decisions regarding what to privatize undermined governmental mandates to ensure that basic human needs are met. While this reflected a critical need for *structural adjustment* in many economies, it is relevant that the IMF was heavily influenced by the policies of its largest donor, the United States, which, until the landmark ruling of the Supreme Court in 2012 (referred to earlier), had not upheld the principle of universality in health care.

This history notwithstanding, three health care principles have always been critical to healthy populations: effectiveness, efficiency, and equity. In the presence of competition, it is often held that the private sector will be more efficient, especially in relation to ancillary services (e.g., supplies, laundry, catering). Regarding pharmaceuticals, the private sector penetrates more deeply, due to superior marketing strategies and a relative lack of successful public sector pharmaceutical initiatives. The private sector also is assumed to be more effective in achieving its performance objectives, often attributed to better governance and accountability, although objectives and measures used to determine this may differ substantially between public and private sectors. For example, products unrelated to disease burden, public priorities, or even product efficacy may still meet commercial objectives. But fundamentally the private sector has no mandate to ensure that basic human needs are met; nor can it respond to health equity as a human right.[18]

In 1998, the Director-General of WHO advocated greater collaboration with the private sector in the context of a global trend toward privatization and declining public sector funding.[19] Despite controversy on the merits of this, especially with regard to roles and motives of commercial entities and their operational methods, partnerships between WHO and commercial entities are now *fait accompli*. Furthermore, the value of an involved private sector is recognized in the Bangkok Charter for Health Promotion (chapter 4).[20]

However, while such arrangements offer new opportunities for enhanced global health funding, they also pose significant risks for public health. As a company's first duty is to its shareholders, potential for conflict of interest arises, along with the need to ensure safeguards to protect the public interest. Corporate strategies used to influence public health policies have been identified within the following categories: public relations, distortion of science, political influence, financial tactics, legal and regulatory tactics, products and services.[21] The potential for conflict may be simple or complex: it should be understood by everyone that private sector interests may differ from the public interest, so one must remain alert to the potential for conflict, whether real or perceived. Nonetheless, recognizing the higher goal of addressing human needs more effectively than in the past, even humanitarian organizations now promote private investment as critical. While civil society and public infrastructures remain essential, both international and national development initiatives increasingly embrace a vibrant private sector.

In several Asian countries, health reform has involved the private sector, sometimes in dramatic ways. That this sector may uplift people in a manner not achieved by the public sector, is illustrated by 2006 Nobel Peace Prize awarded to Muhammad Yunus and the Grameen Bank, Bangladesh, for "efforts to create economic and social development from below" through micro-credit services to the poor[5]. In transitioning from a centrally-planned to a market economy, Vietnam involved the private sector in safe motherhood and family planning by amending policy and regulatory frameworks, while reviving a commune-level public health system to meet basic needs. In the Central Asian Republics and Mongolia, formerly socialist regimes, the creation of a private health sector is now a priority, with programs for family physicians in group practices, effective referral systems in rural areas, and autonomous boards managing hospitals and contracting services. Taiwan has introduced a national health insurance scheme providing universal coverage. By contrast, in the United States, where the private sector has long dominated the health care system, the challenge now is how to meet the health care needs of some 50 million noninsured people, almost 20% of the population. The Patient Protection and Affordable Care Act of the Obama administration (previously discussed) is a big step in this direction although it remains to be seen how this will be implemented.

In developed countries, P3 arrangements now exist across a diverse spectrum: joint policy development and advocacy to advance public health; leadership and management training; quality of care initiatives; integrating health and social care for vulnerable groups; and hazardous waste management. In developing countries, while the impact of P3s requires ongoing evaluation, genuinely good work is emerging: subsidized products, distribution assistance, educational initiatives, and disease control ventures (e.g., Global Alliance for Vaccines and Immunization or GAVI; Medicines for Malaria Venture). In some instances, health services are strengthened (e.g., Gates Foundation/Merck Botswana Comprehensive HIV/AIDS Partnership). WHO-facilitated P3s generally emphasize specific disease interventions, while other P3 models seem better at health systems and community development (e.g., BRAC, formerly Bangladesh Rural Advancement Committee, a people-centered NGO, developed an integrated multidimensional health program, successfully linking foundations, governments and communities).

It is now accepted in many countries that successful ethical private sector co-investments in public health are achievable. Although the private sector may promote inequalities through its typical reliance on market principles, with proper incentives and working within a public sector framework, it may also be harnessed to improve access to and utilization of preventive and curative care. However, for government to succeed in managing this process, policy frameworks and enabling environments must be developed to nurture these P3 synergies to improve health outcomes. Regulatory functions (e.g., licensing and performance monitoring) need to be designed and implemented so as to facilitate service coverage, promote quality of care, and exercise control over costs to clients. If properly designed, private sector participation within public sector frameworks has the potential to complement the public sector, to create or strengthen infrastructure and also to favorably influence market practices.

We close this section with a cautionary note about *regulatory capture,* a risk that may be inherent in P3s. This refers to a phenomenon by which regulatory agencies can come to be dominated by the very industries they were charged with regulating. Recent work points to measures that can be designed to reduce this risk, thereby to safeguard the independence, effectiveness and efficiency of regulation.[22] Regulation needs to be based on the best independent and scientifically objective evidence; while industrial interests are relevant, those interests should follow, not lead.

Organization of Public Health Services within Countries

In the national interest, all countries, even those with a dominant private health sector, publicly finance and operate "public health services" as defined in legislation. Key public health functions are also complemented internationally in the mandates of multilateral health agencies working under the auspices of the United Nations. Public health services thus may be viewed as critical subsystems of larger systems, put in place to protect populations from common or shared threats to their health. While in some settings, aspects of public health may be contracted out (e.g., information systems development, monitoring, and evaluation), it is a responsibility of all nations to ensure that their people are protected from a range of health threats.

Essential public health services have been defined for various jurisdictions from local to international; the following set is taken from the United States:[23]

- Monitor health status to identify community health problems
- Diagnose and investigate health problems and health hazards in the community
- Inform, educate, and empower people about health issues
- Mobilize community partnerships to identify and solve health problems
- Develop policies and plans that support individual and community health efforts
- Enforce laws and regulations that protect health and ensure safety
- Link people to needed personal health services and assure the provision of health care when otherwise unavailable
- Assure a competent public health and personal health care workforce
- Evaluate effectiveness, accessibility, and quality of personal and population-based health services
- Research for new insights and innovative solutions to health problems

Local Public Health: Under a designated health officer with a mandate for publicly financed preventive services at municipal or community level, local public health emphasizes health promotion and protection from health threats arising in or near local settings, such as environmental and microbial hazards; it also entails coordination with other levels of the public health system in the event of threats that involve other jurisdictions from regional to national to global (e.g., influenza, hazardous products).

The organization of local public health services is usually separately administered from that of health care institutions and medical care, and local public health officers are most often accountable instead to a regional or provincial/state authority. Such arrangements help to protect the smaller public health budgets from intrusion by the imperative of treating the sick, and reflect the underlying vision and mandate of public health services as having longer range aims and objectives, dealing mostly with population risk assessment and preventive programming. For example, local public health agencies have a lead role in population based disease prevention and protective services, such as immunization, maternal and child health, elder care and other community oriented programs. In practice, there are overlapping boundaries with most other components of the health care system, and relationships with hospitals and medical care must be managed. In some jurisdictions, separate administration of local public health services has given way to integrated regionalized models that attempt to coordinate all services within one overarching administrative structure, while retaining the integrity of budgets and professional leadership appropriate to the objective(s) being sought.

In many developing countries, the role of a public health physician may also include administration of treatment facilities, even public hospitals, in addition to responsibilities for health promotion and protection from health threats. While this is not usually a desirable set-up, it is sometimes rendered necessary due to public sector resource limitations and higher level policy decisions made ostensibly in favor of acute care often without reference to more fundamental health needs and public health priorities.

Regional Level: In some countries a public health organizational layer is interposed between local and provincial/state levels that mirrors the "regionalization" applied to some other public services. As an operational approach in the hospital sector this works well for diagnostic and treatment services that cannot be justified at local level, but must be within reach of everyone (e.g., costly equipment, specialized cancer treatment). Similarly, for public health referral services, depending on disease burden considerations and availability of expertise, regional services make more sense than building local capacity everywhere (e.g., public health laboratory services, regional waste management, specialized disease control services). In France, followed by the UK, regional public health observatories were set up to serve a range of information and intelligence functions, justified by the need for advanced health situation analysis and related expertise at this level.[24]

As a policy, regionalization requires establishing an intermediate governance structure that assumes functions previously met by state/provincial or local government.[25]

It must therefore develop new capacities at this level such as accountability for democratizing decision making, enhancing responsiveness to public needs, ensuring the fairness of resource distribution among regions, developing a more comprehensive approach to health problems, using resources more efficiently and improving continuity of care.[26] If it is not able to achieve these qualities, it may not be justifiable. A decision to regionalize may be influenced by considerations of geography, cost, efficiency, accountability, and responsiveness. While a few countries have innovated with this approach (e.g., Australia, Canada, New Zealand), most countries have not followed suit (e.g., the United States still functions mostly with a system of national, state, and local public health, although several states have adopted regional models to ensure that every resident receives services).

The potential merits and demerits of "regionalized" public health services remain open to debate and often depend on political decisions regarding whether or not to decentralize governance, fiscal authority and other services to this level. Regionalization is still a new idea for what might be termed "general public health services" and subject to evaluation where it is being tried. In parts of Canada where local boards of public health were replaced by regional health authorities with responsibility for all health services, there was loss of local accountability, leadership and participation in public health issues and the direct link between local and provincial level was lost.[27] Accountability issues arose between regional boards and provincial Ministries of Health, including the extent to which aspirations for a stronger population health focus, and improved continuity of care were achieved.[28] Nonetheless, regionalization offers potential to enhance integration of public health with other health system components (e.g., hospitals and medical care).

In summary, experience with regionalized public health services needs to be monitored with attention to context. Lessons learned may be instructive for the evolution of public health services not only in countries where it is being tried, but in other countries as well. While it is very unlikely to be applicable everywhere (e.g., it is generally inapplicable to small states), the idea may be useful in more settings than it exists currently.

State/Provincial Level: This level applies in countries that differentiate specific authorities, roles and responsibilities between national and state/provincial levels. Normally roles such as foreign policy and defense are assigned to the national level, but much authority for internal affairs is often delegated to the next level. In most federally organized countries, greater authority and capacity for provision of health services falls within state/provincial jurisdiction, usually operating within a national framework but with only limited federal involvement in operating health services, and with varying degrees of cost-sharing. The state/provincial level exercises a major influence on policies, programs and resources allocations for health services at local level. This is presided over by a state/provincial Minister of Health (or equivalent) with responsibility for a system of administration known as a Ministry or Department of Health. The scope of state/provincial health departments can be very broad and diverse, reflecting how governmental responsibilities and resources may be allocated. However, within this there exists a set of core public health functions. These are similar across jurisdictions, with variation depending on priority considerations. For illustrative purposes, Figure 8-1 shows the core functions for British Columbia, Canada's western-most province.[29]

This diagram shows how these core functions are interrelated. The main components of the framework are as follows: (1) Core programs—long-term programs, representing the minimum level of public health services that health authorities would provide in a renewed and modern public health system. These are organized to improve health, and can be assessed ultimately in terms of improved health and well-being and/or reductions in disease, disability, and injury. (2) Core public health strategies—strategies by which core programs are implemented. The Populations and Inequalities "lenses" are intended to ensure that the health needs of specific population groups are addressed. (3) Core public health capacity—health information systems, quality management, research and knowledge development, staff training and development capacity needed to apply public health strategies and implement core programs. The development and implementation of core public health functions is guided by a provincial steering committee.

National Level: health in all countries is politically represented at the national level. This is normally a cabinet post, mostly known as the Minister of Health or equivalent (e.g., Secretary of Health in the United States). A national ministry or department usually reports to this individual (e.g., in the United States this is the Department of Health and Human Services, DHHS). Roles at this level are set out in legislation and usually include policy development, particular areas of priority programming (e.g., reference level public health laboratory services), and other reference functions such as national standards, quality assurance, immigration health, and other specialized services.

Countries vary substantially in how national public health capacities are organized. In some, it is politically, technically and economically feasible to support core public health capacities at the national level through large purpose-designed institutions, such as Finland's National Institute for Health and Welfare, whose work has been studied by many small to mid-sized countries due to Finland's great success in fostering integrated health promotion and disease prevention initiatives (see chapters 4 and 6).

Internationally the best known national public health entity is the US Centers for Disease Control and Prevention (CDC), which is located administratively within

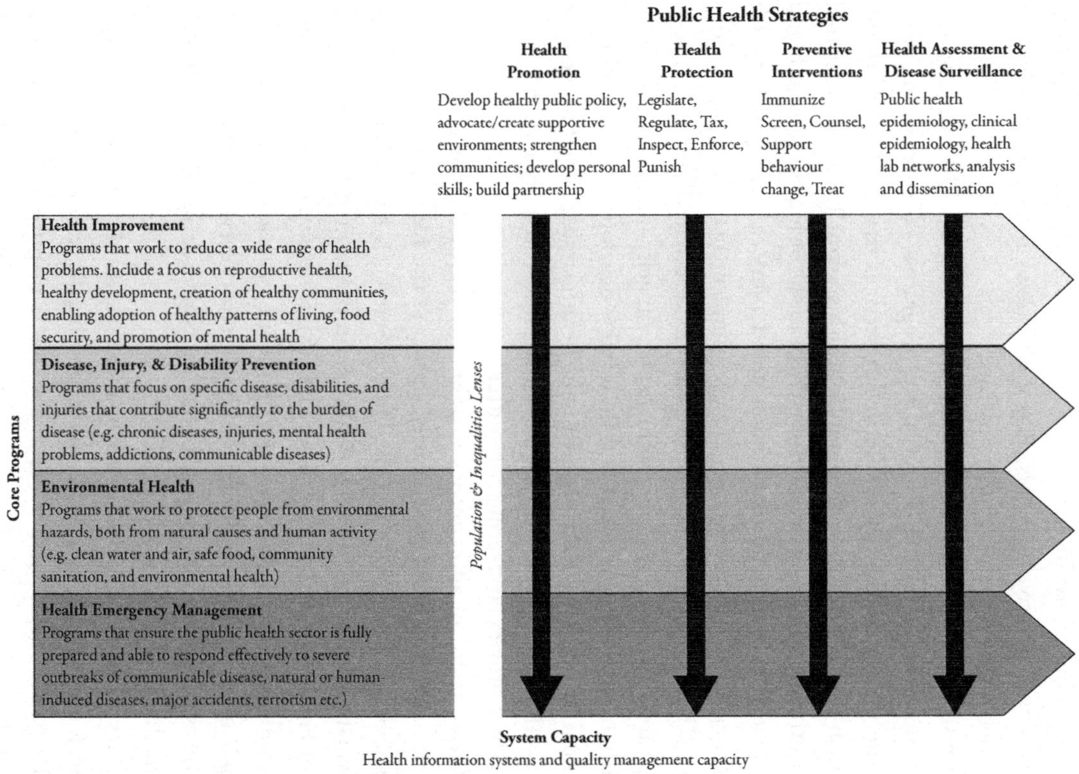

Public Health Strategies

Health Promotion	Health Protection	Preventive Interventions	Health Assessment & Disease Surveillance
Develop healthy public policy, advocate/create supportive environments; strengthen communities; develop personal skills; build partnership	Legislate, Regulate, Tax, Inspect, Enforce, Punish	Immunize, Screen, Counsel, Support behaviour change, Treat	Public health epidemiology; clinical epidemiology, health lab networks, analysis and dissemination

Population & Inequalities Lenses

System Capacity
Health information systems and quality management capacity

Core Programs

Health Improvement
Programs that work to reduce a wide range of health problems. Include a focus on reproductive health, healthy development, creation of healthy communities, enabling adoption of healthy patterns of living, food security, and promotion of mental health

Disease, Injury, & Disability Prevention
Programs that focus on specific disease, disabilities, and injuries that contribute significantly to the burden of disease (e.g. chronic diseases, injuries, mental health problems, addictions, communicable diseases)

Environmental Health
Programs that work to protect people from environmental hazards, both from natural causes and human activity (e.g. clean water and air, safe food, community sanitation, and environmental health)

Health Emergency Management
Programs that ensure the public health sector is fully prepared and able to respond effectively to severe outbreaks of communicable disease, natural or human-induced diseases, major accidents, terrorism etc.)

FIGURE 8-1 A core public health functions framework. Example from British Columbia.

Source: Copyright © Province of British Columbia. All rights reserved.

Reprinted with permission of the Province of British Columbia. www.ipp.gov.bc.ca

the Department of Health and Human Services (DHHS). CDC works primarily to support state health departments and other organizations to develop and sustain capacities for health promotion, disease prevention, occupational safety and health, and environmental health. CDC maintains a full array of reference level public health laboratories within its own organizational structure and budget. It also houses some national capacities that are so prominent in their own right that they seem almost like separate organizations (which they once were before being brought into this unified structure). For example, the National Institutes of Occupational Safety and Health (NIOSH), which is responsible for surveillance, research, and advisory roles regarding the prevention of work-related injury and illness, is part of CDC, as is the National Center for Health Statistics (NCHS). Separately organized under the Department of Labor, the United States also has an Occupational Health and Safety Administration (OSHA). The roles of NIOSH and OSHA are complementary: NIOSH charged with providing the scientific evidence base needed to develop regulations, OSHA responsible for developing health and safety regulations.

However, few countries can afford to maintain such complex organizations as CDC, and must devise alternative approaches. For example, in the United Kingdom, when the need for public health reference laboratories was recognized many decades ago, a decision was taken to recognize where such expertise already existed and to coordinate this within a network designed to respond whenever the reference function was needed.[30] Thus, a Public Health Laboratory Service was established under the 1946 National Health Service Act with the aim of protecting the population from infection through detection, diagnosis, surveillance, prevention and control of infection and communicable diseases. It achieved this through a network of microbiology laboratories, epidemiology and field investigation services, research and development, and education and training programs. This required collaboration with the British National Health Service, local authorities, universities, and other institutions, supported by a headquarters based in London that included a Central Public Health Laboratory. In 2003, this time-honored network was incorporated within a national Health Protection Agency.

Similarly, given the need for a unified approach within the European Union, a European Agency for Safety and Health at Work (EU-OSHA) was set up in Spain in 1996 with the mission "to make Europe's workplaces safer, healthier and more productive. This is done by bringing together and sharing knowledge and information, to promote a culture of risk prevention."[31] The availability of this shared capacity means that individual member countries do not have to replicate it, although "the provisions adopted shall not prevent any Member States from maintaining or introducing more stringent measures for the protection of workers."[32]

This approach to pooling resources for the common good is not unique to the industrialized world and can be found in other parts of the world with much more limited resources. By way of illustration, the health ministries of small Caribbean countries have for decades pooled resources to achieve specialized functions (e.g., since 1974, the Caribbean Epidemiology Centre (CAREC), a common disease control reference capacity for 21 member nations, has operated within the administrative structure of PAHO/WHO).[33] Further organizational development is underway: in 2011 a new Caribbean Public Health Agency (CARPHA) was legally constituted by Caribbean Community Member States. CARPHA will combine the functions of several regional institutes (CAREC and four others [the Caribbean Environmental Health Institute, the Caribbean Food and Nutrition Institute, the Caribbean Health Research Centre, and the Caribbean Research and Drug Treatment Laboratory]) within a single agency. The new agency becomes operational in 2013. It will be better placed to provide integrated public health leadership on behalf of Caribbean residents and visitors.[34]

The important lesson from all this is not that there is any system that necessarily works better than any other, but that all countries must find a way that works for them to ensure that essential national public health services are as effective and efficient as possible.

To conclude this section on another promising new development: national public health institutes are now reaching out among themselves, by affiliating with a recently formed International Association of National Public Health Institutes (IANPHI).[35] IANPHI spearheads improvements in national public health systems through peer-assistance evaluation, grant support and efforts focused on advocacy, collaboration, and sustainability. It provides direct funding to governments in low-resource countries to build and strengthen national public health capacity through development of National Public Health Institutes (NPHIs). It does this through grants to support NPHI to NPHI evaluations, capacity building initiatives, and seed grants to assist research agendas.

Organization of Public Health between Countries—
International and Global Health

Before examining the structure and function of international public health agencies, it is important to define our terms.[36] The field of International Health is a public health enterprise with origins in the health situation of developing countries and the efforts of developed nations and the multilateral system to assist. While closely linked to development assistance (commonly known as "aid"), its scope includes issues of direct interest to developed countries: imported disease, trade in hazardous products, immigration health, quarantine regulations. Increasingly today, however, "international health" emphasizes *technical cooperation* among countries to achieve mutually desired goals such as common norms and standards for disease surveillance, mutually acceptable international health regulations, and operationally effective health systems development. By contrast, the new and rapidly evolving field of Global Health represents the public health perspective on and response to "globalization." Global Health overlaps with, and is partly an outgrowth of international health in synergy with health promotion: its main aim is to achieve global co-operation for solutions to problems that have worldwide health impact. Beyond national and/or regional actions, these require global advocacy and policy frameworks (e.g., tobacco and narcotics, food security, health human resources, hazardous wastes, trans-boundary pollution, and human rights).

Because developing countries are resource challenged and need to build their capacities, they are eligible for enhanced support from international health agencies. These agencies are of four types: multilateral, bilateral, nongovernmental, and other.

MULTILATERAL AGENCIES

Funded primarily by a large number of member governments (hence the term "multilateral"), those with health-related mandates are listed in Table 8-2, along with their websites. The remainder of this section will focus on WHO.

The World Health Organization is the leading multilateral health agency of the United Nations system. Launched in 1948, WHO is governed by a World Health Assembly (WHA) with representatives from almost 200 Member States. The main role of the WHA is to review and approve WHO's policies, program initiatives, and budgets, which are developed by WHO technical staff in consultation with staff of national health ministries and of specialized institutions (public and private) around the world. Highly networked, WHO is primarily a coordinating agency, promoting technical cooperation among countries while facilitating policy development, capacity building, training, and other forms of technical assistance. WHO also assembles health data from member countries; these are analyzed in a standard manner and the resulting information disseminated globally. Collaborative programs with member countries are performed by a Secretariat, supported by six regional offices with representatives in most countries.

Globally, WHO is most visibly associated with such policy and programmatic initiatives as the Framework Convention on Tobacco Control, the Global Burden of Disease project, the International Health Regulations, surveillance of infectious disease of global importance, and disease-specific eradication programs. Many of

TABLE 8-2

International agencies with health-related mandates

Acronym	Agency	Websites
WHO	World Health Organization	http://www.who.int/en/
UNICEF	United Nations Children's Fund	http://www.unicef.org/
UNDP	United Nations Development Programme	http://www.beta.undp.org/undp/en/home.html
WB	The World Bank	http://www.worldbank.org/
UNAIDS	Joint United Nations Programme on HIV/AIDS,	http://www.unaids.org/en/
FAO	Food and Agricultural Organization	http://www.fao.org/
UNFPA	United Nations Population Fund	http://www.unfpa.org/public/
UNHCR	United Nations Refugee Agency	http://www.unhcr.org/cgi-bin/texis/vtx/home
UNFDAC	United Nations Office for Drugs and Crime	http://www.unodc.org/unodc/index.html?ref=menutop

these functions are coordinated by six regional offices in a decentralized manner: while conforming to a broad strategic framework for WHO as a whole, each enjoys sufficient autonomy as to be able to determine priorities based on regional situation analyses. Accordingly, structures, relationships and even terminology for organizational units and posts vary across WHO regions, reflecting diversity in organizational subcultures and priorities, and taking into account member country perspectives.

WHO operates according to the principles of *results based management*—an evolving model for planning, budgeting, monitoring and evaluation. All six Regional Offices remain consistent with WHO's global goals and objectives. For example, for the current six year period (2008–2013), WHO set out a Medium-Term Strategic Plan (MTSP) based on a General Programme of Work, input from various Country Cooperation Strategies and resolutions of WHO Governing Bodies (WHA and equivalent regional bodies). Since the health situation and priorities of each region and member country vary, each Regional Office contributes to this plan in different ways. For each biennium, strategic objectives, targets and approaches are identified as a basis for budget development. WHO also addresses cross-cutting priorities such as gender, ethnicity, aboriginal health, ethics, and NGO development: these themes are interwoven across all WHO programs.

This approach to strategic and operational planning in support of its program of work applies to all WHO levels, with mutually compatible expected results: organizationwide, regionwide, and country-specific. Biennial, annual, and subannual monitoring is carried out to track progress with regard to action plans. Evaluation of the MTSP itself is carried out through medium-term and end-of-term evaluations. In addition, independent evaluations are also carried out by donors; for example, the Multilateral Organisation Performance Assessment Network (MOPAN)[37] is a network of 16 donor countries with a common interest in assessing the organisational effectiveness of the major multilateral organisations they fund, including WHO. A recent MOPAN evaluation reveals that WHO is achieving ongoing management reforms, such as strengthening its results-based management framework, and new management systems to facilitate technical and financial integration and operational risk management across the organization.[38]

Arguably the most critical work of WHO is done on a day to day basis by WHO Country Offices. These offices work in close coordination with national ministries of health to help establish and maintain country-specific health priorities and to develop operational plans to deal with them. From this joint effort emerges the Country Cooperation Strategy (CCS). To obtain an overview of any given CCS, one may simply visit the WHO website for the country. The scope of work is typically broad; for example, WHO Bangladesh lists the following core program clusters: communicable diseases, noncommunicable diseases, family and community health, sustainable development and health environment, health technology and pharmaceuticals, evidence and information for policy.[39]

In general, the more capacity a country has to develop and deliver its health policies and programs, the less likely there will be a national role for WHO, and the more likely it will be seen mostly as a force for global health. This reflects the reality that countries with advanced health science capacities have no WHO country offices per se and relate instead to the regional office and/or to Geneva (e.g., United States, Canada, most European countries). By contrast, resource challenged nations often have large WHO country offices, some with capacities greater than their own health ministry. Between these extremes WHO may focus on special areas of need so as to complement national capacities.

Countries in greatest need of assistance depend substantially on the planning and technical cooperation of their WHO Country Office to help get the job done. Although the WHO Country Representative must represent WHO's global priorities, they must also advocate and support nationally determined ones. To some extent however, this may result in a resource mismatch between the two categories: mirrored in the much greater level of international donor support available for global versus local health priorities that receive less international recognition and support than they should. For example, endemic malnutrition (due to lack of food security) and gastroenteritis (due to inadequate access to potable water) pose much larger burdens of disease in most countries of south Asia than HIV/AIDS, malaria and tuberculosis combined. Yet there is a donor-supported Global Fund for AIDS, Tuberculosis and Malaria (GFATM) but, aside from the Global Alliance for Improved Nutrition (GAIN),[40] which operates projects to fortify foods with micronutrients (chapter 7), no equivalent global fund exists to address the larger issues of malnutrition or diarrhea. Underlying this dichotomy in recent decades, extra-budgetary sources (grants, contracts, donations) have exceeded WHO's regular budget that was historically based on quota contributions from its members. While this diversification protects WHO against unstable government funding, extra-budgetary support—often driven by public-private partnerships—is mostly restricted to specialized initiatives, which has the potential to influence or distort priorities and thereby reduce WHO's organizational capacity for independent decisions regarding resource allocation.

BILATERAL AGENCIES

In addition to supporting multilateral agencies, most developed nations also provide aid on a "country-to-country" basis, attempting to match recipient needs with the donor's objectives and capacity to assist. This is called "bilateral aid." Some smaller donors are geographically selective (e.g., Australia emphasizes its Western-Pacific neighbors). The Netherlands emphasizes its expertise in water technologies. Some follow historical links (e.g., France emphasizes its former colonies). Others both receive and donate international aid (e.g., Cuba, China). The United States links aid to democratic reforms and human rights.[36]

Donor countries often rely on their own expertise through competitive bidding to design, implement and monitor projects funded under bilateral agreements, sometimes requiring that the donor's own products and services be used. Thus, a significant proportion of aid budgets may be recycled within a donor's economy; this is referred to as "tied aid." In reality about half of official aid is invested in the donor countries themselves, and not genuinely available to the recipient although nonetheless counted as such. As each donor has its own motivation, priorities and management style, competition and conflict can arise in some settings, revealing a need to improve donor coordination.

An important step was taken in 2005 with the Paris Declaration on Aid Effectiveness,[41] which recognizes the following principles for both multilateral and bilateral aid:

- Ownership—*Developing countries set their own strategies for poverty reduction, improve their institutions and tackle corruption.*

- Alignment—*Donor countries align behind these objectives and use local systems.*
- Harmonization—*Donor countries coordinate, simplify procedures and share information to avoid duplication.*
- Results—*Developing countries and donors shift focus to development results and results get measured.*
- Mutual accountability—*Donors and partners are accountable for development results.*

Despite popular misconceptions, the track record of wealthy countries in contributing to official development assistance (ODA) is modest.[42] In recent years, ODA comes to about $70–100 billion annually. While superficially impressive, this pales in comparison with (for example) the $350 billion that the United States, Europe, and Japan spend annually on their own farm subsidies, thereby undercutting potential agricultural export markets for developing countries. Four decades ago, wealthy nations promised to allocate 0.7% of Gross National Product for ODA.[43] By 2009, only five (Table 8-3) had met this target (using a similar measure: Gross National Income; GNI), although several others have pledged to reach it by 2015. It is critical for developing countries that ODA targets are honored, effectively placed and fairly counted, so as to help to build sustainable capacities for all the world's people. The Millennium Development Goals and the Paris Declaration should make a difference; but whether such global initiatives to improve performance and accountability will actually do so requires ongoing monitoring and evaluation.

INTERNATIONAL NONGOVERNMENTAL ORGANIZATIONS

International NGOs are increasingly active in development and help to compensate for shortfalls in official multilateral and bilateral aid. For example, US private giving

TABLE 8-3

Official development assistance
OECD Nations in Rank Order by Net ODA as Percent of GNI 2009.[73]

1 Sweden 1.2	7 Finland 0.54	13 Germany 0.35	19 United States 0.2
2 Norway 1.06	8 Ireland 0.54	14 Austria 0.3	20 Greece 0.19
3 Luxembourg 1.01	9 United Kingdom 0.52	15 Canada 0.3	21 Japan 0.18
4 Denmark 0.88	10 Switzerland 0.47	16 Australia 0.29	22 Italy 0.16
5 Netherlands 0.82	11 France 0.46	17 New Zealand 0.29	23 Korea 0.1
6 Belgium 0.55	12 Spain 0.46	18 Portugal 0.23	

is more than double that of its ODA. Such people-to-people aid is often highly focused (e.g., the Helen Keller Foundation strives to prevent blindness and deafness by advancing research and education in combating trachoma, the leading infectious cause of blindness globally).[44] Others have broader motivation: for example, the mission of the Carter Center, while leading specific initiatives such as guinea worm eradication, emphasizes its "fundamental commitment to human rights and the alleviation of human suffering;... to prevent and resolve conflicts, enhance freedom and democracy, and improve health."[45]

Supported mainly by subscriptions or donations, some international NGOs also act under contract to governments or other agencies. The largest NGO is the International Red Cross and Red Crescent Movement, which has national counterparts in most countries. It is mandated under the Geneva Conventions to assist persons affected by armed conflicts, including an important watch-dog role: visiting detainees and providing independent information on prisoners and war victims. Other well-known international NGOs are OXFAM, CARE, Save the Children, World Vision, Medecins Sans Frontieres (doctors without borders). Smaller international NGOs also make valuable contributions, many operating alongside national NGOs and more numerous Community Based Organizations (CBOs) (as discussed in chapter 4). Many exercise key advocacy roles (e.g., to prevent violent conflicts, promoting gender equity). Despite good intentions, international NGOs sometimes have conflicting priorities and mandates, and compete among themselves for political favor and resources. Just as applies to official development agencies of donor countries, better coordination would help them become more effective. As noted in chapter 4, a network of internationally-active NGOs recently adopted a Code of Conduct for Health Systems Strengthening, which reflects this move toward improved working practices.[46] This promising development needs to be monitored and evaluated.

OTHER AGENCIES

Many other institutions, universities, laboratories, and consulting groups are active in bilateral and multilateral initiatives. Several philanthropic bodies contribute substantially to international health (e.g., Bill and Melinda Gates Foundation, Robert Wood Johnson Foundation, David and Lucille Packard Foundation, Aga Khan Development Network).

Strategic Leadership and Management in Public Health Services

To achieve success, public health services must work cooperatively, and include effective community representation in the process. Uncertain political environments in most jurisdictions make this an ongoing challenge. Good intentions are never enough to deliver good outcomes: also needed are policy frameworks, appropriate organizational structures, and functional management, guided by strategic and operational plans. WHO illustrates a commitment to these elements with its approach to results based management (discussed earlier). We now explore the underlying principles in greater depth.

Simply put, to achieve success requires answers to these strategic questions (see also Chapter 5: Linking Health Situation Analysis to Public Health Action): *Where are we? Where do we want to be? How are we going to get there? How will we know we are getting there?* For sound development of public health services, evidence-based strategic thinking combined with community participation are key ingredients in answering each of these questions. Put more formally, what we are referring to here is how to bring together such disciplines as needs assessment, priority setting, policy development, planning, financing, monitoring and evaluation, in a manner that produces effective, responsive and sustainable public health programs for which communities feel some degree of ownership. However, to achieve this, leadership is essential, this being "the capacity to influence others to work together to achieve a common purpose."[47] In other words, evidence by itself is not enough to generate action.

Priority setting in health services planning is not a new challenge but is one of growing importance, especially in publicly financed systems where constrained resources and increasing demand are leading policy makers to address this need more directly than in the past.[48] Similarly, while the term "evidence-based" has gained caché in recent years, taking such an approach to planning public health services is really not a new concept. The logical process is time-honored and, while methods vary across time and place, the generic steps are as follows:

- Assess the situation ("health situation analysis")
- Identify and define problems ("problem analysis")
- Prioritize with regard to the following (evidence-based) criteria
  - Disease burden
  - Intervention effectiveness
  - Economic analysis
  - Operational feasibility

Each of these criteria may be quantified in a way that can assist in ranking different conditions for priority setting purposes. However, setting priorities is not only a quantitative exercise, but must take into account such qualitative considerations as social and political acceptability, and a diverse spectrum of unlike hazards to population health. A priority setting exercise thereby brings into play considerations of a complex and sometimes judgmental nature. For example, the consequences of low probability natural hazards such as flood or earthquake could be catastrophic in the short term; by contrast, high frequency but perceived low risk events could produce considerable ongoing public health burden, such as constant exposure to toxic contaminants in food or water. It is in such contrasts where concepts introduced earlier come into play, such as the choice of relevant indicators (chapter 5) and the "prevention paradox" (see chapter 6).

In other words, public health services must plan for human needs and events with probabilities and consequences across a wide range of real or potential experiences, as well as consider issues of prevention effectiveness and acceptability of alternative interventions. To achieve this, it must call upon its component disciplines, such as health situation analysis, problem analysis and prioritization as a basis for planning how each entity should then be represented in capacity development. Having taken this approach, we are then better placed to move to the next steps in the planning sequence:

- Design and/or adjust program plans accordingly
- Budget/allocate resources in line with the plan
- Monitor the process and evaluate the outcomes
- Recommence the planning, monitoring and evaluation cycle

This approach just outlined may be viewed as public health's version of what is more commonly known as a management cycle; this approach is generally followed in other mature areas of health services planning as well. A version of this approach developed for community based program development is given in Figure 8-2.

RESULTS BASED MANAGEMENT FOR SUCCESSFUL PUBLIC HEALTH PROGRAMS

Setting priorities and making good decisions are major steps, but do not in themselves ensure that successful actions or effective programs will result.[49] This is where

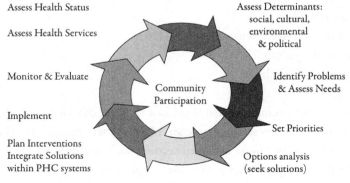

FIGURE 8-2 Planning cycle for a community health system[72].

n assist, by elaborating the critical steps and assumptions thereby
"logic model kelihood that public health initiatives will be effective in achieving
to increas tcomes, and efficient in their delivery. Such approaches also provide
their d thin which initiatives can be monitored to ensure that inputs, activi-
fram and expected results are taking place as planned, and may contribute
ti to determine how much measured change in impact and/or outcome
buted to the intervention. Taken collectively, this is often referred to as
d *management.*

ne early 1990s, logic models have been increasingly applied in public health
for project and program planning, monitoring and evaluation. This resur-
due in part to efforts to improve aid effectiveness following disappointments
rnational development practices during the 1980s, including the failure of
MF structural adjustment policies to address health and social impacts. As a more
constructive alternative, the discipline inherent in logic models quickly became a
requirement for funding from virtually all international development agencies (it
had been advocated by USAID since the 1970s), and has also become accepted practice domestically in donor countries. At the core of logic models is the exercise of
logical framework analysis (LFA) or equivalent. This useful discipline (especially
if facilitated and applied in a participatory environment) can help to generate all
essential elements of planning, monitoring and evaluation. Adopting a participatory approach with stakeholders (both those who will be charged with implementing the initiative, and its beneficiaries) contributing to an LFA exercise promotes
ownership and is also more likely to result in critical assumptions being recognized.
The discipline, when properly practiced, requires policy makers and practitioners to
move away from arbitrary objectives (unsupportable aspirations) and to ensure that
all operational objectives are scientifically sound and managerially feasible, so as to
increase the chances of success.

By "scientifically sound," we refer to evidence of acceptable rigor that the intervention can lead to change at the population level within the proposed timeframe;
this requires a prior body of existing operational research, usually including testing
of the intervention or its components in a real population setting (e.g., demonstration projects). By "managerially feasible" we refer to such considerations as organizational capacity including a budget and other resources sufficient to carry out the
intervention at the scale and length of time required to achieve the expected result;
that the people affected are supportive and willing to accommodate the intervention; and that the necessary political commitment is sufficient to see the process
through, and sustain it for the long haul.

In summary, the use of logic models that take into account good science and good
management is widely recommended to ensure the adoption of feasible operational

objectives and indicators for monitoring and evaluation across a ra[...] and outcomes. This discipline includes identifying critical assumptio[...] *processes* mitigating them if they cannot be dealt with in advance. To develop a[...] *ys of* model is a rigorous undertaking that aims to inform policy makers and p[...] to whether and how a desired outcome may be reached. An LFA matrix is il[...] in Table 8-4.

In applying LFA to monitoring and evaluation, it is important to select indic[...] sparingly. Collecting too much information can reduce data quality, increase co[...] and delay feedback to management, even rendering such feedback irrelevant to dec[...] sion making. Constructing a useful and feasible array of indicators is therefore an important area of planning: it is desirable to select relatively few that are measurable, independently verifiable, and that can be monitored easily and regularly at various levels of an initiative.

There are many useful formulations of LFA, all with variations on terminology and technique. An excellent online review for those unfamiliar with this approach is available from the Australian Agency for International Development (AusAID), as cited.[50]

MONITORING AND EVALUATION AS COMPLEMENTARY DISCIPLINES IN PUBLIC HEALTH

Monitoring and evaluation (often referred to as M&E) are closely linked and complementary disciplines. For our purposes three levels are relevant: process, impact and outcome. *Process* refers to how a given intervention is carried out, including the resource inputs, activities and whom these are reaching. Its purpose is to yield information on policy and intervention designs that will assist in improving their demonstration, dissemination and potential for scaling up (discussed in chapter 4). *Outcome* refers to whether the intervention has resulted or is resulting in changes in an ultimate target of the intervention (e.g., a shift in disease burden). *Impact* falls midway between process and outcome, referring to early or intermediate effects, such as target behaviors or other risk factors that may signal progress toward meeting the project goal.

There are important distinctions between monitoring and evaluation. *Monitoring* refers to the ongoing or periodic review of project inputs and operational milestones to determine whether (or not) it is proceeding according to plan. Although monitoring may be done independently by a third party, good management practice normally requires that managers themselves are monitoring the performance of their programs, especially at the level of process. This is an important component of accountability: given their mandate and requisite resource inputs, public health

TABLE 8-4

A log frame matrix: structure and content

Hierarchical Objective	Indicators	Means of Verification	Assumptions
Goal The long term development impact (policy goal) to which the project contributes.	How achievement of the Goal will be measured—including appropriate targets specified by quantity, quality and time.	Sources of information on the Goal indicator(s)—including who will collect it and how often	Assumptions linking the Purpose to Goal
Purpose The medium term result(s) that the project aims to deliver. Note: Everything within this is considered to be within the "manageable interest" of the project—it is what the project can be held accountable for.	How achievement of the Purpose will be measured—including appropriate targets specified by quantity, quality and time.	Sources of information on Purpose indicator(s)—including who will collect it and how often	
Expected Results (Component Objectives) This level in the hierarchy of objectives can be used to provide a clear link between outputs and outcomes (particularly for larger multi-component activities)	How achievement of Expected Results will be measured—including appropriate targets specified by quantity, quality and time.	Sources of information on the Component Objectives indicator(s)—including who will collect it and how often	Assumptions linking Component Objectives to Purpose or Outcome

(continued)

TABLE 8-4 (Continued)

Hierarchical Objective	Indicators	Means of Verification	Assumptions
Outputs The products or services that the activity will deliver	How the achievement of the Outputs will be measured—including appropriate targets specified by quantity, quality and time.	Sources of information on Output indicator(s)—including who will collect it and how often	Assumptions linking Output to Component Objective
Lower order objectives include Activities and (below this) Tasks.	Indicators, Means of Verification and Assumptions can be identified at activity and task levels also, but this is not usually done depending on operational complexity.		

Note: Terminology varies: what is fundamental is respect for the logic of the process.

program managers are normally held responsible for meeting operational targets (e.g., defined tasks and activities).

While monitoring may identify changes in process, impact or even outcomes, generally it does not permit assessment as to whether or how much this apparent change is attributable to the intervention. For example, monitoring of a local intervention to reduce diarrheal disease incidence by improving hygiene (Figure 8-3A), may not be able to take into account background improvements due to other influences e.g., improving health literacy and access to information; evaluation must take that background improvement into account in order to attribute any amount of change to the intervention itself (Figure 8-3B).[51] Herein lies the distinction from evaluation: *evaluation* attempts to go further, and is normally carried out at strategically important times, such as mid-project or end of project. Evaluation is concerned not only with how things were done, and whether milestones were met, but also the extent to which change is attributable to the intervention. Evaluation is often best carried out by a third party, to ensure independence and freedom from conflict of interest, and requires more scientifically rigorous methods.

Important lessons must be learned from monitoring and evaluation. It is not enough to know simply that an intervention actually worked or didn't in producing improved outcomes in a given setting. To be of value in disseminating the intervention or scaling up, it is critical to know *how* it worked, what could be done to make it work better, and whether operational or contextual factors were keys to its success. This is why monitoring and evaluation are complementary disciplines; Figure 8-4 illustrates how they are situated within an LFA planning process.

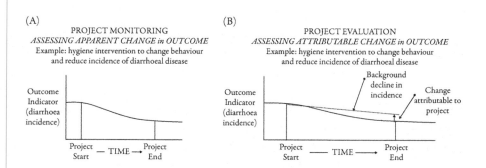

FIGURE 8-3 Comparing apparent change and attributable change.

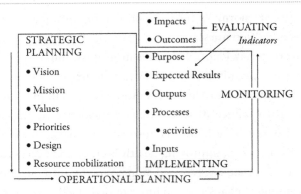

FIGURE 8-4 Where planning, monitoring and evaluation fit within a results-based logic model.

It is relevant to conclude this introduction to M&E with a note on the use of "balanced scorecards." These are a selection of indicators that represent criteria for attaining specified objectives: they focus on key operations and processes, should be adequate for assessing progress toward objectives, and must be objectively verifiable. These are usually derived from the indicators developed from an initial logic model, then embedded within a management information system in a way that renders program monitoring feasible on a continuous basis (e.g., using a "dashboard" of indicators that can be shown on a computer monitor or printed out as ongoing or periodic reports). While the balanced scorecard is a simple and convenient application of a logic model, it will not necessarily answer all evaluation questions, especially with regard to attributing change to an intervention. More purpose designed evaluations may still be necessary periodically.

Public Health Goals and Objectives at Societal Level

Beyond the requirements of specific programs, public health initiatives around the world increasingly reveal the incorporation of health goals and objectives within broader public agendas, collaboration of government with private and voluntary sector participation, encouragement of coalitions, demonstrations with emphasis on integrated approaches at community level, commitment to evaluation (process and/or outcome) and international collaboration. It is important to learn from the emerging experience of such developments as they represent a trend toward more complex initiatives.

Unfortunately, in pursuing broader agendas, many jurisdictions underestimate critical epidemiological and management considerations in the evidence base for goal setting, thereby increasing the likelihood of under-performance or even failure.

For example, the Canadian province of British Columbia (BC) in 2006 announced a bold health promotion initiative called Act Now. Mindful of da Vinci's dictum that "Practice must always be founded on sound theory," our view is that some of the Act Now targets to be met by 2010 from a 2003 baseline were evidence-based and achievable (e.g., a 10% reduction in tobacco use), while others were arbitrary and more aptly viewed as "aspirational" (e.g., a 20% reduction in overweight and obesity). There is no evidence from anywhere in the world that such an ambitious population objective for overweight and obesity could ever be achieved within this timeframe: complex chronic conditions that take decades to develop in a population cannot be so promptly reduced. Taking a longer view, Act Now's potential to reduce disease burdens depends on its sustainability well beyond 2010: a political challenge for successive governments.[48]

Other examples of societywide health objectives are also instructive, the most ambitious being the US Health and Human Services initiative Healthy People 2010 (HP2010). HP2010 was built around two over-arching goals: *the first goal* to increase quality and years of healthy life, challenging the nation to address the complex interactions of health, disease, disability, and early death. The emphasis here is on outcomes, and commitment to implementing effective prevention and health promotion interventions to facilitate progress within the decade. *The second goal* of eliminating health disparities is arguably a more complex challenge that depends more on health systems development in the United States. A mid-course review revealed that disparities were not declining, that it may be more difficult and costly to implement effective prevention and health promotion programs for some populations and, unless greater reductions occur for those with the highest rates of morbidity, large disparities will remain.[52]

With 507 objectives and sub-objectives monitored, HP2010 is the most comprehensive population health vision of any jurisdiction in the world. In addition to health promotion domains, numerous disease-specific domains are included. To illustrate just one area of objective setting, we show the example of food security in Box 8-A.

There is a history to this experience. HP2010 originated from a similar exercise (HP2000) that set out in 1991 specific health goals and targets to be achieved by 2000, using health promotion and disease prevention strategies and tactics. This outlined roles and responsibilities of government agencies, the health sector, industry, other social sectors, and individuals.[53] The experience was considered so relevant and successful that it was reformulated as HP2010 and has become, in effect, a rolling exercise of national health goals and targets that may be extended to 2020 and beyond.[54] Nonetheless, it is difficult to advocate a model that puts forward hundreds

BOX 8-A

EXAMPLE OF SETTING AN OBJECTIVE RELATED TO NUTRITION

Objective: Increase food security among US households and in so doing reduce hunger.

Target: 94%.

Baseline: 88% of all US households were food secure in 1995.

Target setting method: 6 percentage point improvement (50% decrease in food insecurity; consistent with the US pledge to the 1996 World Food Summit).

Data source: Food Security Supplement to the Current Population Survey, US Department of Commerce, Bureau of the Census.

of objectives as realistic for any jurisdiction outside the US. Even within the US, this is more like a "menu" when viewed by state health departments, which have the authority and responsibility for most health services development, and who must translate such objectives in the context of their own health situation, priorities, and existing performance against the indicators.

According to the US National Academy of Sciences, Institute of Medicine (IOM), "despite leading the world in health expenditures, the United States is not fully meeting its potential in health status and lags behind many of its peers." While HP2010 is impressive from a planning perspective, the failings of the US health system are well-recognized domestically and internationally (revisit Table 8-1). The IOM report states:[55] "...the vast majority of health care spending,...is directed towards medical care and biomedical research. However, there is strong evidence that behavior and environment are responsible for over 70% of avoidable mortality, and health care is just one of several determinants of health. Furthermore, the benefits of our current investments in health care are inaccessible to many due to lack of insurance or access to services." Given this analysis, the IOM Committee on Assuring the Health of the Public in the 21st Century embraced the vision articulated in HP2010 as it offers the US a way forward that reflects its systemic realities.

Although the US still has much work to do, the Patient Protection and Affordable Care Act upheld by the Supreme Court on June 28, 2012 (discussed earlier), holds new promise for correcting many of these deficiencies. Among its provisions (under Title IV: Prevention of Chronic Disease and Improving Public Health)[56] are new measures such as the Prevention and Public Health Fund and a National Prevention Strategy.

At global level there are also notable efforts at setting public health goals and objectives. The most historic of these is the WHO coordinated Global Eradication of Smallpox (case study, chapter 2) and WHO is now moving toward other eradication objectives (e.g., poliomyelitis, guinea worm, trachoma). However, most major causes of global disease burden are not amenable to eradication; yet these too benefit from initiatives that invoke evidence-based setting of goals and objectives. Taking diabetes as an example, there have been several regional efforts involving partnership between WHO, the International Diabetes Federation (IDF), individual countries, and industry to promote coherent, evidence-based, and integrated programming to address the global pandemic of type 2 diabetes: first the St Vincent Declaration (1989), which addresses European countries, then the Declaration of the Americas or DOTA (1996), the Western Pacific Declaration on Diabetes (WPDD 2000), and most recently the Declaration and Diabetes Strategy for Sub-Saharan Africa (2006). The declarations were accompanied by action plans with varying levels of detail; for example, for the WPDD this includes a rolling process of planning, monitoring and evaluation.[57] These in turn fostered the development of national diabetes programs,[58] and contributed to an emerging new foundation for a more broadly based approach to the pandemic of NCDs as a whole (chapter 6).

The St Vincent's, Western Pacific and Africa initiatives remain fully in force, but DOTA was discontinued as a joint operational venture of PAHO/WHO and IDF after two 5 year planning and implementation periods; nonetheless it achieved some successes and helped guide a new initiative designed to address a wider range of noncommunicable diseases.[59] It met its short term targets in most countries: designation of national focal points, preparation of national estimates of disease burden, development and implementation of national strategies and plans to deal with diabetes, and recognition of diabetes as a public health problem. The initiative stimulated the development of national guidelines for improving diabetes control in clinical management, diabetes education and nutrition, the defining of minimum acceptable standards of care, enhanced regional training and information sharing, and the implementation in several countries of a quality of care management system.[60] A number of lessons emerged: the relevance of process-related targets to achieve short to medium term success; the value of broadly based participation in gaining recognition of a major cause of disease burden at national health policy level; wide acceptance of an integrated program model; and the critical role of having a Ministry staff member designated in each country as a managerial focal point.[61]

It may also be concluded that recognition by WHO of regionally based policy actions, co-sponsored by an international NGO (in this instance the International Diabetes Federation), with significant industry financial support for related initiatives, adds visibility and enhances commitment to evidence-based approaches and accountability for performance. The resulting gains to implementing organizations and other stakeholders can be attributed to the enhanced cooperation surrounding a mutual challenge and the opportunity for participation in setting goals and objectives. As major risk factors for diabetes are common to most other chronic conditions, interventions in this area, guided by scientifically sound and managerially feasible objectives applied at the level of communities as well as individuals, will positively impact on population health. Ongoing monitoring and evaluation of such initiatives will continue to generate useful lessons for the development of larger and potentially more complex international public health initiatives.

The Issue of Vertical versus Horizontal Program Assistance

There is a long-standing debate in the public health community about the relative merits of so-called "vertical" (categorical or discrete) and "horizontal" programs. This debate is slowly receding as integrated models emerge, which incorporate elements of both types of program. Nonetheless, it is important to recognize the issues at stake.

The debate has been ongoing since the Alma Ata Declaration on Primary Health Care (1978), as discussed in chapter 4. Vertical programs characteristically focus on a specific demographic group, disease, or health issue, usually with specified, measurable objectives within a defined time-frame; their activities are often designed without reference to, and tend to by-pass, broadly based primary health care (PHC) activities. Although now less apparent in developed countries, examples of vertical programming still have a dominate role at all levels of service in development settings, such as special initiatives to address HIV/AIDS, tuberculosis and malaria (see chapter 5 for discussion of the Global Fund). By contrast, horizontal programs focus on providing integrated health care for interrelated health problems for entire populations, and are organized within broadly based public health and primary health care systems. Historically, vertical programs have been favored by the donor community, while horizontal programs remain for in-country jurisdictions to design, develop, and deliver without external assistance.

Vertical programs do offer advantages: targeting resources to health issues deemed to be a priority (much therefore depends on who makes this decision and how it is done). With well-defined (although relatively narrow) operational objectives, vertical programs encourage greater accountability. Some have been highly successful; for example, smallpox eradication, major progress in polio and onchocerciasis, and encouraging advances in tobacco control. Most attractive to donors is the potential for a highly visible return on investment; this reflects well on their own accountability to taxpayers in donor countries.

However, their disadvantages are numerous: they can distort development priorities; they compete inequitably for staff (who are paid much more and enjoy international prestige); they may weaken local health infrastructures, especially primary care; they may duplicate capacities, thereby reducing overall resource efficiencies; their unique organizational structures and reporting requirements are not always suitable for local, broader, and more sustainable uses. They have been criticized for contributing to fragmented health care, delaying development of more broadly based health systems, and for delaying attention to other specific conditions that arguably are of higher priority in terms of disease burden but more difficult to address and/or not so well favored by the donor community (e.g., endemic diarrheal disease in children, and its underlying determinants).

Some vertical programs show success in particular settings, but are difficult to scale up and to sustain. Tuberculosis is a good example, in light of limited overall success despite a high level of global investment. A recent review revealed numerous shortcomings: structures of both in-country health care systems and international donor programs were found sub-optimal for effective delivery of TB treatment, especially for drug-resistant forms, in many high-burden countries. Problems include underdeveloped public health systems, overemphasis on institutionalized care, fragmented funding and service delivery, inadequate training and expertise, inconsistent and sporadic technical assistance, ineffective diagnostic and referral networks, limited information technology and data collection, and inadequate financial resources.[62] To correct most of these deficiencies requires attention to more broadly based health systems support than can be justified or delivered within the framework of a single disease initiative.

Several related issues were presented in chapter 6, especially with regard to how most people actually experience disease through the life-course and the appropriateness of developing integrated approaches and strengthening health systems as a whole. With vertical programs, gains in specific disease control are achieved mostly in mainstream (easy-to-reach) populations, with continuing disadvantages for higher risk groups experiencing barriers to their health. In chapter 6, we noted that these deficiencies are only recently being recognized by donor agencies, and efforts finally being made to correct them by allocating greater program assistance to health systems strengthening.

Based on the foregoing observations, the general case for more integrated policy and management appears strong, whereby all programs are developed and implemented within an overall framework so as to be mutually supportive. Despite this, the continued need for vertical programming remains legitimate in particular instances; for example, as a short-term measure in fragile states, for the control of some epidemics and the management of some emergencies, and so that appropriate services can be provided for specific client groups such as commercial sex workers, drug addicts or prisoners.

There remain the issues of scaling up from locally successful interventions, and sustainability. Wider implementation requires caution, especially for vertical programs, given the limitations just outlined. At this stage, the reader may wish to revisit the section in chapter 4 dealing with "Scaling Up: When Does It Apply, and How Can We Do It?"

The Role of Public Health in Reducing the Impacts of Disasters

What is a disaster? The United Nations defines it as "serious disruption of the functioning of a society, causing widespread human, material, or environmental losses which exceed the ability of the affected society to cope using its own resources." By this definition, only those events where losses exceed a society's ability to cope and external aid is required constitute a disaster.[63] Most classifications identify two main types: natural and human-made. Natural disasters are sub-classified as sudden impact (floods, earthquakes, tidal waves, tropical storms, volcanic eruptions, landslides), slow-onset (drought, famine, environmental degradation, deforestation, pest infestation, and desertification), and epidemic infectious diseases; human-made disasters include two classes: industrial/technological disasters (associated with pollution, spillage of hazardous materials, explosions, and fires) and complex emergencies (e.g., war, internal conflict).

Most natural and human-made disasters occur suddenly and unexpectedly, disrupting normal social and health care systems.[64] Although there is an important role for rapid assessment of damage and risk to human life and health immediately following a disaster, once it has occurred is too late for comprehensive planning: this must be done in advance. All public health jurisdictions therefore need to conduct risk assessments and participate in disaster planning in normal times so as to anticipate and be able to respond to them.

Features of physical and social geography, climate and industrial development are the keys as to where to start. For example, seismically unstable areas are prone to earthquake, low lying areas are susceptible to hurricanes and floods, coastal areas are susceptible to tsunamis, those susceptible to drought are prone to bush fires, human settlements in mountainous areas may be susceptible to avalanche, and so on. Similarly, the proximity of industries may set up an area for increased risk of particular occurrences, either due to the intrinsic risk of some industries or in combination with natural disasters: examples include chemical plants, and other power generating facilities, toxic waste transportation systems and so on. The impact of the 2011 tsunami on Japan is a case in point—a tragedy compounded by damage and meltdown of nuclear power plants affected because they had been sited on the coast, virtually at sea level (see chapter 9 for related discussion).

In addition to physical geography, the potential for natural phenomena to adversely affect people is influenced by size and proximity of populations, quality of building construction, sustainability of utilities (e.g., water, electricity, waste disposal, telecommunications), transportation, and other infrastructure considerations. Time of year also impacts on the risk and even survivability of populations, especially the most vulnerable (e.g., mid-winter in a cold country is not a good time to become homeless).

Experience reveals that mistakes are more often made in the absence of prior recognition of risk, and preparation of organizations and staff to respond in accordance with a predesigned plan, or when relief and/or rescue operations are not efficiently directed or coordinated, and when public communications in response to the disaster are not well considered or well controlled. Similarly, some communities remain at high risk because the lessons of past disasters are not always followed by remedial action (e.g., inadequate building practices may continue unchanged).

Disasters are being reported more frequently in recent decades, proportionally more of the increase being attributed to those which are climate related (e.g., floods, drought), as distinct from those which are not (e.g., earthquake). We return to this global issue in chapter 9. Table 8-5 lists the top ten disasters in 2010, in terms of number of victims.[65]

The World Conference on Disaster Reduction held in Hyogo, Japan, in 2005, pledged to reduce the risks facing millions of people exposed to natural disasters.[66]

TABLE 8-5

Top ten disasters in 2010 by number of victims

Rank	Type of Disaster	Country	Victims (Millions)
1	Flood, May-August	China People's Republic	134.0
2	Flash Flood, July-August	Pakistan	20.4
3	Flood, October-December	Thailand, Cambodia*	9.0
4	Drought, March-August	Thailand	6.5
5	Flood, June-August	China People's Republic	6.0
6	Earthquake, January	Haiti	3.9
7	Flood, September	India	3.3
8	Earthquake, February	Chile	2.7
9	Drought, February-December	Somalia	2.4
10	Flood, April-December	Colombia	2.2
TOTAL			190.3

*Thailand (8,970,911 victims), Cambodia (8 victims).

Source: Guha-Sapir D, Vos F, Below R, with Ponserre S. Annual Disaster Statistical Review 2010: The Numbers and Trends. Brussels: CRED; 2011, as cited in reference #66.

The "Hyogo Framework for Action: 2005–2015" aims to strengthen the capacity of disaster-prone countries to address risk and invest in disaster preparedness. It also recognizes the relationship between disaster reduction, sustainable development and poverty reduction, and calls for an integrated multihazard approach for sustainable development to reduce the incidence and severity of disasters. Implementation is being monitored globally.[67]

It follows from this that public health organizations at all levels should be engaged in relevant aspects of disaster response planning, preparedness, multisector cooperation, coordination and communications. Public health professionals can contribute skills that derive from their competence in such areas as health situation analysis, disease surveillance and rapid assessment techniques, as well as their abilities to lead, manage and work within teams. To be effective, team members should know their roles and practice them: emergency and disaster simulations are a useful way to test the system.

There are aspects of disasters where the health threat is critical. For example, waterborne disease following flooding may represent a major challenge (chapter 7). Conversely, there are issues of emergency shelter and essential food supplies that usually go beyond the capacity of public health organizations: overall responsibility for these is often designated to a dedicated emergency response agency (e.g., in the United States this is FEMA, the Federal Emergency Response Agency, which has its counterparts at state and municipal levels).[68] There are also designated roles for uniformed services (e.g., police, fire fighters, and the military). Similar arrangements are found in other nations. The work of public health agencies must closely coordinate with the work of other elements of the health system (e.g., hospitals must have their own disaster response plans). However, when disasters occur in developing countries, they are more likely to overwhelm local capacities both logistically and financially: this then become a focus for international relief agencies, donor agencies and NGOs. This is true even within developed countries, where local jurisdictions must depend on state and federal response capacities, such as occurred following the impact of Hurricane Katrina on New Orleans in 2005.

Further discussion of complex humanitarian emergencies, including those related to conflict, social breakdown and displacement of people, and the global need for better emergency planning and action on such planning, can be found in chapter 9.

Health Human Resources

It is appropriate to close this chapter by observing that the most important resource in the labor intensive health sector is its people, and that this applies fully to the public health field. That personnel account for most health expenditures virtually everywhere, renders this of major fiscal importance to politicians, funding agencies, accountants and taxpayers. However, greater salience is found in the reality that health (along with education and social services) is a major domain of human service in both public and private sectors. While health is a highly technical field, requiring facilities, equipment, transport, vaccines, drugs, supplies, transport and information infrastructure (all of which also require funding), ultimately everyone depends on intelligent decisions regarding application (or nonapplication) of these resources for their health status, whether assessed at population or personal level. Investing in health to a large extent means investment in human resources: well-trained, well-motivated people who know what they are doing. Health is a "knowledge-based" field, and part of the "knowledge economy."

Health human resources (HHR) is defined by the World Health Organization as "all people engaged in actions whose primary intent is to enhance health." This includes both providers and those who do not deliver services directly but who are essential to effective health system functioning, including many people in public health: policy makers, program coordinators, planners, epidemiologists, health information scientists, environmental inspectors, economists, academicians, administrators, and others. As a field, HHR addresses all aspects of the human resource that are essential to a functional health system: the demographic, social, educational, economic, organizational and policy attributes that influence need, supply and demand, and how these characteristics affect key performance components, such as access, quality, equity, and who bears the cost.

Research capacity pertaining to HHR has been actively expanding in recent years, and related activities can now be found across many government, academic institutions, international organizations, and donor agencies. This is needed in all parts of the world: to foster effective and sustainable health performance at all levels so that people get an essential range of services when needed, from local to national, from developed to developing country settings. The research agenda includes all aspects of HHR noted in the previous paragraph. To take the example of core competencies for public health professionals in the United States (chapter 2), these will continue to evolve in response to evaluation and a growing body of related research, and mirrored by comparable work in other parts of the world in response to their own requirements and circumstances.

Raising awareness of the critical role of HHR in strengthening health system performance and improving health outcomes is high on the global health agenda, and there is a growing body of research literature pertaining to HHR that is relevant to particular global issues.[69] For example, migration of health professionals away from countries in greatest need, often in response to drives by recruitment firms based in developed countries, is extensively studied, and is a serious issue with ethical implications. In 2010, the World Health Assembly issued a Global Policy of Practice on the International Recruitment of Health Personnel.[70] Although nonbinding on Member States and recruitment agencies, the Code promotes principles and practices for the ethical international recruitment of health personnel. It advocates the strengthening of health personnel information systems to support effective health workforce research, policy, and planning in member countries.

As this closing section is just a brief introduction to health human resources, the reader may wish to seek more comprehensive discussion from sources such as the WHO reference cited.[71]

Conclusion

In this chapter we tried to show how community foundations, health situation analysis, health promotion, disease prevention and disaster response, all fit within the context of organization and function of public health from local to global levels. To be fully effective team players, practitioners must also be able to relate their work to how larger health systems are designed and operate, the challenges facing them. And, of course, they must have a sound knowledge of public health organizations, structures and functions, the comparative merits of particular program designs, the importance of a well-trained, well-motivated human resource, and the over-arching importance of sound priority setting, planning, monitoring and evaluation in order to assure longer term success.

The purpose of this chapter is to consider issues of global concern that have major implications for the future, such as climate change, lifestyle expectations, population dynamics and disaster response. As custodians of our planet, our ecological footprint is cause for concern: there is a clear need for new ethical leadership that is more respectful of and in tune with our environment as a core human relationship. The chapter therefore opens with a focus on the planet, moving then to health and population issues. We examine the impacts of climate change on distribution of disease vectors and the displacement of peoples, and discuss what we can do about these trends at the level of public policy and as individuals. Also presented are new shifts in public health education in response to the need for greater health literacy. Our intent in laying out these ideas is to illustrate the importance of forward thinking in assessing our health futures.

9

GLOBAL ECOLOGY AND EMERGING HEALTH CHALLENGES

The Ever-Changing Environment of Planet Earth

PLANET EARTH CAME into existence about 4.5 billion years ago. Variations in the composition of our atmosphere began with those geophysical origins, including the influence of cosmic impacts, including various forms of radiation, especially solar. With the infusion of this energy, the development of air, water and the substances that were to become early forms of food, became key ingredients for the origins of life. The fossil record suggests that the earliest life forms, primitive microorganisms, appeared about 3.5 billion years ago. Complex vegetative and animal species evolved through adaptation to changing environments, and this process in itself influenced environmental change, contributing to such phenomena as the oxygen and nitrogen cycles and the development of soil. Meteor impact and consequent massive dust storms are thought to explain the abrupt disappearance of dinosaurs, and such a catastrophe today would have similar impact on distribution and abundance of living organisms. Natural environmental variations continue in such forms as volcanic activity, wind erosion, dust storms, chemical reactions, and forest fires. For example, volcanic activity around the world, from the Azores[1] to Vanuatu,[2] can produce sudden or ongoing impacts on air, earth and water, with impacts on health and population migrations.

Although the geological record shows that the earth's climate has been influenced over countless millions of years by volcanic eruptions, variations in ocean currents, and changes in Earth's axis, some recent variations are anthropogenic.[3] For example, traces of lead in the Greenland ice have been linked to atmospheric pollution two millennia ago, mostly attributed to Roman smelting in the Rio Tinto region of Spain.[4] Lead levels of that era were about four times the natural background level. This illustrates not only the long distance transportation of air pollutants, half a world from their point of origin, but also the persistence of some of them in the environment. The Greenland ice cap also reflects the impact of North American industrial emissions over the past century, during which substantial increases have been recorded for: sulphates, ammonium, nitrates, fluoride, formaldehyde, halocarbons, hydrogen peroxide, and carbon monoxide. Along with a massive increase in lead content (250 times pre-industrial levels), other heavy metals (zinc, copper, cadmium) also show increases although these are more moderate (2.3, 2.7 and 9-fold, respectively). The impact of policies and laws requiring the removal of lead from gasoline is reflected in recent lead reductions in ice core measurements.[5] Evidence of anthropogenic impacts can be found today in virtually all environments, from the polar regions to coral reefs.

Over the past two centuries, human activity (directly, or indirectly through other species, e.g., overgrazing) has substantially modified natural emissions and their impacts, and produced new ones. Illustrating the former are the 1997–1998 forest fires in Indonesia, among the largest in history, and attributed mostly to "slash and burn" practices for clearing forests to make space for agriculture. This event produced an air pollution disaster, and vividly illustrated the major problem of trans-boundary air pollution and the need for national, regional and global policies to prevent and mitigate such impacts. Research into the event revealed that much of the smoke (airborne particulate matter) came from burning peat marsh biomass. The severity and extent of air pollution was unprecedented, affecting some 300 million people across Southeast Asia, with major health impacts. The economic costs due to this environmental disaster were enormous and yet to be fully determined. Among the important sectors severely affected were air and land transport, shipping, construction, tourism, and agro-based industries.[6]

The phenomenon of developing new emissions over the past two centuries is illustrated by the industrialization that led to a proliferation of "smokestack industries," first in western Europe, then in North America, now around the world, such that air pollution has become a global concern. *Air pollution disasters* in the mid-20th century (Meuse Valley, Belgium 1930, Donora, Pennsylvania 1948, and London, England 1952), in which thousands perished within days from the acute effects of intense smog, drew attention to this alarming trend, and provoked the introduction of Clean Air legislation, first in the United Kingdom (1956), then in the United States (1970) and other countries.[7] While extreme exposures appear to have abated in developed countries, due mostly to regulatory actions and self-interest (most people do not want to breathe dirty air, and many industries wish to be disassociated from it), severe air pollution now occurs in large cities in many developing countries (e.g., Kathmandu, Shanghai, Beijing, Sao Paulo, Mexico City), and a resulting global threat is emerging from the accumulating emissions worldwide. Until the recent forest fires in Indonesia, many observers thought that air pollution disasters were a thing of the past; but now we recognize that we may be on the verge of a new wave of such events, given the extent with which unsustainable environmental practices affect all parts of the world.

The Intergovernmental Panel on Climate Change (IPCC) is the leading international body for the assessment of climate change. It was established by the United Nations Environment Programme (UNEP) and the World Meteorological Organization (WMO) to provide the world with a scientific view on the current state of knowledge in climate change and its potential environmental and socioeconomic impacts.[8] The relatively sudden increase in average global air temperature over the past century has been linked by the IPPC to the increase in atmospheric "greenhouse gases" due to the burning of fossil fuels, land clearing, and other human activities. Effects include rising sea levels and changes in climate, weather patterns, and air quality. The process is hazardous to people, domestic and wild animals, and cultivated and wild plant life, through the associated occurrence of violent storms, floods, droughts, heat-waves, smog, geographic extension of insect-borne diseases, and other impacts such as desertification. The term "greenhouse gases" (GHGs) refers to emissions that permit passage of solar radiation to reach Earth's surface, but that impede the escape of longer wave-length radiation, thereby trapping heat in the atmosphere (the "greenhouse effect"). GHGs include carbon dioxide (released by burning fossil fuels), methane (from digestion or decomposition of vegetation, including from cattle, estimated 1.5 billion globally), nitrous oxide, and a mixture of chlorinated fluorocarbons (CFCs), perflurocarbons (PFC) and sulfur hexafluoride (SF), and other gases.

The Health Impacts of Climate Change

Among the wide range of issues that have been addressed by the IPCC is the potential adverse health effects related to climate change. The global burden of disease has already been impacted by climate change through changing weather patterns (temperature, precipitation, sea level rise, more frequent extreme weather events) and changes in ecosystems such as water, air, food quality, have also impacted agriculture, industry, settlements, and the economy.

Recent extreme weather events (hurricanes, floods, and heat waves) have provided evidence that adaptive capacity to respond to adverse health impacts needs to be improved even in developed countries.[8] This calls for increased capacity to respond to disasters and increased preparedness to identify and protect vulnerable populations. Adverse impacts are expected to be greatest for low income countries, urban poor, elderly and children, subsistence farmers and coastal populations.[8] Mass migration of people is often driven by environmental causes, such as coastal flooding and newly forming deserts. Such possibilities were speculative until recent decades, but are now the focus of intense research and have policy implications that require timely action.

According to the Union of Concerned Scientists, people bear unequal health risks from climate change for several reasons.[9] *Climate impacts differ by region:* People who live in floodplains are more likely to see river or coastal flooding; those who live in regions with poor air quality today are at greater risk from poor air quality in the future; those who live in regions more susceptible to the climate change induced ingress of disease vectors, will contract those diseases. *Some people are more vulnerable to illness or death:* Young children, the elderly, and those already ill are less able to withstand heat and poor air quality; temperature extremes and smog hit people with heart and respiratory diseases heavily. *Wealthy nations are more likely to adapt to projected climate change and recover from climate-related disasters than poor countries:* even within nations, the less economically fortunate are more vulnerable—less likely to have air conditioning and well-insulated homes; fewer resources to escape danger. These are not theoretical risks: such impacts are happening now and will increase as the future unfolds.

Increased morbidity, mortality, and hospital visits related to heat waves have been reported from Australia, Belgium, Canada, the Czech Republic, Finland, France, Germany, Japan, The Netherlands, New Zealand, Portugal, Spain, Tajikistan, Switzerland, the United Kingdom, and South Asia.[8] In France, a parliamentary inquiry concluded that the 2003 epidemic of heat-related deaths was unforeseen due to inadequate heat-related surveillance and that the limited public health response was due to limited capacity within the public health system and lack of communication between public organizations.[8] In 2004, in response, numerous initiatives were launched: national and local action plans, reevaluation of care of the elderly, building modifications in residential facilities (e.g., adding cool rooms), and improved health and environmental surveillance.[8] Similar changes have been implemented in other European countries but developing countries potentially severely affected have greater resource limitations that renders proposed interventions of this type much less feasible in those settings.

Gradual increases in daily temperatures without the profound heat wave incidents just discussed have impacted indigenous populations. Changes in animal populations related to climate change will influence hunting patterns. Access to some hunting and fishing areas is dependent on the presence or absence of snow and ice.[10] Subsistence hunting and fishing are linked with ecological and environmental conditions and many practices are particularly vulnerable to climate change.[10] In Russia, spring weather and sea ice conditions are strongly correlated with timing of hunting walrus and whales.[10] In Barrow, Alaska, goose hunting is carried out inland, followed by whale hunting that is dependent on sea ice. Earlier snow melt results in an earlier hunting season for geese, which conflicts with whale hunting season and increases time pressure for subsistence hunters.[10] Both food insecurity and the risk of injuries may increase as hunters and fishers experience increased time pressure. Further, for villages that use a traditional food cache for meat storage and drying during the fall and winter months, a decrease in the length of cold weather may lead to increased spoilage of food, which would increase economic distress.[10]

There are concerns that climate change is beginning to impact the distribution of specific disease conditions, as demonstrated by the link between emissions of Chlorinated Fluorocarbons (CFCs—a GHG) and increased incidence of malignant melanoma (see "Case Study of an Indirect Health Effect of a Greenhouse Gas," chapter 2), and by the following example of dengue fever.

Dengue is now the world's leading arboviral disease, estimating 100 million cases of dengue fever annually, 250,000 of dengue hemorrhagic fever (DHF), and 25,000 deaths.[11] Reported from over 100 countries, 2.5 billion people now live in endemic areas. Dengue threatens populations around the world due to the expanding distribution of the virus and its mosquito vectors, co-circulation of serotypes, and the emergence of more complex and life-threatening forms of the disease in new areas. Mathematical models simulating climate change were reported by Johns Hopkins University researchers in 1998,[12] projecting that rising global temperatures will increase the range of mosquitoes that transmit dengue fever. Researchers showed that epidemic potential increases with only a relatively small temperature rise: fewer mosquitoes are necessary to maintain or spread dengue in a vulnerable population. Predicted areas of encroachment were mostly temperate regions bordering on endemic zones, where humans and the mosquito *Aedes aegypti* (principal vector), often co-exist, but where lower temperatures until then had suppressed transmission. Global warming would not only increase the mosquito's range but also reduce the size of larva and, ultimately, adult size. Since smaller adults feed more frequently to develop eggs, warmer temperatures boost the frequency of double feeding and increase transmission potential. Also, virus incubation inside mosquitoes is shortened at higher temperatures; this also can promote higher transmission rates.

It is not possible so far to confirm that climate change has produced this trend, as many factors go into the occurrence of vector-borne diseases. However, since those forecasts were published, the dengue situation has become more serious in many parts of the world. Because (as noted in chapter 6) it now involves co-circulation of three serotypes, the potential for disease burden is enhanced because a primary infection does not immunize against subsequent infection from another strain; to the contrary, it sets up a complex immune response that may result in more serious disease (e.g., dengue hemorrhagic fever and dengue shock syndrome). Although there has been ample warning of this increasing threat, diminished attention to health in many countries (e.g., education and mosquito abatement) and deteriorating infrastructures (e.g., drains and ditches, ideal for mosquito breeding) have weakened health protection. Increasingly dengue is also reported in travelers returning from infected areas. However, concerns for the impact on tourism have led to reluctant recognition by the political establishment in some countries. This is self-defeating because ultimately any nation failing to take action is more likely to have dengue become endemic. The major risk is of course for the people of the affected countries, especially those who live in heavily mosquito-afflicted areas, most often the poor who typically have limited political representation. The adequacy of health care systems may not be sufficient to cope with epidemic surges. Clearly the appropriate response is to refocus on prevention.[13]

Beyond the concern about dengue fever, as just reviewed, future climate change is anticipated to impact the distribution of other vector borne diseases (e.g., West Nile virus, malaria). However, whether it will do so remains not only to be seen, but also to be scientifically determined: it is important to emphasize that other factors (e.g., changes in land use, population density, human behavior) can also change the distribution of vectors and the extent of vector-borne diseases. The potential impacts of climate change may also vary within and between countries.

While there is need therefore for appropriate scientific caution regarding the interpretation of evidence, public health authorities must stay alert to new information as it emerges. To quote Major Greenwood, author of "Epidemics and Crowd Diseases" (1936)[14] and a famous pioneer in our field: "the scientific purist, who will wait for medical statistics until they are nosologically exact, is no wiser than Horace's rustic waiting for the river to flow away."[15] Our translation for the context of climate change and human health impacts: there is a fine line between being scientifically correct, and too late to have taken timely, effective action.

In this spirit, we take note of the IPCC Fourth Assessment Report (2007),[16] which finds that climate change has already altered the distribution of some disease vectors. Among their referenced examples: ticks have extended their range north in Sweden and Canada and into higher altitudes in the Czech Republic; in northeastern North America, there is evidence of recent micro-evolutionary (genetic) responses of the mosquito species *Wyeomyia smithii* to increased average land surface temperatures and earlier arrival of spring in the past two decades. Although not a vector of human disease, this species is closely related to important arbovirus vector species that may be undergoing similar evolutionary changes; and some bird migration patterns have changed, which may be relevant to issues such as the global reach of conditions such as avian influenza. As the saying goes: to be forewarned is to be forearmed.

What Can Be Done?

One of the wisest critics of prevailing economic theories in the 20th century, E.F. Schumacher (1911–1977), famously said that *"There is no substitute for energy… It is not 'just another commodity' but the precondition of all commodities, a basic factor equal with air, water, and earth."* Schumacher was an advocate for global reconfiguration of economies around the principle of local sustainability.[17] While atmospheric pollution, GHG accumulation, and climate change are larger existential issues than public health *per se*, the health implications are becoming steadily clearer. A key responsibility of public health leaders therefore includes engaging with others on the common goal of achieving balance between human activity and that of our natural world. However, while this is by no means a revolutionary idea, it is one that threatens some current political and industrial leaders who seem unable to grasp the vision, and are bent on resisting change. We all have vested interests, but the largest vested interest for everyone surely should be healthy survival on our planet, the only world we will ever know. The technological future does not require that we move back wholesale into the days of sail, water wheels and windmills, let alone caves, but we surely must find new ways to move intelligently toward increasing the use of renewable sources that do not pollute or warm the planet, and restoring ecological balance wherever this is still possible.

With this in mind we have selected three illustrative areas where our actions might make the largest difference: energy practices, land use management and lifestyle expectations. We also need to consider how to mitigate or contain adverse impacts where damage is already done.

Energy: Recognizing that for a long time into the future, largely because of the scale of investment already made in existing industrial and transportation infrastructures, we will remain dependent on fossil fuels. However, as the IPPC has determined, our current phase of climate change is largely attributable to this, and if we are to be responsible custodians of our planet, we must find cleaner, more efficient methods of combustion. This applies at all levels from large scale power generation and transportation to how people cook in their homes. For example, keeping in mind that about two-thirds of all health effects from air pollution are due to indoor sources in less developed countries (chapter 7), more efficient domestic stoves offer the immediate dual advantages of lower emissions and reduced human health effects.[18] In developed countries, it is often more convenient for individuals to point to heavy industry as the only major culprit, but we are all ultimately responsible in the individual decisions we make: for example in transportation and recreation choices. Clearly, we need research, development and implementation of renewable forms of energy, such as solar and wind power. While practical alternatives are already emerging at local community level, industry and transport also need to find ways to apply these technologies on a large scale. The recent trend toward hybrid and electric vehicles is encouraging. Switching from coal or oil to natural gas is a good interim solution: although this too is a fossil fuel, it burns more cleanly. Ultimately though, industry must move to emissions-free sources as the major category of energy supply. As public health professionals we must participate in this effort, technically and as citizens.

Alternative power sources need to be reexamined in a dispassionate manner.[19] For example, despite the fears and local health impacts generated by such events as the meltdown of reactors in Fukushima, Japan (2011) and the earlier more harmful experience of Chernobyl, Ukraine (1986), nuclear power remains one of the safest options available to meet the energy demands of many nations. By contrast, fossil fuels are by far the most hazardous to human health (premature deaths caused by inhaling fossil fuel emissions are estimated at 288,000 annually), and endanger the planet through global warming. Hydroelectricity appears safe (although the worst accident from any energy related source is the Banqiao/Shimantan dam failure in China: ~30,000 people killed in 1975), but new opportunities are limited. Biofuels, wind, and tidal power also entail trade-offs (e.g., crops for food versus fuel, aesthetic impacts of wind power, disruption of fish migration and bird habitats, silt build-up with tidal power). However, these options may offer more potential than now realized as technologies advance: true also for solar and geothermal power. In conclusion, risks are associated with every energy source and decisions must be made in every context regarding the viability of available choices. As an OECD report pointed out:[20] there is little value in rejecting one source if that which replaces it presents even greater hazards.

Land Use Management: As already discussed in the context of forest fires in South East Asia, uncontrolled burning for agricultural and forestry purposes recently produced one of the largest air pollution disasters in recorded history, with widespread and almost immediate health and economic impacts. From the standpoint of climate change, there are also long term impacts. The release of GHGs from "slash and burn"` practices damages the atmosphere; this is compounded by deforestation itself, diminishing the role of trees in the removal of carbon dioxide, thereby contributing to its build up in the atmosphere. The solution to this, supported by on-going research so that we can understand the situation better, is to improve land-use management.

An even more serious situation has been happening in the Amazon basin, which accounts for over half the world's rain-forests. Most of this is located in Brazil, where extensive slash and burn practices have been under way for decades, with consequent reduction in forested areas that are visible by naked eye from space, accompanied by the forced displacement of indigenous peoples, itself a human rights travesty. Nonetheless, there is cause for cautious optimism: for example, the Pilot Program to Conserve the Brazilian Rain Forest (PPG7)[21] is a multilateral initiative of the Brazilian government, civil society and the international community aimed at developing innovative tools and methodologies for conserving Brazil's rain forests.

The objective of PPG7 is to maximize the environmental benefits of rain forests through the implementation of projects that contribute to reduction of the deforestation rate in Brazil. Launched in 1992, results so far are promising: the demarcation of indigenous lands respects the autonomy of indigenous peoples and their land rights, while establishment of community-managed extractive reserves and increased adoption of certified forest management rendered a more sustainable local economic development. The initiative has fostered a participatory approach to biodiversity at local level, funding over 200 community projects that experiment with new models of forest conservation and the sustainable use of natural resources. Stronger public institutions have emerged with enhanced capacity for environmental management; this includes participation of civil society in policy debates, and led to new political constituencies and stronger civil society networks linking more than 700 NGOs. Thousands of community leaders have been trained in fire prevention and control; this saves lives. Not least, while much of this effort is directed at ecological issues, a sound approach to ecology is a foundation for global public health: protection of indigenous rights, community participation and strengthening of civil society institutions all offer avenues for strengthening public health at community level.

In conclusion, the value of trees as a source of lumber or wood is highly specific: whether for housing or fuel, survival depends on them in many parts of the world. Similarly, the land they stand on is sometimes viewed as more valuable than the trees themselves, such that they are sacrificed for the purpose of opening up agriculture. Such decisions are based mostly on short-term economic considerations, without global perspective. By contrast, the long-term value of forests as a "carbon sink" for absorbing carbon dioxide and regenerating oxygen is critical to preserving biodiversity and preventing global warming. These considerations are critical to our eventual survival as a species. Out of these competing values emerged the field of environmental ethics (chapter 3): a discipline in philosophy that studies the moral relationship of human beings to, and also the value and moral status of, the environment and its nonhuman contents.[22] Under the "cap and trade" provisions of international treaties (e.g., the Kyoto protocol), industrialized nations lacking the ability to expand their own forests may partially compensate for their GHG emissions by paying for the establishment and maintenance of forests in other countries. Similarly, "cap and trade" could be applied by investing in certain agricultural practices in developing countries: for example, agricultural emissions of methane (a GHG), may be reduced by adjusting water management, crop rotation and tillage practices. So far however, major industrialized nations are not cooperating: it runs counter to their perceived economic interests.

Lifestyle Expectations: In 1987, the World Commission on the Environment and Development (often referred to as the Bruntland Commission, after its chairperson, Dr Gro Haarlem Brundtland, a public health physician, former Prime Minister of Norway and subsequently Director-General of the World Health Organization) defined *sustainable development* as "that which meets the needs of the present without compromising the ability of future generations to meet their own needs." The commission promoted the precautionary principle (chapter 3) that if an action or policy has a suspected risk of causing harm to the public or to the environment, in the absence of scientific consensus that it is harmful, the burden of proof that it is *not* harmful falls on those taking the action. This clearly applies to the issue of climate change, just as it does for emissions that can cause direct health effects, either for the worker or for the community exposed to air, soil or water pollution. While the Commission focused mostly on the key role of industry in relation to GHG emissions, there is a greater role for the individual in all this than usually accorded, much of which is also synergistic with healthier lifestyles. Besides, we must "own the problem" we share responsibility for, before we also can be expected to deal with it.

The cultures and habits of billions of people have a major impact on climate change. However, because individual behavior is determined largely by the social environment (social-ecological model, chapters 4 and 6), if a community chooses to lower or remove barriers to change, individual behavior change can become more achievable and sustainable. Individual choice thus may be facilitated by public policies including tax policy; examples include the provision of designated HOV (high occupancy vehicle) and bicycle lanes on roads, improved public transportation, greater public investment in pedestrian paths and hiking trails, and tax incentives in favor of more fuel-efficient vehicle and transportation choices. At the individual level, related decisions are made when considering fuel costs, time, distance and enjoyment involved, not to forget the positive ethic of contributing to global solutions by acting locally. Thus individuals may be encouraged to opt for vehicle sharing, improved public transport, or a more active mode transport such as walking or using a bicycle.[23] Remember also, time spent in physical activity repays through reduced risk of heart attacks and other diseases. Other time and energy efficient alternatives include choosing closer options for routine business or shopping, and teleconferencing. To achieve this type of change at societal level, where it is not already taking place, requires a culture shift: talk with your family, neighbors and associates about it.

The Brundtland Commission was followed in 1992 in Rio de Janeiro, by a Conference on the Environment and Development, where the *"polluter pays"* principle was widely accepted. This holds that the full costs associated with pollution should be met by the organization responsible for it.[24] In practice, it is often assumed that this is intended for industry. However, consider for a moment a hypothetical scenario in which the "polluter pays" principle is applied to individuals: we as citizens would have to pay the full costs associated with our own pollution, such as from vehicles, appliances, garden equipment, or smoke from inefficient domestic wood-stoves. If we had to pay *the full cost of the environmental and health impact* personally, it is likely that we would favor less damaging choices. There is a role here for more active citizen advocacy because, so far, the consumer is generally not held directly accountable for such choices.

Recent studies show that urban sprawl is associated with increased use of private vehicles, higher per-capita fuel consumption, reduced physical fitness and adverse health effects. Existing sprawl may be reduced through innovative urban redevelopment (e.g., "in-fill" housing) that attract people to live and work in closer proximity and thus make it cost-effective for providers of goods and services to locate closer to their consumers, while preventing future sprawl by improved urban planning. In support of this, municipalities could review their urban development plans with intent to reduce present and future sprawl, and encourage developers to give more attention to the concept of "compact communities" less dependent on the use of private vehicles, better served by public transport: more environmentally friendly and healthier places in which to live. Private sector policies also need to be environmentally friendly. For example, many organizations subsidize parking for their senior staff, yet offer no incentives for anyone (senior staff or otherwise) who takes public transport; developing modern, efficient and comfortable public transport is a key to reducing the environmental footprint of Earth's 7 billion people.

Human Population Issues

Population dynamics (chapter 5) including population increases, changing age structures, fertility and mortality and migration, impact every aspect of human, social and economic development and have major implications for public health needs.

Consider now the following statement from UNICEF (2011):[25]

Globally, people are living longer and healthier lives, and couples are choosing to have fewer children. However, because so many couples are in, or will soon be entering, their reproductive years, the world population is projected to increase for decades to come. Meeting the needs of current and future generations presents daunting challenges.

Whether we can live together equitably on a healthy planet will depend on the choices and decisions we make now. In a world of 7 billion people, and counting, we need to count each other.

In 2011 the world population exceeded 7 billion people, up from 2.5 billion in 1950. Half of the 7 billion are women and girls. Of the 7 billion people, 1 billion are illiterate and of these 66% are women. Female literacy is strongly associated with the overall health of a country.[26] Key health indicators such as life expectancy, infant survival and maternal mortality are all associated with educational attainment; maternal household behaviors are believed to influence the health and well-being of families. A greater understanding of the complex interface between general literacy and health literacy has emerged in analysis of the HIV/AIDS epidemic in Africa; development of a health literacy index as a composite measure of the outcome of health promotion and prevention activities may lead to documenting competencies that need to be developed to improve health status of countries, communities, and vulnerable groups.[27]

The number of people living in poverty is estimated to be 1.2 billion; 70% are women and children. Absolute poverty and unemployment are widely recognized as contributing to ill health. The material determinants of health appear to exercise their effects through psychosocial pathways such as social affiliations, early emotional development, and social status:[28] income inequality influences the proportion of a population who are insecure about their personal dignity, worth, and competence. People vulnerable to feelings of shame are more likely to use violence to gain respect; their use of drugs and alcohol also leads to increases in unintentional as well as intentional injuries. Further, such feelings are powerful and recurrent sources of chronic stress, thus increasing vulnerability to infections and cardiovascular diseases.[29] Acknowledging that poverty and inequality contribute to ill health should not neglect the contribution of the social environment and psychological welfare that accompany disadvantage worldwide.

A 2007 World Bank report, *Population Issues in the 21st Century: Role of the World Bank*,[30] noted that family size can also greatly affect women's jobs in the workplace. One cross-national survey suggests that the percentage of women in the labor force is inversely related to national birth rates. In Bolivia, there were strong links between women using contraception and having jobs outside of the home. In the Philippines, the average income growth for women with 1–3 pregnancies was twice that of women who had been pregnant more than seven times. The globe's highest birth rates are found in Sub-Saharan Africa, where average fertility remains above five children per woman. The low status of women often poses a barrier because in many societies, women lack the power to make their own decisions about using contraceptives or using other reproductive healthcare. Educating girls, improving economic opportunities for women, while giving them control over the design, management, and oversight of reproductive health programs, are critical ways of encouraging better access to these essential health programs.

Public health professionals and their organizations can make a difference: by advocating more attention to the structural determinants of the social environment to diminish the overall burden of disadvantage through policies addressing gender, employment, incomes, education that reduce the proportion of the population who fall behind and the distance between population groups.[31]

Migration: In 2005 there were over 191 million people living outside their country of origin, 3% of the total world population.[32] Although a relatively small percentage of the total number of migrants (9.2 million in 2005) were fleeing armed conflict, natural disaster and persecution, these numbers can increase rapidly over short periods. Economic migrants are the largest growing segment of the migrating population and, with increases in economic problems worldwide, this trend is likely to continue and can be associated with human rights issues in the recipient country (see chapter 5). Of particular concern for less developed countries is the emigration of skilled workers seeking higher incomes elsewhere. For example, migration of health care professionals from developing to developed countries places a significant burden on the health care systems of countries already struggling to meet the needs of their populations.

Another change that has implications for public health is the increase in the number of women who are migrating. Women constitute half of the migrating population and in some countries 70–80%.[34] Migrant women often end up as low paid service workers in jobs that are unregulated such as domestic work and may at much higher risk of exploitation, violence and abuse including human trafficking. These result in long term problems for women including increased number of unplanned pregnancies, sexually transmitted diseases, and often rejection by their family of origin if they wish to return home. Public health professionals need to be engaged in understanding these issues as they occur in their communities. The public health needs of immigrants give rise to a wide range of issues that require intercultural sensitivity as well as language skills that have not been traditionally part of public health professional education.

A global response to these increasingly pressing issues is developing through an International Organization for Migration (IOM). IOM is committed to the principle that humane and orderly migration benefits migrants and society.[33] As the leading international organization for migration, IOM acts with its partners in the international community: to assist in meeting the growing operational challenges of migration management; to advance understanding of migration issues; encourage social and economic development through migration; and to uphold the human dignity and well-being of migrants. Their approach includes attention to human rights in accordance with international law, including combating migrant smuggling and trafficking in persons, in particular women and children. They are involved in examining root causes of migration and promoting best practices, and participating in humanitarian responses to emergency and post-crises situations. Finally they are committed to undertake programs that facilitate the voluntary return and reintegration of refugees, displaced persons, migrants and other individuals in need of international migration services, in cooperation with other relevant international organizations as appropriate, and taking into account the needs and concerns of local communities. They are also mandated to address labor migration, in particular short term movements, and other types of circular migration. Although IOM has no legal protection mandate, the fact remains that its activities contribute to protecting human rights, having the effect, or consequence, of protecting persons involved in migration.

Returning briefly to the issue of climate change, there is an ever growing link between this and migration: as deserts expand and sea levels rise, a new category of migrant is emerging: climate refuges. Consider the following expression of angst from a spokesperson for the small Pacific island nation of Tuvalu:

We don't want to leave this place. We don't want to leave, it's our land, our God given land, it is our culture, we can't leave. People won't leave until the very last minute.[34]

Looking ahead, what chance has Tuvalu in the face of climate change, no part of it over four meters above sea level? Which industrialized nations will take in Tuvaluans when forced to flee from rising waters? But Tuvalu is not alone: it belongs to the Alliance of Small Island States (AOSIS), a 42 member coalition drawn from all oceans and world regions. They share similar development challenges and concerns about vulnerability to the effects of global climate change. AOSIS is an advocate for global sanity: an impressive 5% of the global population, 350 million people (ten times Canada)—now under an existential threat not of their own making.[35]

Migration of Health Professionals: As already noted in this chapter and in chapter 8, migration of health care workers from developing to developed nations places a burden on those countries; rural areas are particularly vulnerable. For example, the population of Sub-Saharan Africa totals over 660 million, with a ratio of fewer than 13 physicians per 100,000. The continent bears 24% of the global disease burden but has only 3% of the health care workforce and 1% of the world's financial resources.[36] Nonetheless, due to economic conditions, wage differentials, rapid population growth among young people, and conflict, significant numbers of African-trained health workers migrate every year to developed regions, leaving behind severely depleted health systems.[37] That some of this is in response to incentives and recruitment by "first world countries" constitutes "third world aid to first world countries."

The shortage of health professionals derives from a combination of underproduction, internal maldistribution and emigration of trained workers. According to recent WHO estimates, the current workforce in some of the most affected countries in sub-Saharan Africa would need to be scaled up by as much as 140% just to attain international health development targets such as those in the Millennium Declaration.[38] Beyond this, many African countries cannot meet widely accepted basic standards for health care coverage by physicians, nurses and midwives: an additional 2.4 million physicians, nurses and midwives are needed, along with an additional 1.9 million pharmacists, health aides, technicians and other auxiliary personnel.[37] Data from the Least Developed Countries Report 2007 demonstrated that the percentage of doctors practicing in the US relative to the total number of doctors in the home country ranges from 43% in Liberia to 10% in Zambia.[39] This would not be a problem if the number of doctors remaining in their country of origin was sufficient to meet population needs, but this is not the case. For example, Zambia has only seven doctors per 100,000 people, compared with the US level (approaching 300). Even though the actual number of professionals from the poorest nations working abroad may be small, the impact on services in the home nation can be severe.

Many of the efforts to retain health professionals are focused on the health care system itself. For example, Swaziland provides HIV/AIDS services for health care workers who, practicing in high-prevalence areas with minimal resources for safety measures, are at an increased risk for occupational exposure.[40] Other efforts build on the belief that providing workers with needed resources for care motivates them to stay and work in their home countries. Improved wages are also a key to retention. Salary support can help motivate health care workers to remain in their countries, even if it means working with fewer resources. Other types of inducements have been offered, such as lunch allowances, care loans and affordable housing. Some countries have begun to recruit trainees from rural areas. In South Africa, local students can receive scholarships for health care training on the condition they agree to return to their home district to practice. A study of the program found that trainees from rural areas were three to eight times as likely as those from urban areas to practice in rural regions after graduation.

The good news: the critical shortage of health care workers in many parts of the developing world is beginning to receive attention from donors and international agencies. Donors are increasingly realizing that without enough trained workers to deliver drugs, vaccines and care, funding projects will not have the desired effects. This documented shortage of indigenous health care workers inspired the American Public Health Association to pass a policy statement on "Ethical Restrictions on International Recruitment of Health Professionals to the United States."[41] The policy recognizes the role of the US in exacerbating the international crisis, calling on employers to adopt voluntary codes for ethical recruitment and on the government to contract only with employers who have done so. Similar codes of conduct have been passed by comparable organization in several other countries. The future of global health services in the 21st century lies to a large extent in the management of this crisis in human resources for health.

Migration has long been part of human activity and an ongoing challenge is how best to expand the positive contributions of international migration—especially when it comes to poverty reduction and development—while mitigating the health and social risks for all involved.

Changing Patterns of Health Risk

Food Security and World Hunger: The Food and Agriculture Organization of the United Nations (FAO) estimates that 1.02 billion people were undernourished in 2009—about 100 million more than in 2008. As a result, reaching the World Food Summit target (chapter 7) and the *Millennium Development Goal* for hunger reduction (chapters 6 and 7) looks increasingly out of reach.[42] Poor harvests were not to blame. The FAO estimated that total cereal production in 2009 was only slightly below the record high set in 2008. Instead, *the increase in hunger is mainly a result of poor people's inability to afford the food that is produced.* Many drew down savings during the food price crisis and have now lost jobs as a result of the global economic crisis. Food prices increased considerably in developing countries during the 2006–8 world food crisis and were still high when the economic crisis started. Domestic prices of staple foods were typically 17% higher at the end of 2008 than two years earlier, after adjusting for inflation. This seriously hurt the *purchasing power* of poor consumers, who often spend 40% of their income on staple foods. Thus, the global economic crisis hit developing countries at a very bad time. It further reduced access to food by lowering employment opportunities, remittances from abroad, development aid, foreign direct investment, and export opportunities. *How can hunger be eliminated?* [43] Improving world food security calls for both immediate relief and fundamental structural changes. In the short term, safety nets and social protection programs must be improved to reach those most in need. In the medium and long term, *the structural solution to hunger lies in increasing agricultural productivity to increase incomes and produce food at lower cost, especially in poor countries.* The importance of longer-term measures is evidenced by the unacceptably high number of people who did not get enough to eat before the crises and are likely to remain hungry even after the food and economic crises have passed. In addition, these measures must be coupled with better *governance and institutions* at all levels.

Desertification and Food Security: Deserts are among the most beautiful of landscapes, but their aridity renders them able to sustain only the hardiest forms of plant and animal life. Desertification refers to the degradation of dry lands, due to climate change and human activity: the conversion of arid or semi-arid land, usually by overgrazing, deforestation, overextraction of groundwater, drought, overplanting, or some combination of these. As dry lands are home to about 2 billion people, increasing desertification is a global problem, with major impacts on all species.

The international community has focused on this challenge in the form of a United Nations Convention to Combat Desertification (UNCCD),[44] one off-spring of the 1992 Rio Conference already referred to. At a UNCCD conference in 2009 in Argentina, its executive secretary, warned that action is urgent: *"If we cannot find a solution ... in 2025, close to 7% [of the planet's soil] could be affected ... There will not be global security without food security."*[45]

That conference offered both warnings and potential solutions. For example, dryland populations are already some of the planet's most vulnerable: about 90% of these are in developing countries. However, the process of desertification may be possible to halt: for example, soil experts are working with native plant species in susceptible regions to restore bio-diversity and soil quality through a process of revegetation. Relevant to the global search for carbon-capture methods, dryland soils may have enormous potential for carbon sequestration, which may offer a longer term economic solution if carbon trading can be established: long-term sustainable management of soil must be given priority over the short-term gains.[46]

While research intensifies into how to reverse the process, the immediate need is to ensure that cultivation techniques are ecologically sound: to prevent desertification before it starts. Practices that contribute to soil degradation include removing crop residue for cheap fodder, fuel and fencing; removing topsoil for making bricks; and using animal waste for cooking rather than returning it to the soil as natural fertilizer. These practices can be changed through education.

Food Safety and Globalization: As discussed in chapter 7, unsafe food can give rise to a range of problems from short to long term.[47] The potential for international concerns arises because the food distribution system has become globalized: increasingly long distances now exist between producers and consumers. Responsibility for food safety in many countries is shared across numerous agencies whose general lack of integration in itself is a potential global hazard. This is turn has motivated the development of new approaches to better coordinate strategy for the mitigation of foodborne disease. Globalization of food production and trade lead to the development of an international food safety network called the International Food Safety Authorities Network (INFOSAN), which is a joint effort between the Food and Agricultural Organization of the United Nations (FAO) and WHO. Such an approach relies mainly on the Hazard Analysis Critical Control Point System (HACCP), which has been advocated by WHO for nearly 20 years.[48] The full potential of this program has not been realized. Further strengthening of preventive and emergency operations related to food safety is needed.

Obesity and Noncommunicable Diseases: Changes in diet and declines in physical activity associated with rural-urban population drifts have given rise to increasing overweight and obesity in many nations for virtually all epidemiological transition variants (chapter 5). These are among the key risk factors for noncommunicable diseases (NCDs, chapter 6) (e.g., type 2 diabetes, circulatory disease, and musculoskeletal problems) that now dominate the disease burden globally. The obesity pandemic is a challenge for both developing and developing countries alike. Few nations, if any, can claim to have dealt with it effectively: it is now a challenge everywhere. For developing countries with already overstretched health care systems, it is of potentially greater concern: they must now cope with a "double burden"—in addition to an "unfinished agenda" of widespread undernutrition and infectious diseases, an emerging burden of NCDs associated with overnutrition. It is important to take note of this issue again in this chapter as it constitutes an emerging global health challenge: in addition to physical activity norms, it brings into focus issues related to standards for food quality and nutrition, as well as issues of food labeling, marketing and even commercial trade practices, not to forget health literacy as a population health goal; it is likely that the solution will have to be a global one.

Disaster Risk Reduction

The role of public health in disasters was introduced in some detail in chapter 8, where reference was made to the WHO Collaborating Centre for Research on the Epidemiology of Disasters (CRED). We now examine some of the longer term implications of their work.

Since 1988 CRED has maintained an Emergency Events Database (EM-DAT), which was created with initial support from WHO and the Belgian Government. EM-DAT contains data on the occurrence and effects of over 18,000 mass disasters in the world from 1900 to present.[49] The database is compiled from various sources, including UN agencies, nongovernmental organizations, insurance companies, research institutes and press agencies. Figure 9-1 is a graph of the number of natural disasters that have been reported. In order to be entered into the database at least one of the following criteria has to be met: (1) ten or more people were reported killed; (2) one hundred or more people were reported to be affected; (3) a state of emergency was declared; (4) there was a call for international assistance.

Data are collected on the number of disaster events, the country where the disaster occurred; the type of disaster (natural, technological, complex); the month, day, and year the disaster occurred; the number of people killed or missing; the number of people injured; the number of people needing immediate assistance for shelter; the number affected, which includes those needing immediate assistance and those who were displaced or evacuated; and the estimated damages (in US dollars). Data are provided to assist disaster and relief agencies in mitigating the impact of disasters

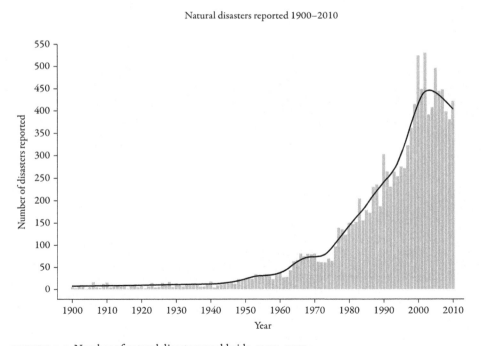

FIGURE 9-1 Number of natural disasters worldwide, 1900–2010.

Source: EM-DAT: The OFDA/CRED International Disaster Database—www.emdat.be— Universite Catholique de Louvin—Brussels—Belgium.

on vulnerable populations and to assist the integration of health components into development and poverty alleviation programs. Figure 9-1 shows the increasing number of natural disasters reported during 1900–2010. Figure 9-2 shows the increasing number of people affected and the decline in overall deaths attributed to disasters despite the increasing occurrence. Attention to developing capacity to mitigate loss of life may have had a profound influence on reducing this loss; given this favorable trend, continued attention to such capacity development is warranted into the future.

In 1999, the United Nations International Strategy for Disaster Reduction was established for the coordination of disaster reduction and to ensure synergies among disaster reduction activities.[50] Core areas of work include ensuring that disaster risk reduction is applied to climate change adaptations, to increase investment in disaster risk reduction, to build disaster resilient cities, schools and hospitals and to increase the international system for disaster risk reduction. These programs clearly have potential to protect the health of vulnerable populations into the future by increasing awareness, building disaster resilient communities, and recognizing the responsibility of all sectors to address increased capacity to

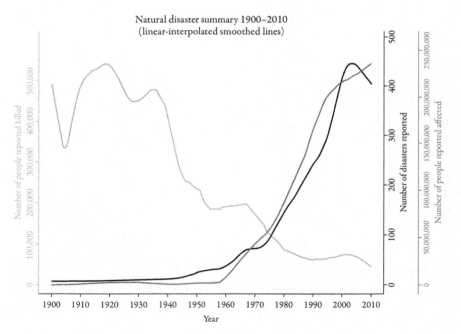

FIGURE 9-2 Summary of the number of natural disasters, number of people reported killed and number of people affects, 1900–2010.

Source: EM-DAT: The OFDA/CRED International Disaster Database—www.emdat.be— Universite Catholique de Louvin—Brussels—Belgium.

respond to disasters and to assist affected communities. The work of this group is closely linked with increased understanding of how countries need to adapt to climate change. Since climate change leads to gradual changes in average temperature, sea level, and the timing and amount of precipitation, it will also contribute to more frequent, severe and unpredictable hazards such as cyclones, floods and heat waves. Therefore adapting to climate change can be understood as adapting development to such gradual changes and managing risks associated with severe and unpredictable weather events.[51]

The physical infrastructures of regional economies, including urban centers, being mostly fixed spatially, cannot be easily relocated. Adapting their ongoing development to changing climatic conditions such as reduced or increased water availability and sea level increases therefore requires substantial long-term investment. This can be of critical importance in some situations: new urban drainage systems may be needed to adjust for changes in precipitation and similar investments may be required for locally sustainable agriculture. In the city of Vancouver, Canada, climate change related plans are emerging for dikes, flood control gates and sacrificial first floors. This is not unique: many world cities have been making preparations for many years; some (e.g., Amsterdam) are expert at it.[35] There have also been notable failures to make adequate preparation despite increasing evidence of risk, for example for New Orleans, where ecosystem restoration and levee improvements had been advised for decades, devastating inundation followed Hurricane Katrina in 2005 with enormous impact on people and the local economy.[52]

However, as introduced in chapter 8 (section entitled "The Role of Public Health in Reducing the Impacts of Disasters") extreme hazards are not always associated with commensurate population risks as risk variations depend on the proximity and vulnerability of people to the hazard. As noted by the United Nations Office for Disaster Risk Reduction,[51] countries with small and vulnerable economies have significant difficulty absorbing and recovering from disaster impacts. Those that rely heavily on agriculture are more vulnerable to climatic variability and changes in precipitation and temperature. Ecosystem decline, poverty and badly managed urban growth also contribute to the possibility of rapidly increasing number of losses in disasters.

Because increasing climate change disaster losses inhibit the achievement of Millennium Development Goals (chapter 5), some countries (e.g., Viet Nam, Philippines Colombia, South Africa) are integrating disaster management with national climate change response planning.[51] While progress in coordinating disaster risk reduction and climate change adaptation has been slow, such efforts help to make investment in national development more cost-effective, thereby also benefiting schools, hospitals, water, sanitation, and poverty reduction.

TABLE 9-1

Examples of adaptations used to reduce climate risks

Reactive	Emergency response, disaster recovery, mitigation.
Proactive	Crop diversification, seasonal climate forecasting, early warning systems (e.g. famine, tsunamis), water storage, insurance, supplemental irrigation, community education regarding action in the event of a disaster.

The International Strategy for Disaster Reduction classifies adaptations used to reduce climate risk as reactive or proactive as illustrated in Table 9-1.[51] A case study (discussed later in the chapter) about the project Horn of Africa Risk Transfer for Adaptation, which is a collaborative program between Oxfam America and local and international partners, describes one proactive risk reduction activity that is currently active in Ethiopia and expanding to Senegal: monitoring reports to date document the promise this program has for reducing vulnerability of subsistence farmers to weather-shocks.

The Educated Citizen and Public Health

Undergraduate education programs in public health have grown rapidly in the first decade of the 21st century, and represent a new approach.[53] While other undergraduate health programs have existed for many years (health education, environmental health and health administration) they have focused primarily on professional training. Personal health and wellness courses have also been popular undergraduate courses. A number of principles have been developed that differentiate the new approach, called the educated citizen and public health, from these programs.

Consider now this statement from the Association of American Colleges and Universities:[54]

An understanding of public health is a critical component of good citizenship and a prerequisite for taking responsibility for building healthy societies. At its best, the study of public health combines the social sciences, sciences, mathematics, humanities, and the arts. At the same time, it serves as a vehicle for the development of written and oral communication skills, critical and creative thinking, quantitative and information literacy, and teamwork and problem solving. It incorporates civic knowledge and engagement—both local and global, intercultural competence, and ethical reasoning and action, while forming the foundation for lifelong learning. The study of public health, in other words, models a capacious vision of liberal education.

Public health education, until such developments as this, has focused on relatively advanced professional requirements, taking as core disciplines: biostatistics, community and behavioral health, environmental/occupational health, epidemiology, health care policy and administration. These are reflected in the domains of analytical/assessment skills, policy development/program planning skills, community dimensions of practice skills, public health science skills, financial planning and management skills, and leadership and systems thinking skills. The addition of communication skills and cultural competency skills as central domains for public health professionals has added new dimensions to future training programs that have not yet been fully developed and integrated within most traditional schools of public health; to achieve this calls for partnering with new collaborators to fully develop the needed curricula.

By contrast, the educated citizen and public health approach is designed to satisfy general education requirements for all undergraduate students and may provide the needed impetus to increase health literacy in the population. It includes applied and integrative learning using experiential approaches, incorporating epidemiologic concepts as part of general education and taking a population and global perspective to understanding diseases and other health conditions and developing an appreciation for public health as a field that is grounded in and applies to arts and science disciplines ranging from economics and public policy to chemistry, biology, anthropology, communications, and ethics. As presented in chapter 2, this breadth of vision is also reflected in public health core competencies, although these too are works in progress.

As such developments takes hold, public health professionals will need to become more engaged with undergraduate education for the concept of the educated citizen and public health to become fully realized. Ultimately public health professionals must become involved in all levels of the education system to fully achieve the aims of health literacy in society as a whole.

CASE STUDY: A MULTIDIMENSIONAL RISK REDUCTION
APPROACH TO CLIMATE CHANGE

Horn of Africa Risk Transfer for Adaptation (HARITA)[55,56,57]

The HARITA model is a holistic approach to risk management involving three components: risk reduction, risk transfer and prudent risk taking. The program is designed to increase climate change resilience in communities that are marginal in their ability to produce enough food for the community, and who therefore are vulnerable to extreme temperatures, extraordinary rainfall events, and intense prolonged periods of drought and flooding. The program provides disaster insurance and financial credit and provides long term sustainable investments in agriculture. As an adaptation program, HARITA enables farmers to purchase crop insurance by working or directly by payment.

The program began in Ethiopia. In the first year 200 farmers enrolled, by the second year the number increased to 1300 and in 2011 there enrolled 13000 in 43 villages enrolled in the program. Risk reduction activities of farmers who purchase premiums with labor include improved irrigation and soil management practices. Acknowledging that changes in weather will have profound consequences, crop farmers are provided information and time to select more heat-resistant crops, improve water resources and shift planting dates. Risk transfer involves provision of weather indexed insurance where farmers enrolled can work to earn insurance certificates protecting them against rainfall deficits. The final part of the program, prudent risk taking, represents credit designed to diversify the crops being produced, to increase technology in the form of high yield seeds or irrigation, and increase production of high value crops such as spices and vegetables.

This model for sustainable development is founded on principles of collaboration and mutual support by public and private organizations, communities, and government ministries. Expansion to new regions in Ethiopia and beyond (e.g., expansion of the model to Senegal and two other countries is planned) will diversify the risk pool and strengthen the risk management scheme.

Epilogue

As public health scholar-practitioners, we have drawn from our experience an ecological perspective on the role of public health as an evolving social institution of global importance. We have put forward a set of ideas and an array of facts that reflects our synthesis of what public health is about. Ideas are born out of observations and debate, values drive us to explore them, to test them, and out of this may emerge facts. At the heart of this effort lies a desire to assist newcomers to gain an appreciation for the ecological values that underpin our multidisciplinary field. While intimately intertwined with facts, it is the ideas themselves that are more closely aligned with those values. These in turn may cause us to strengthen, reject, or modify our ideas. This process is a lot like the wisdom expressed by Nobel Laureate TS Eliot (1888–1965) in the poem Little Gidding, No 4 of his Four Quartets:

> *We shall not cease from exploration And the end of all our exploring Will be to arrive where we started And know the place for the first time.*

Public health depends on more than good ideas and an evidence base; it calls for a logical way of thinking: awareness that a public health need exists, understanding what causes it, a capacity to deal with it, a sense of values that it matters, and (not least) the political will to rectify it. None of this is achieved by acting on impulse, but by organizational commitments to systematic health situation analysis and surveillance, a relevant research infrastructure, a sound process for making decisions, effective and efficient intervention technologies, competent planning, sufficient resource allocation, good management practices, effective communication and teamwork, and rigorous evaluation. Success requires engaging in dialogue with people from allied and contrary fields and viewpoints, with open minds and generosity: the ability to compromise for the common good. Leadership is an essential ingredient throughout, at all levels.

The 21st century is one of upheaval, with great struggles taking place between competing ideas and values. In the face of such conflict, it is often difficult to determine what weight to place on this or that opinion, especially when there is also so much interest vested by some in keeping things the way they are. But indecision and inertia must give way to vision and the courage to act on it. Having core values such as intellectual honesty is important to all of this: when combined with knowledge that is based on evidence, we can see alternative futures, and thereby derive the opportunity, even duty, to bring about a positive future by acting now, rather than to do nothing. While knowledge is a form of power, how or whether we plan to use it for the benefit of all is the key to that more positive future. If our array of ideas and facts are based on sound evidence and guided by sound values, then it must take even sounder evidence and values to put them aside. It is our belief that promoting a set of public health values to guide this expanding knowledge base, as we have tried to do throughout this work, will help us navigate this complexity to achieve a healthier, more ecologically sustainable future for all.

A looming issue for the future of humankind and all other species on the planet is population growth. Along with economic pressures, the absolute numbers of people on earth have stretched all our resources. Changing our perspective on parenthood is imperative for reframing the discussion about limiting population growth. Consider now the following quotation:

> Biologically, all that I give "my" child is a set of chromosomes. Are they my chromosomes? Hardly. Sequestered in the germinal area long before my birth, my gonadal chromosomes have lived a life of their own, beyond my control. Mutation has altered them. In reproduction, "my" germ plasm is assembled in a new combination and mixed with another assortment with a similar history. "My" child's germ plasm is not mine, it is really only part of the community's store. I was merely the temporary custodian of part of it.
>
> If parenthood is a right, population control is impossible. If parenthood is only a privilege, and if parents see themselves as trustees of the germ plasm and guardians of the rights of future generations, then there is hope for mankind.[1]

In other words, we can choose to be active as advocates for public health by using all scientific knowledge available to provide us with a basis for reframing approaches that have not been successful in tackling difficult and controversial issues. In order to succeed we must also continue to align public health with politics at all levels from local to global: as Rudolph Virchow, founder of modern pathology and one of the founders of Social Medicine (1821–1902) stated, "medicine is a social science, and politics is but medicine writ large."[2]

So all this is "public health." Taking the health impacts of climate change as an example, if we are to contemplate this seemingly daunting future in a creative way, we need to establish a new mindset that promotes a spirit of creative enterprise, not despondent resignation. Those who advocate for "green enterprise" are on the right side of this issue, while those who are fighting a rearguard action, reminiscing over a fossil fuel and smokestack past that we now know holds no sustainable future for the planet, are on the wrong side. In an analogous manner, our current food system has placed a significant burden on soil and water resources while providing us with food that may not provide the nutrition needed for survival, and at the same time it has created an unhealthy population at risk for chronic diseases. The movement away from processed foods holds promise not only to improve the quality of the food supply, but also to support the workers who grow the food. Innovative approaches are being tried throughout the world to support local agriculture, reduce the burden of losses due to drought and flooding, and encouraging better stewardship through crop and seed diversity. The same applies to the underlying realities of economic recessions: the specter of decline needs to be recast as an opportunity to do things differently, for example ensuring more equitable and cooperative health care emphasizing health care as a right, not as a business, and the need to invest creatively in education, as it is our next generations who will find new ways avenues for health and prosperity in a new future. We must not squander these opportunities as we strive to reestablish balance with the natural world.

Thus, in these pages, we have depicted the field of public health as a body of knowledge and practice that respects the ways in which our ecology, natural and manmade, has shaped human development and health. Settings and circumstances from prehistory to the present have offered advantages and disadvantages. As a consequence of our decisions as a species, especially in recent history, people have adversely impacted global, regional, and local ecosystems, with increasingly dire consequences. Not everything has gone awry: in fact we have much good to point to also, such as the Universal Declaration on Human Rights. Yet we continue to be confronted by such contrasts as interplanetary rocket launches while millions starve in the Horn of Africa, pandemic diseases persist as corporate heads and sports stars travel on private jets, and some national economies are perched on the verge of collapse. The need for enlightened and responsible policy actions is more important today than it has ever been. Human beings are currently causing the greatest mass extinction of species since the extinction of the dinosaurs 65 million years ago. If we cannot get along as a species and look after our planet's environment as one that sustains all life as we know it, our own extinction will eventually follow.

Some of our forebears did great service through their ground breaking contributions to the development of public health thinking, as did others in related fields of the health sciences. Public health professionals have acted on their evidence and insights and even gone beyond this to develop systems of evidence and organization that translate information into action, but now we need new leaders who will have the vision to take us into the future with more clarity.

We leave the last word to American urban planner Daniel H Burnham (1846–1912):

Make no little plans; they have no magic to stir men's blood and probably will themselves not be realized. Make big plans; aim high in hope and work, remembering that a noble, logical diagram once recorded will not die.

References

CHAPTER ONE

1. Last J. *Preface. Dictionary of Public Health*. New York, NY: Oxford University Press; 2007.
2. Constitution of the World Health Organization. http://www.who.int/governance/eb/who_constitution_en.pdf. Accessed December 31, 2011.
3. University of Ottawa. Society, the Individual, and Medicine. http://www.med.uottawa.ca/sim/data/Health_Definitions_e.htm. Accessed 10–01–2012.
4. Public Health Agency of Canada. Pan Canadian Public Health Network. Guidelines for MPH Programmes in Canada. 2009. http://www.phac-aspc.gc.ca/php-psp/pdf/guidelines-lignes_directrices_MPH-2009-eng.pdf. Accessed February 8, 2012.
5. Kirch W (ed.). *Encyclopedia of Public Health*. New York, NY: Springer Press; 2008.
6. Benatar S, Brock G (eds.). *Global Health and Global Health Ethics*. Cambridge, UK: Cambridge University Press; 2011.
7. Mays L. A brief history of hydraulic technology during antiquity (special issue). *Environmental Hydraulics*. 2008;*8*(5–6):471–484.
8. Rosen G. *A History of Public Health*. Expanded Edition. Baltimore, MD: Johns Hopkins University Press; 1993.
9. Printz, D . The role of water harvesting in alleviating water scarcity in arid areas. Keynote lecture. Proceedings, International Conference on Water Resources Management in Arid Regions. March 23–27, 2002. Kuwait: Kuwait Institute for Scientific Research; 2002;*3*: 107–22. http://www.ipcp.org.br/References/Agua/aguaCapta/WaterHarvesting.pdf. Accessed December 31, 2011.
10. Code of Hammurabi. http://www.fordham.edu/halsall/ancient/hamcode.asp. Accessed December 31, 2011.

11. Robinson DL. *Brain, Mind and Behavior* (2nd ed.). Ballina, Ireland: Pontoon Publications; 2009.

12. WHO History of International Classification of Diseases http://www.who.int/classifications/icd/en/HistoryOfICD.pdf. Accessed November 21, 2011.

13. Knibbs GH. The International Classification of Disease and Causes of Death and its revision. *Med J Australia.* 1929;*1*:2–12.

14. Graunt J. *Bills of Mortality 1662.* http://www.neonatology.org/pdf/graunt.pdf. Accessed November 21, 2011.

15. Bertillon J. Classification of the causes of death (abstract). *Transactions of the 15th International Congress on Hygiene Demography.* Washington DC; 1912.

16. White F. Community health sciences and the legacy of Ibn Ridwan at the Aga Khan University. *East Mediterran Health J.* 2001;*7*:1–3.

17. White F. De Re Metallica: treatise of Georgius Agricola Revisited. *Ann R College Phys Surg Canada.* 1994;*27*:163–166.

18. Klassen, CD, Watkins JB. *Casarett & Doull's toxicology: The basic science of poisons.* Companion handbook (5th ed.). Toronto: McGraw Hill; 1999.

19. Ramazzini B. *de Morbis Artificum* (Diseases of Workers, Rosen G, trans.) New York, NY: NY Academy of Medicine Library/Hafner Publishing Co.; 1964.

20. White FMM. Nosocomial infection control: scope and implications for health care, a historical view. *Am J Infect Control.* 1981;*9*:61–69.

21. van Leeuwenhoek A. (1632–1723) http://www.ucmp.berkeley.edu/history/leeuwenhoek.html. Accessed December 10, 2011.

22. Schultz M, Smith T . Emerging Infectious Diseases. www.cdc.gov/eid. 14(12); December 2008.

23. Harrison G. *Mosquitoes, Malaria and Man: A History of the Hostilities since 1880.* New York, NY: E.P. Dutton; 1978.

24. Packard, R.M . *The Making of a Tropical Disease: A Short History of Malaria.* Baltimore, MD: Johns Hopkins University Press; 2007.

25. US Centers for Disease Control and Prevention. History of Quarantine. http://www.cdc.gov/quarantine/HistoryQuarantine.html. Accessed November 29, 2011.

26. Hanan E. The pools of Sepphoris: Ritual baths or bathtubs? They're not ritual baths. *Biblical Archgy Rev.* 2000;*26*,4:42–45.

27. Von Furstenberg D. *The Bath.* New York, NY: Random House; 1993.

28. Snow J. *Snow on Cholera.* New York, NY: The Commonwealth Fund/ Oxford University Press; 1936.

29. *On the Mode of Communication of Cholera,* 8 volumes, London, 1849; 2nd ed. 1855.

30. Riedel S. Edward Jenner and the history of smallpox and vaccination. *Baylor Univ MedCenter Proc.* 2005;*18*,1:21–23.

31. Edward Jenner (1749–1823). The Three Original Publications on Vaccination Against Smallpox. The Harvard Classics; 1909–1914. http://www.bartleby.com/38/4/1.html. Accessed December 11, 2011.

32. James Lind: A treatise of the scurvy, 1753 http://inspire.stat.ucla.edu/unit_04/scurvy.pdf. Accessed December 11, 2011.

33. Takaki (TK). The preservation of health amongst the personnel of the Japanese Navy and Army. Three lectures delivered at St Thomas's Hospital, London on May 7, 9, 11, 1906. Exerpted from Lancet. (1906): 1369–1371; 190. Reprinted in: Buck C, Llopis A, Najera E,

Terris M (eds.). *The Challenge of Epidemiology: Issues and Selected Readings*. Scientific Publication No. 505. Washington DC: Pan American Health Organization. 1988; 75–79.

34. Zimmerman MB. Research on iodine deficiency and goiter in the 19th and early 20th centuries. *J Nutrition*. 2008;*138*:2060–2063. http://jn.nutrition.org/content/138/11/2060. full. Accessed December 14, 2011.

35. Jean Baptiste Boussingault—A Biographical Sketch (February 2, 1802—May 11, 1887). *J Nutrition*. 1964;*84*:1–9. http://jn.nutrition.org/content/84/1/1.full.pdf. Accessed December 14, 2011.

36. Carpenter KJ. David Marine and the problem of Goitre. *J Nutrition*. 2005;*135*:675–680. http://jn.nutrition.org/content/135/4/675.full. Accessed December 14, 2011.

37. International Council for the Control of Iodine Deficiency Disorders (ICCIDD). History of Salt Iodization. http://www.iccidd.org/pages/protecting-children/fortifying-salt/history-of-salt-iodization.php. Accessed Dec 14, 2011.

38. Terris M. *Goldberger on Pellagra*. Baton Rouge, LA: Louisiana State University Press; 1964.

39. Bollet A. Politics and pellagra: the epidemic of pellagra in the U.S. in the early twentieth century. *Yale J Biol Med*. 1992;*65*:211–221.

40. Dr Joseph Goldberger and the War on Pellagra. http://history.nih.gov/exhibits/goldberger/docs/intro_2.htm. Accessed December 10, 2011.

41. Bates DV, Caton RB. *A Citizen's Guide to Air Pollution* (2nd ed.). Vancouver, BC: David Suzuki Foundation; 2002.

42. Chadwick E (1843). *Report on the Sanitary Condition of the Labouring Population of Great Britain. A Supplementary Report on the results of a Special Inquiry into The Practice of Internment in Towns*. London: R. Clowes & Sons, for Her Majesty's Stationery Office. https://play.google.com/store/books/details?id=2IYIAAAAQAAJ&rdid=book-2IYIAAAAQAAJ&rdot=1. Accessed November 8, 2009.

43. Attewell A. Florence Nightingale (1820–1910) http://www.ibe.unesco.org/fileadmin/user_upload/archive/publications/ThinkersPdf/nightingalee.PDF. Accessed December 31, 2011.

44. Distinguished Women of Past and Present. Alice Hamilton (1869–1970). http://www.distinguishedwomen.com/biographies/hamilton-a.html. Accessed June 11, 2012.

45. Accreditation Criteria—Public Health Programs (amended June 2011). Council for Education on Public Health. Washington DC. 2011. http://www.ceph.org/pdf/PHP-Criteria-2011.pdf. Accessed January 4, 2011.

CHAPTER TWO

1. Canadian Tuberculosis Committee. An Advisory Committee Statement (ACS-9). Housing conditions that serve as risk factors for infection and disease. *Canada Communicable Dis Rep*. 2007;*33*:1–13.

2. van den Bos GAM, Triemstra AHM. Quality of life as an instrument for need assessment and outcome assessment of health care in chronic patients. *Quality in Health Care*. 1999;*8*:247–252.

3. Pickett KE, Wilkinson RG. Inequality: an under-acknowledged source of mental illness and distress. *Br J Psychiatry*. 2010;*197*(6):426–428.

4. Brownson RC, Baker EA, Leet, TL, Gillespie KN (eds.). *Evidence-Based Public Health*. New York, NY: Oxford University Press; 2003.

5. Briss PA, Brownson RC, Fielding JE, Zaza S. Developing and using the Guide to Community Preventive Services: Lessons learned about evidence-based public health. *Annu Rev Public Health*. 2004;*25*:281–302.

6. Hausman AJ. Implications of evidence-based practice for community health. *Am J Community Psychol*. 2002;*30*(3):453–467.

7. World Health Organization. *Prevention of Mental Disorders—Effective Interventions and Policy Options*. Geneva. 2004. http://www.who.int/mental_health/evidence/en/prevention_of_mental_disorders_sr.pdf. Accessed January 16, 2012.

8. Global Forum on Health Research. *The 10/90 report on health research 1999*. Geneva: World Health Organization; 1999.

9. White F. Global Journal of Public Health (inaugural editorial) *GJMEDPH*. 2012;*1*(1):1–2. http://www.gjmedph.org/uploads/Editorial.pdf. Accessed June 15, 2012.

10. Daniels M, Hill AB. Chemotherapy of pulmonary tuberculosis in young adults. An analysis of the combined results of three Medical Research Council trials. *Br Med J*. 1952;*1*:1162.

11. National Collaborating Centre for Methods and Tools. McMaster University http://www.nccmt.ca/. Accessed January 16, 2012.

12. Minkler M, Wallerstein N. *Community-Based Participatory Research for Health*. San Francisco, CA: Jossey-Bass; 2003.

13. Agency for Healthcare Research and Quality. Community-based Participatory Research—assessing the evidence. AHRQ Publication No. 04–E022-2 July 2004. http://www.ahrq.gov/downloads/pub/evidence/pdf/cbpr/cbpr.pdf. Accessed June 15, 2012.

14. Core Competencies for Public Health in Canada. http://www.phac-aspc.gc.ca/php-psp/ccph-cesp/about_cc-apropos_ce-eng.php. Accessed December 3, 2011.

15. Birt C. Towards a European Framework for Public Health Competencies. Andrija Stamper School of Public Health. January 17, 2011. Ppt. https://docs.google.com/viewer?a=v&q=cache:qONIvfTo4kAJ:www.epha.org/IMG/ppt/Zagreb_ASPHER_EPHA_2_170111.ppt+Towards+a+European+Framework+for+public+health+competencies&hl=en&pid=bl&srcid=ADGEESgNAbqANxVMolrqHHcstjKL49F_WBrTIiHP7TfVSv9gWsB1AOZXqaw7zahCuv7BI_yROduJPORx9OCABaiOYtck5eIGesvYRu7dLUaQtDYrWj9JUDbQuE9CdlpotOFVN-PjEfD5&sig=AHIEtbTOhMOur4_IQEpZwwNa6xn4zm2JjA. Accessed February 9, 2012.

16. Council on Linkages between Academia and Public Health Practice. Core Competencies for Public Health Professionals. Adopted May 3, 2010. http://www.phf.org/programs/council/Pages/default.aspx. Accessed January 16, 2012.

17. Association of Schools of Public Health. MPH Core Competency Model. Updates September 9, 2010. http://www.asph.org/document.cfm?page=851. Accessed January 16, 2012.

18. Fenner F. The Florey Lecture, 1983: Biological control, as exemplified by smallpox eradication and myxomatosis. *Proc R Soc London B*. 1983;*218*:259–285.

19. World Health Organization Media Centre. Anniversary of Smallpox Eradication. http://www.who.int/mediacentre/multimedia/podcasts/2010/smallpox_20100618/en/. Accessed January 16, 2012.

20. The control and eradication of smallpox in South Asia. Smallpox History. The Wellcome Trust Centre for the History of Medicine at UCL. http://www.smallpoxhistory.ucl.ac.uk/. Accessed November 23, 2011.

21. Cueto M. *Cold War, Deadly Fevers: Malaria Eradication in Mexico, 1955–1975*. Baltimore MD: Johns Hopkins University Press; 2007.

22. Harrison G. *Mosquitoes, Malaria and Man: A History of the Hostilities since 1880*. New York, NY: E.P. Dutton; 1978.

23. Packard RM. *The Making of a Tropical Disease: A Short History of Malaria*. Baltimore, MD: Johns Hopkins University Press; 2007.

24. WHO Global Malaria Programme. World Malaria Report 2011. http://www.who.int/malaria/world_malaria_report_2011/9789241564403_eng.pdf. Accessed Jan 5, 2012.

25. Diederen BMW. Legionella spp. and Legionaires' disease. *J Infect*. 2008;*56*:1–12. Doi: 10.1016/j.jinf.2007.09.010.

26. Fraser DW, Tsai TR, Orenstein W, Parkin WE, Beecham HJ, Sharrar RG, et al. Legionnaires' disease: description of an epidemic of pneumonia. *N Engl J Med*. 1977;*297*:1189–1197.

27. CDC Childhood Lead Poisoning Prevention. *National Center for Environmental Health*. Centers for Disease Control and Prevention. Atlanta GA. March 12, 2003.

28. Schmitt N, Brown G, Derkin EL, Larsen AA, Saville JM, McCausland ED. Lead poisoning in horses. An environmental health hazard. *Arch Environ Health*. 1971;*23*(3):185–195.

29. Snowball AF. Development of an air pollution control program at Cominco's Kimberley Operation. *J Air Pollut Control Assoc*. 1966;*16*(2):59–62.

30. Neri LC, Johansen HL, Schmitt N, Pagan RT, Hewitt D. Blood lead levels in children in two British Columbia communities. In: Hemphill DD (ed.). *Trace Substances in Environmental Health—XII*, proceedings of the University of Missouri's 12th Annual Conference on Trace Substances in Environmental Health, 6–8 June 1978, Columbia, MO. Columbia: University of Missouri, 1978; 403–409.

31. Schmitt N, Philion JJ, Larsen AA, Harnade KM, Lynch AJ. Surface soil as a potential source of lead exposure for young children. *Can Med Assoc J*. 1979;*121*(11):1474–1478.

32. Hertzman C, Ward H, Ames N, Kelly S, Yates C. Childhood lead exposure in Trail revisited. *Can J Public Health*. 1991;*82*(6):385–391.

33. Ames N. Acceptable level of human health risks resulting from smelter contaminants in the Trail area. Kootenay Boundary Community Health Services Society; May 2001.

34. Hilts SR, Bock SE, Oke TL, Yates CL, Copes RA. Effect of interventions on children's blood lead levels. *Environ Health Perspect*. 1998;*106*(2):79–83.

35. Hilts SR. Effect of smelter emission reductions on children's blood lead levels. *Sci Tot Environ*. 2003;*303*:51–58.

36. Air Quality in British Columbia: a Public Health Perspective. Provincial Health Officer's Annual Report 2003. Ministry of Health Services. British Columbia. http://www.health.gov.bc.ca/pho/pdf/phoannual2003. pdf. Accessed January 6, 2012.

37. Trail Health and Environmental Committee. Annual Fall Blood Testing Results 2007. http://thec.ca/?page_id=8/. Accessed January 6, 2012.

38. Green A, Whiteman D, Frost C, Battistutta D. Sun exposure, skin cancers and related skin conditions. *J Epidemiol*. 1999;*9*(6 Suppl):S7–S13.

39. Armstrong BK. Stratospheric ozone and health. *Int J Epidemiol*. 1994;*23*:873–885.

40. Canadian Cancer Society/National Cancer Institute of Canada: Canadian Cancer Statistics 2007. Toronto, Canada, 2007.

41. United States Environmental Protection Agency. The Montreal Protocol on Substances that Deplete the Ozone Layer. Adopted September 16, 1987. http://www.epa.gov/ozone/intpol/. Accessed January 6, 2012.

42. Last JM. *Public Health and Human Ecology*. 2nd ed. Stamford, Connecticut: Appleton & Lange; 1998.

43. Marrett LD, Nguyen HL, Armstrong BK. Trends in the incidence of cutaneous malignant melanoma in New South Wales, 1983–1996. *Int J Cancer*. 2001;*92*:457–462.

44. President's Cancer Panel. Reducing Environmental Cancer Risk. What We Can Do Now. 2008–2009 Annual Report. National Institutes of Health (US). Bethesda MD: National Cancer Institute. April 2010. http://deainfo.nci.nih.gov/advisory/pcp/annualReports/pcp08-09rpt/PCP_Report_08-09_508.pdf. Accessed January 6, 2012.

45. The International Agency for Research on Cancer Working Group on artificial ultraviolet (UV) light and skin cancer. The association of use of sunbeds with cutaneous malignant melanoma and other skin cancers: A systematic review. *Int J Cancer*. 2007;*120*(5):1116–1122.

46. World Health Organization. *WHO Report on the Global Tobacco Epidemic 2009: Implementing Smoke-Free Environments*. Geneva: WHO Press; 2009.

47. Shafey O, Dolwick S, Guindon GE (eds.). *Tobacco Control Country Profiles*. 2nd ed. Atlanta, GA: American Cancer Society; 2003.

48. World Health Organization. Tobacco Free Initiative http://www.who.int/tobacco/en/. Accessed 10/2011.

49. World Health Organization. *Tobacco Industry Interference with Tobacco Control*. Geneva: WHO Press; 2008.

50. World Health Organization. *Tobacco Industry and Corporate Responsibility: An Inherent Contradiction*. Geneva: WHO Press; 2004.

51. Resnicow K, Soler R., Braithwaite RL. Cultural sensitivity in substance abuse prevention. *J Community Psychol*. 2000;*28*(3):271–290.

CHAPTER THREE

1. Pinker S. *The Better Angels Of Our Nature*. New York, NY: Viking; 2011.

2. Coughlin SS, Soskolne CL, Goodman KW. *Case Studies in Public Health Ethics*. Washington DC: American Public Health Association; 1997.

3. The Drafters of the Universal Declaration of Human Rights. http://www.un.org/en/documents/udhr/drafters.shtml. Accessed December 1, 2011.

4. Declaration of Human Rights. http://www.un.org/en/documents/udhr/. Accessed December 1, 2011.

5. Beauchamp T, Childress J. *Principles of Biomedical Ethics*. New York, NY: Oxford University Press; 1979.

6. Heymann DL. *Control of Communicable Diseases Manual*. 19th ed. Washington DC: American Public Health Association; 2008.

7. Weed DL, McKeown RE. Science and social responsibility in public health. *Environ Health Perspect*. 2003;*111*(14):1804–1808.

8. Weed DL, McKeown RE. Epidemiology and virtue ethics. *Int J Epidemiol*. 1998;*27*:343–349.

9. Plane passengers sue TB patient. CNN Health, 2007. http://articles.cnn.com/2007-07-12/health/tb.suit_1_andrew-speaker-tb-patient-tb-tests?_s=PM:HEALTH. Accessed December 1, 2011.

10. Man in 2007 TB scare sues CDC over privacy. *Denver Post.* 2009. http://www.denverpost.com/news/ci_12258920?source=pkg. Accessed December 1, 2011.

11. 2009 H1N1 Flu http://www.cdc.gov/h1n1flu/. Accessed January 18, 2012.

12. Behind China's Aggressive Stance on Swine Flu. http://www.time.com/time/world/article/0,8599,1913384,00.html. Accessed December 2, 2011.

13. DHHS.CDC. Building capacity to fluoridate. *Literature Review.* June 2003.

14. United Nations Conference on Environment and Development 1992. Rio Declaration on Environment and Development. http://www.un.org/documents/ga/conf151/aconf15126-1annex1.htm. Accessed June 16, 2012.

15. Marchant G. From general policy to legal rule: aspirations and limitations of the precautionary rule. *Environ Health Perspect.* 2003;*111*(14):1799–1803.

16. Artificial sweeteners and cancer. http://www.cancer.gov/cancertopics/factsheet/Risk/artificial-sweeteners. Accessed June 17, 2012.

17. The flawed 1976 National "swine flu" influenza immunization program. http://www.whale.to/vaccine/flawed_1976.html. Accessed June 17, 2012.

18. Environmental Ethics. http://plato.stanford.edu/entries/ethics-environmental/#EarDevEnvEth. Accessed January19, 2012.

19. Ross LF. Mandatory versus voluntary consent for newborn screening? *Kennedy Institute of Ethics Journal.* 2010;*20*(4):299–328.

20. Pawlikowkski J, Sak J, Marczewski K. The analysis of the ethical, organizational and legal aspects of Polish biobanks activity. *Eur J Public Health.* 2009;*6*:707–710.

21. Little J, Potter B, Allanson J, Caulfield T, Carroll JC, Wilson B. Canada: public health genomics. *Public Health Genomics.* 2009;*12*:112–120.

22. P3G. Public population project in genomics. http://www.p3g.org/secretariat/index.shtml. Accessed January 1, 2012

23. Purcell M. Raising healthy children: moral and political responsibility for childhood obesity. *J Public Health Policy.* 2012;*31*(4):433–446.

24. Convention on the Rights of the Childhttp://www2.ohchr.org/english/law/crc.htm. Accessed December 3, 2011.

25. Petrini C. Triage in public health emergencies: ethical issues. *Intern Emerg Med.* 2010;*5*:137–144.

26. Singer PA, Benetar SR, Bernstein M, Daar AS, Dickens BM, MacRae SK, et al. Ethics and SARS: lessons from Toronto. *Br Med J.* 2003;*327*:1342–1344.

27. Ng JM. Ethical issues encountered during the SARS Crisis. *The Meducator.* 2012;*1*(4):12–14. http://digitalcommons.mcmaster.ca/cgi/viewcontent.cgi?article=1047&context=meducator. Accessed May 31, 2012.

28. Emanuel EJ. The Lessons of SARS. *Ann Intern Med.* 2003;*139*:589–591.

CHAPTER FOUR

1. White F, Nanan D. Community health case studies selected from developing and developed countries—common principles for moving from evidence to action. *Arch Med Sci.* 2008;*4*(4):358–363.

2. Institute of Medicine. *The Future of the Public's Health in the 21st Century*. November 2002. National Academy of Sciences. Washington DC; 2003.

3. Jacobs J. [1961] *The Death and Life of Great American Cities* (Modern Library edition). New York: Random House 1993.

4. Lenaway D, Halverson P, Sotnikov S, Tilson H, Corso L, Millington W. Public health systems research: setting a national agenda. *Am J Public Health*. 2006;*96*(3):410–413.

5. International Network of Indigenous Health Knowledge and Development. Hosted by James Cook University. http://www.inihkd.org/. Accessed Nov 10, 2011.

6. United Nations Covenant on Economic, Social and Cultural Rights. http://www.hrweb.org/legal/escr.html. Accessed January 21, 2012.

7. White F. A voluntary perspective on health promotion—the role of non-governmental organizations, particularly in the voluntary sector. *Health Promotion*. 1986;*1*(4):429–436.

8. Health Alliance International. The NGO Code of Conduct for Health Systems Strengthening Initiative. http://ngocodeofconduct.org/. Accessed January 21, 2012.

9. Nayani P, White F, Nanan D. Public-private partnership as a success factor for health systems. *Medicine Today*. 2006;*4*:135–142. http://www.phabc.org/files/Nayani_White_Nanan_Public-Private_Partnership-pg135–142.pdf. Accessed January 21, 2012.

10. Prince M. Tax policy as social policy Canadian tax assistance for people with disabilities. *Canadian Public Policy*. 2001;27:4487–4501.

11. Asian Development Bank. Health sector reform in Asia and the Pacific: an overview. In: *Health Sector Reform in Asia and the Pacific: Options for Developing Countries*; Manila: Asian Development Bank; 1999: 4–14.

12. Ullah ANZ, Newell JN, Ahmed JU, Hyder MKA. Islam a government-NGO collaboration: the case of tuberculosis control in Bangladesh. *Health Policy and Planning Health Policy Plan*. 2006;*21*:143–155.

13. Ketsela T, Habimana P, Martines J, Mbewe A, Williams A, Sabiiti J, et al. Integrated Management of Childhood Illness (IMCI). Chapter 5 In: *Opportunities for Africa's Newborns*. World Health Organization on behalf of The Partnership for Maternal Newborn and Child Health. 2006;. 91–100. http://www.who.int/pmnch/media/publications/aon-sectionIII_5.pdf. Accessed July 4, 2012.

14. Lamb R. *Hybrid Organization*. University of Hawaii, Manoa. June 17, 2004. http://www.vfh.fh-brandenburg.de/vfh/gastvorlesungen/gastvortrag_05.pdf. Accessed January 21, 2012.

15. Menard C. The Economics of Hybrid Organizations. Presidential address to the annual conference of the International Society for New Institutional Economics, MIT, September 27–29, 2002. *J Institutional and Theoretical Econ*. 2004;*160*:345–376. http://www.econ.kobe-u.ac.jp/~yanagawa/Economics_of_Hybrids—JITE-2004.pdf. Accessed July 4, 2012.

16. Executive Summary. The emerging fourth sector—a new sector of organizations at the intersection of the public, private and social sectors. The Fourth Sector Network, the Aspen Institute and the W.K. Kellogg Foundation. 2009. Washington DC. http://www.cornerstoneondemand.org/assets/resources/4thsectopaper.pdf. Accessed January 21, 2012.

17. Last JM (ed). *A Dictionary of Public Health*. New York, NY: Oxford University Press; 2007.

18. Alma Ata Declaration on Primary Health Care. http://www.who.int/hpr/NPH/docs/declaration_almaata.pdf. Accessed January 21, 2012.

19. John TJ, White F. Public health in South Asia. In: Beaglehole R (ed.). *Global Public Health: A New Era.* New York, NY: Oxford University Press; 2003; 172–190.

20. People's Health Movement. People's Charter for Health. http://www.phmovement.org/sites/www.phmovement.org/files/phm-pch-english.pdf. Accessed July 4, 2012.

21. United Nations Development Programme. Human Development Report 2003. *Millennium Development Goals: A Compact Among Nations to End Human Poverty.* New York: Oxford University Press; 2003.

22. UN General Assembly. 65th Session Agenda Items 115. Special Session on the MDGs. Outcome Document: New York. September, 2010.

23. The Bangkok Charter of Health Promotion in a Globalized World. http://www.who.int/healthpromotion/conferences/6gchp/hpr_050829_%20BCHP.pdf. Accessed January 21, 2012.

24. de Leeuw E, Tang KC, Beaglehole R. Ottawa to Bangkok—health promotion's journey from principles to *"glocal"* implementation. *Health Promot Int.* 2006;*21*(suppl 1):1–4.

25. Raeburn J, Akerman M, Chuengsatiansup K, Meija F, Oladepo O. Community capacity building and health promotion in a globalized world. *Health Promot Int.* 2006;*21*(suppl 1):84–90.

26. Ottawa Charter for Health Promotion. First International Conference on Health Promotion Ottawa, 21 November 1986—WHO/HPR/HEP/95.1 http://www.who.int/hpr/NPH/docs/ottawa_charter_hp.pdf. Accessed January 21, 2012.

27. Hill M, Carroll S. Health Promotion, health education, and the public's health. In: Detels R, Beaglehole R, Lansang MA, Gulliford M (eds.). *Oxford Textbook of Public Health.* Vol 2. 5th ed. New York, NY: Oxford University Press; 2009; 752–766.

28. White F. De la evidencia al desempeno: como fijar prioridades y tomar buenas decisiones. Current Topics. *Pan Am J Public Health.* 1998;4:69–74.

29. Krieger N. Theories for social epidemiology in the 21st century: an ecosocial perspective. *Int J Epidemiol.* 2001;*30*(4):668–677. http://ije.oxfordjournals.org/content/30/4/668.long. Accessed November 9, 2011.

30. Centers for Disease Control and Prevention. Injury Center: Violence Prevention. The Social Ecological Model—A Framework for Prevention. Page last updated: September 9, 2009. http://www.cdc.gov/violenceprevention/overview/social-ecologicalmodel.html. Accessed January 21, 2012.

31. Dahlberg LL, Krug EG. Violence—a global public health problem. In: Krug E, Dahlberg LL, Mercy JA, Zwi AB, Lozano R (eds.). *World Report on Violence and Health.* Geneva, Switzerland: World Health Organization; 2002; 1–56.

32. African Medical and Research Foundation. A Very African Journey. Nairobi, 2007. http://64.176.64.243/A%20Very%20African%20Journey.pdf. Accessed January 21, 2012.

33. Karimuio J, Ilako F, Gichangi M. Trachoma control using the WHO adopted "safe with azithromycin." *East Afr Med J.* 2007;*84*:127–135.

34. Bailey R, Lietman T. The SAFE strategy for the elimination of trachoma by 2020: will it work? *Bull World Health Organ.* 2001;*79*:233–236.

35. White F. Capacity building for health research in developing countries: a manager's approach. *Rev Panam Salud Publica.* 2002;*12*:165–172.

36. White F. The Urban Health Project, Karachi. *Bull World Health Organ.* 2000;*78*:565.

37. Rabbani F. The Aga Khan University and the Urban Health Project. In: Blumenthal DS, Boelen C . *Universities and the Health of the Disadvantaged.* Geneva: World Health Organization; WHO/EIP/OSD/2000.10; 2001.

38. Rabbani F, Shaikh BT, Mahmood Q, Khan KS, Israr SM, Memon Y. Medical education and training: responding to community needs. *Med Sci Monit.* 2005;*11*:SR21–SR25.

39. Zaidi S. Rural Community Development Project: conceptual dimensions. In: *Health, Population and the Environment: Knowledge, Lessons and Challenges.* Islam A, Tahir MZ (eds). Karachi: Aga Khan University/ City Publishers; 2000; 59–75.

40. International Finance Corporation (IFC): Environmental Review Summary—Lasmo Oil Pakistan. http://www.ifc.org/ifcext/spiwebsite1.nsf/ProjectDisplay/ERS10408. Accessed January 21, 2012.

41. United Nations Commission on Sustainable Development. Social aspects of sustainable development. In: Mauritius' submission to the 5th Session of the Commission on Sustainable Development, April 1997. http://www.un.org/esa/agenda21/natlinfo/countr/mauritiu/social.htm#health. Accessed October 1, 2012.

42. Dowse GK, Gareeboo H, Alberti KG, et al. Changes in population cholesterol concentrations and other cardiovascular risk factor levels after five years of the non-communicable disease intervention programme in Mauritius. Mauritius Non-communicable Disease Study Group. *Br Med J.* 1995;*311*:1255–1259.

43. Söderberg S, Zimmet P, Tuomilehto J, et al. Increasing prevalence of type 2 diabetes mellitus in all ethnic groups in Mauritius. *Diabet Med.* 2005;*22*:61–68.

44. African Development Bank. Appraisal Report: Support to the National Health Plan Project—Republic of Mauritius.MRS/PSHH/2001/01 OCDE October 2001.

45. WHO Statistical Information System. Available at http://www.who.int/whosis/en/ April 24, 2008.

46. Puska P, Tuomilehto J, Nissinen A, Vartiainen E. *The North Karelia Project—20 Year Results and Experiences.* Helsinki: National Public Health Institute; 1995.

47. CINDI Highlights 2005. WHO Regional Office for Europe. Copenhagen 2006. Available at: http://www.euro.who.int/document/E89308.pdf.

48. Jadue L, Vega J, Escobar MC, et al. Risk factors for noncommunicable diseases: methods and global results of the CARMEN program basal survey [Spanish]. *Rev Med Chil.* 1999;*127*:1004–1013.

49. Policy Development and Implementation Processes in the CINDI and Carmen Noncommunicable Disease Intervention Programmes—a comparative study. World Health Organization 2004. Available at: http://www.phac-aspc.gc.ca/ccdpc-cpcmc/cindi/pdf/cindi_policy_en.pdf.

50. Oxford Health Alliance—Confronting the Epidemic of Chronic Disease. http://www.oxha.org/. Accessed January 21, 2012.

51. Commonwealth Secretariat. Taking up the challenge of non-communicable diseases in the Commonwealth: 17 Good Practice Case Studies. London 2011. http://www.thecommonwealth.org/files/237519/FileName/CSHealthPublicationA5_web.pdf. Accessed July 4, 2012.

52. Galea G, Powis B, Tamplin SA. Healthy Islands in the Western Pacific—International Settings Development. http://heapro.oxfordjournals.org/cgi/content/full/15/2/169. Accessed January 21, 2012.

53. Wisconsin Office of Rural Health. Strong Rural Communities Initiative. UW School of Medicine and Public Health. Available at: http://www.worh.org/SRCIoverview. Accessed January 21, 2012.

54. Miseviciene I. Kaunas City Identity from Health Perspective: Possibilities of Intersectoral Cooperation. University-City Cooperation. 8th BSRUA Seminar. Kaunas. May 11–12, 2007. https://docs.google.com/viewer?a=v&q=cache:XUYpedo6B_wJ:bsrun.utu.fi/tiedostot/Turku_BSUA_presentations/Miseviciene_Kaunas_Medical.ppt+Miseviciene+I. +Kaunas+City+identity+from+health+perspective&hl=en&gl=ca&pid=bl&srcid=A DGEESgczR7pVLomYmHEo4umtYlGNSVLgq-pDcx2wkrQfWFaIvE6LvsMibC8OM 7jS1syo8jURAgytzxjHZs4LBLxZT-qofrL3TeylWbz3-Wmg70cmBVFA51wepobVRDF uSB1SD47x4dn&sig=AHIEtbS-ZX_9u2TZEd4iAva4plvVCZpkJQ. Accessed January 21, 2012.

55. Hepburn L, Miller M, Azrael D, Hemenway D. The US gun stock: results from the 2004 national firearms survey. *Inj Prev.* 2007;*13*(1):15–19. Doi: 10.1136/ip.2006.013607. http:// www.ncbi.nlm.nih.gov/pmc/articles/PMC2610545/pdf/15.pdf. Accessed January 21, 2012.

56. Heath I. Treating violence as a public health problem. *Br Med J.* 2002;*325*:726. Doi: 10.1136/ bmj.325.7367.726; October 5, 2002.

57. Zakocs RC, Earp JAL. Explaining variation in gun control policy advocacy tactics among local organizations. *Health Educ Behav.* 2003;*30*:360–374.

58. First reports evaluating the effectiveness of strategies for preventing violence: firearms laws. findings from the Task Force on Community Preventive Services. *MMWR.* October 3, 2003 / 52(RR14):11–20. http://www.cdc.gov/mmwR/preview/mmwrhtml/rr5214a2.htm. Accessed January 21, 2012.

59. Cowan J, Kessler J. Changing the Gun Debate. DLC Blueprint Magazine, Democratic Leadership Council. July 12, 2001. http://www.dlc.org/ndol_ci.cfm?kaid=119&subid=15 7&contentid=3560. Accessed January 21, 2012.

60. El-Guebaly N. Don't drink and drive: the successful message of Mothers Against Drunk Driving (MADD). *World Psychiatry.* 2005;*4*(1):35–36. http://www.ncbi.nlm.nih.gov/ pmc/articles/PMC1414720/. Accessed January 21, 2012.

61. Asbridge M, Mann RE, Flam-Zalcman R, Stoduto G. The criminalization of impaired driving in Canada: assessing the deterrent impact of Canada's first per se law. *J Stud Alcohol.* 2004;*65*(4):450–459. http://www.madd.ca/english/news/pr/JSA-asbridge-08.pdf. Accessed January 21, 2012.

62. Polacsek M, Rogers EM, Woodall WG, Delaney H, Wheeler D, Rao N. MADD victim impact panels and stages-of-change in drunk-driving prevention. *J Stud Alcohol.* 2001;*62*(3):344–350.

63. Reading J, Elias B. Chapter 2—An Examination of Residential Schools and Elder Health. In: First Nations and Inuit Health Surveys. Published by the National Steering Committee. Health Canada; 1999. http://www.fnigc.ca/sites/default/files/ENpdf/RHS_1997/rhs_ 1997_final_report.pdf. Accessed January 21, 2012.

64. Milloy JS. (1996) Socio-cultural Project Area 7: Residential Schools. "Suffer the Little Children." A History of the Residential School System, 1830–1992. Submitted to the Royal Commission on Aboriginal Peoples. 25 April. As cited in Reading J, Elias B. (1999) Op Cit.

65. Truth and Reconciliation Commission of Canada. For the child taken, for the parent left behind. http://www.trc.ca/websites/trcinstitution/index.php?p=26. Accessed January 21, 2012.

66. Leaders for Life Program. Leadership capabilities for an integrated health system in British Columbia—the BC health leadership framework. http://www.royalroads.ca/NR/rdonlyres/7F061C51-E275-414B-8CE4-D980D2A48271/0/FinalCapabilities_forWeb.pdf. Accessed January 21, 2012.

67. White F. Global Journal of Public Health (inaugural editorial). *GJMEDPH*. 2012;*1*(1):1–2. http://www.gjmedph.org/uploads/Editorial.pdf

68. Yamey G. Scaling Up Global Health Interventions: A Proposed Framework for Success. *PLoS Med*. 2011;*8*(6):e1001049. Doi: 10.1371/journal.pmed.1001049. http://www.plosmedicine.org/article/info:doi%2F10.1371%2Fjournal.pmed.1001049. Accessed January 21, 2012.

69. Hancock T. Healthy communities must also be sustainable communities. *Public Health Reports*. 2000;*115*:151–156.

70. What Is Sustainable Community Development? Centre for Sustainable Community Development. Simon Fraser University. http://www.sfu.ca/cscd.html. Accessed October 9, 2010.

71. Yunus M. *Banker to the Poor*. New York, NY: Public Affairs; 2003.

72. Von Schirnding Y. The World Summit on Sustainable Development: reaffirming the centrality of health. *Globalization and Health*. 2005;*1*:8. Doi: 10.1186/1744-8603-1-8. http://www.globalizationandhealth.com/content/1/1/8. Accessed January 21, 2012.

73. The Budapest Declaration. Building European Civil Society through Community Development. *Community Dev J*. 2004;*39*(4):423–429. Doi: 10.1093/cdj/bsh040.

CHAPTER FIVE

1. Wallace RB. Public health and preventive medicine: trends and guideposts. Chapter 1 In: *Public Health & Preventive Medicine*. 15th ed. New York, NY: McGraw Hill; 2008; 3, 4.

2. Health Canada. *Taking Action on Population Health*. 1998. Ottawa. Cat. No. H39-445/1998E ISBN 0-662-27431-8 http://www.phac-aspc.gc.ca/ph-sp/pdf/tad-eng.pdf. Accessed November 29, 2011.

3. Dunn JR, Hayes MV. Toward a lexicon of population health. *Can J Public Health*. 1999;*90*(suppl 1):S7–S10.

4. Friedman DJ, Starfield B. Models of population health: their value for US public health practice, policy and research. *Am J Public Health*. 2003;*93*(3):366–369.

5. Grundy E. Demography and public health. Chapter 7.2 In: Detels R, Beaglehole R, Lansing M-A, Gulliford M (eds.). *Oxford Textbook of Public Health*. 5th ed. Oxford: Oxford University Press; 2009; 734–751.

6. Kapiszewski A. United Nations Expert Group Meeting on International Migrations and Development in the Arab Region. Arab versus Asian Migrant Workers in the GSS Countries. UN/POP/EGM/2006/02 22 May 2006 http://www.un.org/esa/population/meetings/EGM_Ittmig_Arab/P02_Kapiszewski.pdf. Accessed November 24, 2011.

7. As World Passes 7 Billion Milestone, UN Urges Action to Meet Key Challenges. UN News Service. October 31, 2011. http://www.un.org/apps/news/story.asp?NewsID=40257. Accessed November 20, 2011.

8. 2008 World Population Data Sheet. Population Reference Bureau. http://www.prb.org/pdf08/08WPDS_Eng.pdf. Accessed November 21, 2011.

9. White F, Nanan D. International and global health. Chapter 76 In: *Maxcy-Rosenau-Last. Public Health & Preventive Medicine.* 15th ed. New York, NY: McGraw Hill; 2008; 1252–1258.

10. UNFPA. Sex-ratio Imbalance in Asia: Trends, Consequences and Policy Responses. Executive Summary of Regional Analysis. 4th Asia Pacific Conference on Reproductive and Sexual Health and Rights. Oct 29–31, 2007 Hyderabad, India. http://www.unfpa.org/gender/docs/studies/summaries/reg_exe_summary.pdf. Accessed Nov 29, 2011.

11. Pande R, Malhotra A. Son Preference and Daughter Neglect in India. What Happens to Living Girls? 2006 International Center for Research on Women. http://www.icrw.org/docs/2006_son-preference.pdf. Accessed Nov 29, 2011.

12. Rising sex-ratio imbalance "a danger." Xinhua, China Daily. Updated: 2007-01-23 07:16. http://www.chinadaily.com.cn/china/2007-01/23/content_789821.htm. Accessed Nov 29, 2011.

13. Vogel L. Sex selection migrates to Canada. NEWS January 16, 2012. *Can Med Assoc J.* Doi: 10.1503/cmaj.109-4091. http://www.cmaj.ca/site/earlyreleases/16jan12_sex-selection-migrates-to-canada.xhtml. Accessed January 22, 2012.

14. 2008 World Population Data Sheet. Population Reference Bureau. http://www.prb.org/pdf08/08WPDS_Eng.pdf. Accessed November 21, 2011.

15. Telles EE. Incorporating Race and Ethnicity into the UN Millennium Development Goals. Race Report. Inter American Dialogue. January 2007. http://www.thedialogue.org/PublicationFiles/telles.pdf. Accessed Nov 24, 2011.

16. Rockett IRH. Population and health: an introduction to epidemiology. (fig 2, p. 9). *Population Bulletin.* 1999;54:44.

17. Popkin BM, Gordon-Larsen P. The nutrition transition: worldwide obesity dynamics and their determinants. *Int J Obesity.* 2004;28:S2–S9. Doi: 10.1038/sj.ijo.0802804.

18. US Department of Health and Human Services. Healthy People 2010. http://www.healthypeople.gov/2020/default.aspx. Accessed November 29, 2011.

19. Kroeger A. Kloss-Quiroga B. Module 5: Input—Situation Analysis. In: Kloss-Quiroga B (ed.). *Facilitators Manual. District Health Management Tools.* InWEnt—Public Health Division. Berlin; 2004. https://docs.google.com/viewer?a=v&q=cache:NwwlUNi7oPMJ:www.aidstar-two.org/Tools-Database.cfm?action%3Ddownload%26id%3D447+District+Health+Management+Tools.+InWEnt+%E2%80%93+Public+Health+Division.+Berlin+2004.&hl=en&gl=ca&pid=bl&srcid=ADGEEShlgCtYiJfolE_IopCcK7RiOBA15xM1dVTSVsn5zHoRK2YFbOFyQZoW8OMoUHs_GJ747eXU8tFRmF_LoJk_62uVGzUfxzTdDIbjuYztqgkVK89k8eU1WLxisIQ7WAVUONk9QTY&sig=AHIEtbQd4qD3wKcr5kOw6S3_bnknGscjLQ. Accessed July 4, 2012.

20. The Chief Public Health Officer's Report on The State of Public Health in Canada 2009. http://www.phac-aspc.gc.ca/publicat/2009/cphorsphc-respcacsp/cphorsphc-respcacsp03-eng.php. Accessed Nov 24, 2009.

21. UNICEF. The State of the World's Children 2009. Maternal and Newborn Health. http://www.unicef.org/sowc09/. Accessed Nov 24, 2009.

22. World Health Organization. Roll Back Malaria. Proposed Methods and Instruments for Situation Analysis. WHO/CDS/RBM/99.01.a E. 26 March 1999. http://www.rollback-malaria.org/docs/methodology.pdf. Accessed Nov 24, 2009.

23. Diabetes in Australia. CATI Technical Reference Group. National Public Health Partnership. May 2003. http://www.dhs.vic.gov.au/nphp/catitrg/diabetesbgpaper.pdf. Accessed November 24, 2009.

24. Morris JN. The uses of epidemiology. *Br Med J.* 1955;.2:395–401.

25. Pan American Health Organization. Special Program for Health Analysis. Health indicators: building blocks for health situation analysis. *Epidemiological Bulletin.* 2001;22(4):1–5. http://www.paho.org/english/sha/eb_v22n4.pdf. Accessed July 4, 2012.

26. Ross DA, Hinman AR. Public health informatics. Chapter 5 In: *Public Health and Preventive Medicine.* 15th ed. McGraw Hill; 2008.

27. Bain MRS, Chalmers JWT, Brewster DH. Routinely collected data in national and regional databases—an underused resource. *J Public Health Med.* 1997;19(4):413–418.

28. Kondo N, Sembajwe G, Kawachi I., van Dam R, Subramanian S, Yamagata Z. Income inequality, mortality, and self-rated health: meta-analysis of multilevel studies. *Br Med J.* 2009;339:bmj.b4471. http://www.bmj.com/content/339/bmj.b4471. Accessed November 27, 2011.

29. Subramanian SV. Income inequality and health: what have we learned so far? *Epidemiol Rev.* 2004;26(1):78–91. Doi: 10.1093/epirev/mxh003.

30. Kawachi I. Income inequality and health. In: Berkman LF, Kawachi I (eds.). *Social Epidemiology.* New York, NY: Oxford University Press; 2000; 76–94.

31. Global Burden of Disease (GBD) project, Health Statistics and Health Information Systems. World Health Organization. http://www.who.int/healthinfo/global_burden_disease/en/. Accessed November 27, 2011.

32. Mont D, Loeb M. Beyond DALYs: Developing Indicators to Assess the Impact of Public Health Interventions on the Lives of People with Disabilities. World Bank SP Discussion Paper No. 0815. May 2008. http://siteresources.worldbank.org/SOCIALPROTECTION/Resources/SP-Discussion-papers/Disability-DP/0815.pdf. Accessed November 27, 2011.

33. AvRuskin GA, Jacquez GM, Meliker JR, Slotnick MJ, Kaufmann AM, Nriagu JO. Visualization and exploratory analysis of epidemiologic data using a novel space time information system. *Int J Health Geographics.* 2004;3(26). Doi: 10.1186/1476-072X-3-26.

34. Stallones L, Nuckols JR, Berry JK. Surveillance around hazardous waste sites: Geographic Information Systems and reproductive outcomes. *Environmental Research.* 1992;59:81–92.

35. Xiang H, Nuckols JR, Stallones L. A geographic information assessment of birth weight and crop production patterns around mother's residence. *Environ Res.* 2000;82:160–167.

36. Friss RH, Sellers TA. *Epidemiology for Public Health Practice.* 3rd ed. Boston MA: Jones and Bartlett; 2004.

37. Karimuio J, Ilako F, Gichangi M. Trachoma control using the WHO adopted "safe with azithromycin." *East Afr Med J.* 2007;84:127–135.

38. Bailey R, Lietman T. The SAFE strategy for the elimination of trachoma by 2020: will it work? *Bull World Health Organ.* 2001;79:233–236.

39. Zaidi S. Rural Community Development Project: conceptual dimensions. In: Islam A (ed.). *Health, Population and the Environment: Knowledge, Lessons and Challenges.* Karachi: Aga Khan University/ City Publishers; 2000; 59–75.

40. International Finance Corporation (IFC): Environmental Review Summary—Lasmo Oil Pakistan. http://www.ifc.org/ifcext/spiwebsite1.nsf/ProjectDisplay/ERS10408. Accessed January 21, 2012.

41. United Nations Commission on Sustainable Development. Social aspects of sustainable development. In: Mauritius' submission to the 5th Session of the Commission on Sustainable Development, April 1997. http://www.un.org/esa/agenda21/natlinfo/countr/mauritiu/social.htm#health. Accessed October 1, 2012.

42. African Development Bank. Appraisal Report: Support to the National Health Plan Project—Republic of Mauritius. MRS/PSHH/2001/01 OCDE October 2001.

43. Policy Development and Implementation Processes in the CINDI and CARMEN Noncommunicable Disease Intervention Programmes—A Comparative Study. World Health Organization 2004. Available at: http://www.phac-aspc.gc.ca/ccdpc-cpcmc/cindi/pdf/cindi_policy_en.pdf.

44. Oxford Health Alliance—confronting the epidemic of chronic disease. http://www.oxha.org/. Accessed January 21, 2012.

45. Commonwealth Secretariat. Taking up the challenge of non-communicable diseases in the Commonwealth: 17 Good Practice Case Studies. London 2011. http://www.thecommonwealth.org/files/237519/FileName/CSHealthPublicationA5_web.pdf. Accessed January 21, 2012.

46. World Health Organization. Commission on the Social Determinants of Health. Geneva, August 2008. http://www.who.int/social_determinants/final_report/en/index.html. Accessed November 3, 2009.

47. United Nations Development Programme. About the MDGs: Basics—What Are the Millennium Development Goals? http://www.undp.org/mdg/basics.shtml. Accessed November 30, 2009.

48. Sachs J. *The End of Poverty—How We Can Make It Happen in Our Lifetime.* London: Penguin; 2005.

49. White F. Development assistance for health—donor commitment as a critical success factor. *Can J Public Health.* 2011;*102*(6):421–423.

50. The World Bank. Figure 1a from 2010 World Development Indicators. http://data.worldbank.org/data-catalog/world-development-indicators/wdi-2010. Accessed July 6, 2012.

51. UN General Assembly. 65th Session Agenda Items 115. Special Session on the MDGs. Outcome Document: New York. September, 2010.

52. Ravallion M. A Comparative Perspective on Poverty Reduction in Brazil, China and India. The World Bank Development Research Group—Director's Office Policy Research Working Paper 5080—October 2009 WPS5080. http://www-wds.worldbank.org/external/default/WDSContentServer/WDSP/IB/2009/10/15/000158349_20091015114049/Rendered/PDF/WPS5080.pdf. Accessed Nov 6, 2009.

53. US Centers for Disease Control and Prevention. Guidelines for Evaluating Public Health Surveillance Systems. MMWR Recommendations and Reports. July 27, 2001 / 50(RR13);1–35. http://www.cdc.gov/mmwr/preview/mmwrhtml/rr5013a1.htm. Accessed November 19, 2009.

54. Heyman DL. *Control of Communicable Diseases Manual: An Official Report of the American Public Health Association.* 19th ed. Washington DC: American Public Health Association; 2008.

55. Wallace RB. Epidemiology and public health. Chapter 2 In: *Public Health & Preventive Medicine.* 15th ed. New York, NY: McGraw Hill; 2008; 5–26.

56. Buehler JW, Hopkins RS, Overhage JM, Sosin DM, Tong V. Framework for Evaluating Public Health Surveillance Systems for Early Detection of Outbreaks. MMWR

Recommendations and Reports. May 7, 2004/53(RR05);1–11. http://www.cdc.gov/MMWR/preview/mmwrhtml/rr5305a1.htm. Accessed Dec 23, 2009.

57. World Health Organization. What has changed in the International Health Regulations (2005). http://www.who.int/ihr/revisionchange/en/print.html WHO, 2009. Accessed December 23, 2009.

58. World Health Organization. International Health Regulations (2005). www.who.int/ihr. Accessed November 28, 2011.

59. Wilson K, Tigerstrom B, McDougall C. Protecting global health security through the *International Health Regulations: requirements and challenges. Can Med Assoc J.* 2008;*179*(1):434–438. http://www.cmaj.ca/cgi/reprint/179/1/44.pdf. Accessed December 23, 2009.

60. Eysenbach G. SARS and Population Health Technology. *J Med Internet Res.* 2003;*5*(2):e14. Published online 2003 June 30. Doi: 10.2196/jmir.5.2.e14. http://www.ncbi.nlm.nih.gov/pmc/articles/PMC1550560/?tool=pmcentrez. Accessed November 30, 2009.

61. Reisen WK. Landscape epidemiology of vector-borne diseases. *Ann Rev Entomol.* 2010;*55*:461–483.

62. Gregg MB (ed.). *Field Epidemiology.* New York, NY: Oxford University Press; 1996.

63. Baker MC, Mathieu E, Fleming FM, Deming M, King JD, Garba A, et al . Mapping, monitoring, and surveillance of neglected tropical diseases: towards a policy framework. *The Lancet,* 2010;*375*(9710):231–238. http://www.thelancet.com/journals/lancet/article/PIIS0140-6736(09)61458-6/abstract

64. Haub C. The World at 7 Million. Presentation on: 2011 World Population Data Sheet and Population Bulletin. Population Reference Bureau. http://www.prb.org/pdf11/2011-world-population-data-sheet-presentation.pdf. Accessed November 24, 2011.

65. Population Reference Bureau. Population Data Sheet 2009. http://www.prb.org/pdf09/09wpds_eng.pdf. Accessed November 24, 2011.

66. Population Reference Bureau, analysis of data from U.S. Census Bureau. 2008 World Population Data Sheet. Population Reference Bureau. http://www.prb.org/pdf08/08WPDS_Eng.pdf. Accessed November 21, 2011.

CHAPTER SIX

1. Krieger N. 2001. Theories for social epidemiology in the 21st century: an ecosocial perspective. *Int J Epidemiol.* 2001;*30*(4):668–677. http://ije.oxfordjournals.org/content/30/4/668.long. Accessed November 9, 2011.

2. McMichael AJ. Prisoners of the proximate: loosening the constraints on epidemiology in an age of change. *Am J Epidemiol.* 1999;*149*(10):887–897.

3. U.S. Department of Health and Human Services. *Healthy People 2010.* 2nd ed. 2 vols. Washington, DC: U.S. Government Printing Office; 2000.

4. Heyman DJ (ed.). *Control of Communicable Diseases Manual.* 19th ed. Washington DC: American Public Health Association; 2008.

5. National Center for Biotechnology Information. National Institutes of Health. http://www.ncbi.nlm.nih.gov/mesh/68001523. Accessed June 23, 2012.

6. World Health Organization. Prevention of Mental Disorders—Effective Interventions and Policy Options. Summary Report. Geneva, 2004. http://www.who.int/mental_health/evidence/en/prevention_of_mental_disorders_sr.pdf. Accessed June 22, 2012.

7. Young F, Critchley JA, Johnstone LK, Unwin NC . Globalization and co-morbidity between TB, diabetes, HIV, and metabolic syndrome in sub-Saharan Africa. *Globalization and Health*. 2009;*5*(9). Doi: 10.1186/1744-8603-5-9. http://www.globalizationandhealth.com/content/5/1/9. Accessed June 22, 2012.

8. Barker DJP. Maternal nutrition, fetal nutrition, and disease in later life. *Nutrition*. 1997;*13*:807–813.

9. World Health Organization. International Classification of Functioning, Disability and Health (ICF) http://www.who.int/classifications/icf/en/. Accessed October 1, 2011.

10. Disability and Health. In: HealthyPeople.gov Health People 2010—improving the Health of Americans. http://healthypeople.gov/2020/topicsobjectives2020/overview.aspx?topicid=9. Accessed September 13, 2011.

11. Federman M. What Is the Meaning of The Medium Is the Message? McLuhan Program in Culture and Technology. http://individual.utoronto.ca/markfederman/article_medium-isthemessage.htm. Accessed June 25, 2012.

12. White F, Nanan D . International and global health. Chapter 76 In: Maxcy-Rosenau-Last. *Public Health & Preventive Medicine*. 15th ed. New York, NY: McGraw Hill; 2008; 1251–1258.

13. Omran AR. *The Epidemiological Transition in the Americas*. Washington, DC: Pan American Health Organization and University of Maryland; 1996.

14. Figure 6–1 adapted from Figure 3.19 in: Omran AR. *The Epidemiological Transition in the Americas*. Washington, DC: Pan American Health Organization and University of Maryland; 1996.

15. Nash C, Hoobler CG . *One Man, One Medicine, One Health: The James H Steele Story*. Charleston, SC: Booksurge. 2009.

16. One Health Initiative http://www.onehealthinitiative.com/. Accessed April 26, 2011 .

17. Last JM. (ed.). *A Dictionary of Public Health*. New York, NY Oxford University Press; 2007.

18. Last JM. The iceberg. *Lancet*. 1963;2:28–31.

19. Hetzel BS (ed.). *International Council for Control of Iodine Deficiency Disorders (ICCIDD). Towards the Global Elimination of Brain Damage Due to Iodine Deficiency*. Delhi: Oxford University Press; 2004.

20. Wilson JMG, Jungner G . Principles and practice of screening for disease. World Health Organization; 1968. http://whqlibdoc.who.int/php/WHO_PHP_34.pdf. Accessed December 27, 2011.

21. Rosolowich V. Breast self-examination. Breast Disease Committee of the Society of Obstetricians and Gynaecologists of Canada. *J Obstet Gynaecol Can*. 2006;*28*(8):728–730.

22. Lin K, Croswell JM, Koenig H, Lam C, Maltz A (eds.). Prostate-Specific Antigen-Based Screening for Prostate Cancer: An Evidence Update for the U.S. Preventive Services Task Force. Agency for Healthcare Research and Quality (US); Report No.: 12–05160-EF-1. 2011.

23. World Health Organization. Antiretroviral therapy of HIV infections in infants and children in resource-limited settings: towards universal access. Geneva, 2006. http://www.who.int/hiv/pub/guidelines/WHOpaediatric.pdf. Accessed October 26, 2011.

24. Hammer SM. Antiretroviral treatment as prevention. *N Engl J Med*. 2011;*365*:561–562. http://www.nejm.org/doi/full/10.1056/NEJMe1107487. Accessed December 27, 2011.

25. Beaglehole R, Bonita R, Kjellstrom T . *Basic Epidemiology*. Geneva: World Health Organization; 1993.

26. Barnett DJ, Balicer RD, Blodgett D, et al. The application of the Haddon Matrix to public health readiness and response planning. *Environmental Health Perspectives* 2005;*113*(5):10. http://ehp03.niehs.nih.gov/article/fetchArticle.action?articleURI=info%3Adoi%2F10.12 89%2Fehp.7491. Accessed June 25, 2012

27. Runyan C. Using the Haddon matrix: introducing the third dimension. *Injury Prevention.* 1998;*4*:302–307.

28. Hinman A. Eradication of vaccine-preventable diseases. *Ann Rev Public Health.* 1999;*20*:211–229.

29. Henderson DA. Eradication: lessons from the past. *Bull World Health Organ.* 1998;*76* (suppl 2):7–21.

30. International Task Force for Disease Eradication—Eradication and Elimination Programs Currently Sanctioned by The World Health Organization, as cited by The Carter Center; 2011. http://www.cartercenter.org/health/itfde/who.html. Accessed October 2, 2011.

31. Schemann JF, Guinot C, Ilboudo L, et al Trachoma, flies and environmental factors in Burkina Faso. *Trans R Soc Trop Med Hyg.* 2003;*97*(1):63–68.

32. Rozendaal JA. *Vector Control—Methods for use by Individuals and Communities.* Geneva: World Health Organization; 1997.

33. Meslin FX, Stohr K, Heyman D, et al. Public health implications of emerging zoonoses. *Rev Sci Tech.* 2000;*1*:310–317.

34. Alleyne BC, Orford RR, Lacey BA, White FMM. Rate of slaughter may increase risk of human brucellosis in a meat packing plant. *J Occupational Medicine.* 1986;*28*: 445–450.

35. Gregg MB (ed.). *Field Epidemiology.* New York, NY: Oxford University Press; 1996.

36. Anderson RM, May RM . Age related changes in the rate of disease transmission: implications for the design of vaccination programs. *J Hyg London.* 1985;*94*:365–436.

37. US Centers for Disease Control and Prevention. History and Epidemiology of Global Smallpox Eradication: Slides and Notes. http://www.bt.cdc.gov/agent/smallpox/training/overview/pdf/eradicationhistory.pdf. Accessed June 23, 2012.

38. Kim TH, Johnstone J, Loab M. Vaccine herd effect. *Scand J Infect Dis.* 2011;*43*(9): 683–689.

39. Fine P. Invited commentary on "herd immunity: basic concept and relevance to public health immunization practices." *Am J Epidemiol.* 1995;*141*(3):185–186.

40. Poulin D, Levesque I. Ensuring safe drinking water in First Nations communities in Canada. Article written for the Journal of the International Water Association. Posted on the Health Canada website. http://www.hc-sc.gc.ca/fniah-spnia/promotion/public-publique/sfw-sep-eng.php Posted: 2010-10-06. Accessed October 3, 2011 .

41. Embil J, Pereira L, White F, Garner J, Manuel F . Prevalence of ascaris lumbricoides in a small Nova Scotia community. *Am J Trop Med Hyg.* 1984;*33*:595–598.

42. Coovadia HM, Hadingham J . HIV/AIDS: global trends, global funds and delivery bottlenecks. *Globalization and Health.* 2005;*1*:13. Doi: 10.1186/1744-8603-1-13.

43. West KP, Caballero B, Black RE . Nutrition. Chapter 5 In: Merson MH, Black RE, Mills AJ. *International Public Health: Diseases, Programs, Systems, and Policies.* Gaithersburg MD: Aspen Publishers; 2001; 207–291.

44. White F. Editorial: Climate change and the expanding global reach of dengue fever—warnings unheeded? *Int J Med Public Health.* 2011;*1*(3):1.

45. World Health Organization. Global Burden of Disease Report 2004. Table 13. http://www.who.int/healthinfo/global_burden_disease/GBD_report_2004update_part4.pdf. Accessed September 27, 2011.

46. Rose G. Sick individuals and sick populations. *Int J Epidemiol*. 1985;*14*:32–38.

47. MacMahon S. Blood pressure and the risk of cardiovascular disease. *N Eng J Med*. 2000;*342*:50–52.

48. Stewart A, Burke W, Khoury MJ, Zimmerns R . Genomics and Public Health. Chapter 2.4 In: Detels R, Beaglehole R, Lansang MA, Gulliford M (eds.). *Oxford Textbook of Public Health*. Vol. 1. New York, NY: Oxford University Press; 2009; 137–158.

49. Leonard WR, Sorensen MV, Galloway VA, Spencer GJ, Mosher MJ, Osipova L . Climatic influences on basal metabolic rates among circumpolar populations. *Am J Human Biol*. 2002;*14*:609–620.

50. Childs B. Medical genetics to genomic medicine. *Med Secoli*. 2002;*14*(3):707–721.

51. US Department of Energy and the US National Institutes of Health. Human Genome Project Information http://www.ornl.gov/sci/techresources/Human_Genome/home.shtml. Accessed November 14, 2011.

52. Fodor JG, Frohlich JJ, Genest JJG, McPherson PR . Recommendations for the management and treatment of dyslipidemia. Report of the Working Group on Hypercholesterolemia and Other Dyslipidemias *Can Med Assoc J*. 2000;*162*:10. http://www.cmaj.ca/content/162/10/1441.full. Accessed October 6, 2011.

53. Vineis P, Saracci R . Gene-environment interactions and public health. Chapter 9.1 Volume 3 In: Detels R, Beaglehole R, Lansang M-A, Gulliford M . *The Practice of Public Health. Oxford Textbook of Public Health*. 5th ed. New York, NY: Oxford University Press; 2009; 957–970.

54. Lancaster JM, Powell CB, Kauff ND, et al. Society of Gynecologic Oncologists Education Committee statement on risk assessment for inherited gynecologic cancer predispositions. *Gynecol Oncol*. 2007;*107*(2):159–162.

55. Epstein CJ. Medical genetics in the genomic medicine of the 21st century. *Am J Hum Genet*. 2006;*79*(3):434–438.

56. White F, Nanan D . Community health case studies selected from developing and developed countries—common principles for moving from evidence to action. *Arch Med Sci*. 2008;*4*(4):358–363.

57. Puska P, Tuomilehto J, Nissinen A, Vartiainen E . *The North Karelia Project—20 Year Results and Experiences*. Helsinki: National Public Health Institute; 1995.

58. Vartiainen E, Jousilahti P, Alfthan G, Sundvall J, Pietinen P, Puska P . Cardio-vascular risk factor changes in Finland, 1972–1997. *Int J Epidemiol*. 2000;*29*:49–56.

59. Puska P, Keller I . Primary prevention of non-communicable diseases. Experiences from population based interventions in Finland for the global work of WHO. *Z Kardiol*. 2004;*93*(suppl 2):1137–1142.

60. Puska P, Tuomilehto J, Nissinen A, Vartiainen E . *The North Karelia Project—20 Year Results and Experiences*. Helsinki: National Public Health Institute; 1995.

61. Linnan L, Steckler A . *Process Evaluation for Public Health Interventions and Research*. San Francisco, CL: Wiley/ Jossey-Bass; 2002.

62. "3 FOUR 50 Initiative." Oxford Health Alliance. http://www.3four50.com/. Accessed May 5, 2011 .

63. United Nations General Assembly. Draft Political Declaration of the High Level Meeting on the Prevention and Control of Non-Communicable Diseases. Ratified September 19, 2011. http://www.un.org/en/ga/ncdmeeting2011/pdf/NCD_draft_political_declaration. pdf. Accessed November 14, 2011.

64. World Health Organization. Global Status Report on Noncommunicable Diseases 2010. ISBN 978 92 4 068645 8 (PDF) http://whqlibdoc.who.int/publications/2011/9789240686458_eng.pdf. Accessed Sept 27, 2011.

65. International Diabetes Federation. A Call to Action on Diabetes. 2010. Brussels. http://www.idf.org/webdata/Call-to-Action-on-Diabetes.pdf. Accessed November 13, 2011.

66. Steyn NP, Mann J, Bennett PH, Temple N, Zimmet P, Tuomilehto J, Lindstrom J, Louheranta A . Diet, nutrition and the prevention of type 2 diabetes. *Public Health Nutrition*. 2004;7(1A):147–165.

67. Piwernetz K. DIABCARE Quality Network in Europe—a model for quality management in chronic diseases. *Int Clin Psychopharmacol*. 2001;16(suppl 3):S5–S13.

68. White F, Nanan D . Status of national diabetes programmes in the Americas. *Bull World Health Organ*. 1999;77(12):981–987.

69. Murphy D, Chapel T, Clark C . Moving diabetes care from science to practice: the evolution of the National Diabetes Prevention and Control Program. *Annals of Internal Medicine*. 2004;140(11):978–984.

70. Unwin N, Zimmet P . The epidemiology and prevention of diabetes mellitus. Chapter 9.6 In: Detels R, Beaglehole R, Lansang M-A, Gulliford M (eds.). Volume 3: *The Practice of Public Health. Oxford Textbook of Public Health*. 5th ed. New York, NY: Oxford University Press; 2009; 1068–1080.

71. Sacks JJ, Sniezek JE. Targeting Arthritis: The Nation's leading cause of disability. In: *Promising Practices in Chronic Disease Prevention and Control. A Public Health Framework for Action. Centers for Disease Control and Prevention*. 2003; 5-1–18. http://c.ymcdn.com/sites/www.chronicdisease.org/resource/resmgr/Coordinated_CD_/Coordinated_CD_PromisingPrac.pdf. Accessed October 1, 2012.

72. Wagner EH, Austin BT, Davis C, Hindmarsh M, Schaefer J, Bonomi A . Improving chronic illness care: translating evidence into action. *Health Aff (Millwood)*. 2001;20(6):64–78.

73. McKenna MT, Taylor WR, Marks JS, Koplan JP . Current issues and challenges in chronic disease control. In: Brownson RC, Remington PL, Davis JR, eds. *Chronic Disease Epidemiology and Control*. 2nd ed. Washington, DC: American Public Health Assoc.; 1998; 1–26.

74. Barr VJ, Robinson S, Marin-Link B, Underhill L, Dotts A, Ravensdale D, Salivaras S . The Expanded Chronic Care Model: an integration of concepts and strategies from population health promotion and the Chronic Care Model. *Healthcare Quarterly*. 2003;7(1):73–82.

75. Martin CM. Chronic disease and illness care—Adding principles of family medicine to address ongoing health system redesign. *Canadian Family Physician*. 2007;53(12):2086–2091.

76. National Institute of Mental Health Strategic Plan. NIH Publication No. 08-6368 Revised 2008 http://www.nimh.nih.gov/about/strategic-planning-reports/index.shtml. Accessed September 20, 2011.

77. Mrazek PJ, Haggerty RJ (eds.). Reducing risks for mental disorders: Frontiers for preventive intervention research. Committee on Prevention of Mental Disorders. Washington DC: Institute of Medicine/ National Academy Press; 1994.

78. World Health Organization. Prevention of Mental Disorders—Effective Interventions and Policy Options. Geneva, 2004. http://www.who.int/mental_health/evidence/en/prevention_of_mental_disorders_sr.pdf. Accessed June 24, 2012.

79. Roe DA. Attempts at the eradication of pellagra: a historical review. In: Lilienfeld AM (ed.). *Aspects of the History of Epidemiology—Times, Places, and Persons*. Baltimore, MD: Johns Hopkins University Press; 1980; 62–78.

80. Berger PA. Medical treatment of mental illness *Science*. 1978;*200*(4344):974–981.

81. Gill CJ. Chicago Institute of Disability Research. As cited in: University of Toronto. AccessAbility Resource Centre. http://www.utm.utoronto.ca/~w3access/text%20faculty%20staff.html. Accessed June 28, 2011.

82. Gill CJ. Treating families coping with disability: doing no harm. *West J Med*. 1991;*154*[Rehabilitation Medicine Special Issue]:624–625. Accessed October 7, 2011.

83. Murray CJL, Lopez AD. *The Global Burden of Disease*. Geneva: World Health Organization, Harvard School of Public Health, World Bank; 1996.

84. World Health Organization Revised Global Burden of Disease (GBD) 2002 Estimates. Geneva, 2002. http://www.who.int/healthinfo/global_burden_disease/en/index.html. Accessed October 7, 2011.

85. The Canadian Problem Gambling Index: User Manual. Canadian Centre on Substance Abuse. www.ccsa.ca. Accessed June 14, 2011.

86. Hodgins DC, Stea JN, Grant JE. Gambling disorders. *Lancet*. 2011;*378*(9806):1874–1884.

87. Volberg RA. The future of gambling in the United Kingdom—Increasing access creates more problem gamblers. *Br Med J*. 2000;*320*(7249):1556. http://www.ncbi.nlm.nih.gov/pmc/articles/PMC1127354/?tool=pmcentrez. Accessed October 7, 2011.

88. Wood E, Tyndall MW, Montaner JS, Kerr T. Summary of findings from the evaluation of a pilot medically supervised safer injecting facility. *Can Med Assoc J*. 2006;*175*(11):1399–1404.

89. Marshall BDL, Milloy MJ, Wood E, Montaner JSG, Kerr T. Reduction in overdose mortality after the opening of North America's first medically supervised safer injecting facility: A retrospective population-based study. *Lancet*. Published online April 18, 2011. Doi: 10.1016/S0140-6736(10)62353-7.

90. Petrar S, Kerr T, Tyndall MW, Zhang R, Montaner JS, Wood E. Injection drug users' perceptions regarding use of a medically supervised safer injecting facility. *Addictive Behaviors*. 2006;*32*(5):1088–1093.

91. Fairbairn N, Small W, Shannon K, Wood E, Kerr T. Seeking refuge from violence in street-based drug scenes: Women's experiences in North America's first supervised injection facility. *Soc Sci Med*. 2008;*67*(5):817–823.

92. BC Centre for Excellence in HIV/AIDS. http://www.cfenet.ubc.ca/. Accessed September 2, 2011.

93. Shaikh BT, Kadir MM, Pappas G. Thirty years of Alma Ata pledges: Is devolution in Pakistan an opportunity for rekindling primary health care? *J Pak Med Assoc*. 2007;*57*(5):259–260.

94. Reading J. The Crisis of Chronic Disease among Aboriginal Peoples: A Challenge for Public Health, Population Health And Social Policy. Victoria, BC: University of Victoria; 2010. http://www.cahr.uvic.ca/docs/ChronicDisease%20Final.pdf. Accessed October 1, 2012.

95. Kuh Y, Ben-Shlomo Y, Lynch J, Hallqvist J, Power C. Life course epidemiology. *J Epidemiol Community Health*. 2003 ;*57*:778–783. Doi: 10.1136/jech.57.10.778.

96. Darnton-Hill I, Nishida C, James WPT . A life course approach to diet, nutrition and the prevention of chronic diseases. *Public Health Nutrition.* 2004;7(1A):101–121.

97. Ringheim K, Gribble J, Foreman M . Integrating family planning and maternal and child health care: saving lives, money, and time. Population Reference Bureau. Policy Brief June 2010.

98. Waddington C, Egger D . Integrated Health Services—What and Why? Technical Brief No. 1|7 Geneva: World Health Organization; 2008. http://www.who.int/healthsystems/technical_brief_final.pdf. Accessed October 7, 2011.

99. Centers for Disease Control and Prevention. Recommended immunization schedules for persons aged 0–18 years—United States, 2011. MMWR 2011;60,5. http://www.cdc.gov/mmwr/preview/mmwrhtml/mm6005a6.htm. Accessed June 25, 2012.

100. Figure 3 adapted from Figure 7 in: Hetzel BS (ed.). International Council for Control of Iodine Deficiency Disorders (ICCIDD). *Towards the Global Elimination of Brain Damage Due to Iodine Deficiency.* Delhi: Oxford University Press; 2004. http://www.iccidd.org/pages/towards-the-global-elimination-of-brain-damage-due-to-iodine-deficiency.php. Accessed July 5, 2012.

101. United Nations Administrative Committee on Coordination, Sub-Committee on Nutrition (ACC/SCN) in collaboration with International Food Policy Research Institute (IFPRI). 4th Report on the World Nutrition Situation. Figure 1.1 Geneva UN/ACC/SCN, 2000. http://www.ifpri.org/sites/default/files/pubs/pubs/books/4thrpt/4threport.pdf. Accessed July 5, 2012.

CHAPTER SEVEN

1. U.S. Environmental Protection Agency. Environmental Justice http://www.epa.gov/environmentaljustice/index.html. Accessed June 19, 2012.

2. U.S. Environmental Protection Agency. International treaties and initiatives: Chemicals and Waste. Multinational Environmental Initiatives. http://www.epa.gov/oswer/international/factsheets/200610-international-chemical-hazards.htm. Accessed June 19, 2012.

3. United Nations Framework Convention on Global Climate Change. Background on the UNFCCC: The international response to climate change. http://unfccc.int/essential_background/items/6031.php. Accessed June 4, 2012.

4. Hong S, Candelone J-P, Turetta C, Boutropn C . Changes in natural lead, copper, zinc and cadmium concentrations in central Greenland ice from 8250 to 149,100 years ago: their association with climate changes and resultant variations of dominant source contributions. *Earth Planetary Sci Lett.* 1996;143:233–244.

5. British Columbia Ministry of Health. Services. Air quality in British Columbia, a Public Health Perspective. 2004. http://www.health.gov.bc.ca/pho/pdf/phoannual2003.pdf. Accessed January 2, 2012.

6. World Health Organization 2000 Air Quality and Health. Fact sheet N 313 Updated September 2011. http://www.who.int/mediacentre/factsheets/fs313/en/index.html. Accessed January 7, 2012.

7. Last JM. The iceberg. *Lancet.* 1963;2:28–31.

8. White F. Health risk assessment of pesticides: development of epidemiological approaches. In: Forget G, Goodman T, de Villiers A (eds.). *Impact of Pesticide Use on Health in Developing Countries.* Ottawa: IDRC; 1993; 17–25.

9. Klaassen CD (ed.). *Casarett and Doull's Toxicology—The Basic Science of Poisons*. 6th ed. New York, NY: McGraw-Hill; 2001.

10. United Nations. Millennium Development Goals: Environmental Sustainability. http:// www.un.org/millenniumgoals/environ.shtml. Accessed January 26, 2012.

11. White F, Nanan DJ. International and global health. Chapter 76 In: Maxcy-Rosenau-Last. *Public Health and Preventive Medicine*. 15th ed. New York, NY: McGraw Hill; 2008; 1251–1258.

12. White F. Water: life force or instrument of war? *Lancet*. 2002;[suppl 360]:s29–s30.

13. US Environmental Protection Agency. Drinking Water Pathogens and Their Indicators: A Reference Guide. http://www.epa.gov/enviro/html/icr/gloss_path.html. Accessed January 3, 2012.

14. Water, health and ecosystems. *Health and Environmental Linkages Initiative*. World Health Organization and United Nations Environment Programme. 2012. http://www.who.int/ heli/risks/water/water/en/index.html. Accessed June 19, 2012.

15. International Joint Commission—United States and Canada. 2012. http://www.ijc.org/ en/publications/rpts.htm. Acessed June 19, 2012.

16. Cantor KP, Lynch CF, Hildesheim ME, Dosemeci M, Lubin J, Alavanja M, Craun G . Drinking water source and chlorination by-products i. risk of bladder cancer. *Epidemiology*. 1998;*9*(1):21–28.

17. Kanitz S, Franco Y, Patrone V, Caltabellotta M, Raffo E, Riggi C, Timitilli D, Ravera G . Association between drinking water disinfection and somatic parameters at birth. *Environ Health Perspect*. 1996;*104*(5):516–520.

18. Gallagher M, Nuckols JR., Stallones L., Savitz DA . Exposure to trihalomethanes and adverse pregnancy outcomes in Colorado. *Epidemiology*. 1998;*9*(5):484–489.

19. Marcus PM. Female breast cancer and trihalomethane levels in drinking water in North Carolina. *Epidemiology*. 1998;*9*(2):156–160.

20. Centers for Disease Control. Global Water, Sanitation and Hygiene. http://www.cdc.gov/ healthywater/global/wash_diseases.html. Accessed January 3, 2012.

21. Mutreja A, Kim DW, Thomson NR, Connor TR, Lee JH, et al. Evidence for several waves of global transmission in the seventh cholera pandemic. *Nature*. 2011;*477*:462–465. Doi: 10.1038/nature10392.

22. Cholera Confirmed in Haiti, October 21, 2010. http://www.cdc.gov/haiticholera/ situation/. Accessed January 2, 2012.

23. Nanan D, White F, Azam I, Afsar H, Hozabri S . Evaluation of a water, sanitation and hygiene education intervention on diarrhoea in Northern Pakistan. *Bull World Health Organ*. 2003;*81*:160–165.

24. World Health Organization. Health and Environment Linkages Initiative (HELI) Vector borne disease http://www.who.int/heli/risks/vectors/vector/en/index.html. Accessed January 2, 2012 .

25. Centers for Disease Control and Prevention. Vector or insect-borne diseases associated with water. http://www.cdc.gov/healthywater/global/wash_diseases.html#vector accessed January 2, 2012.

26. Patz JA, Githeko AK, McCarty JP, Hussein S, Confalonieri U, De Wet N . Climate change and infectious diseases. Chapter 6 In: McMichael AJ, Campbell-Lendrum DH, Corvalan CF, Ebi KL, Scheraga JD, Woodward A (eds.). *Climate Change and Human Health:*

Risks and Responses. Geneva: WHO; 2003; 103–132. http://www.who.int/globalchange/publications/climatechangechap6.pdf. Accessed January 24, 2012.

27. World Health Organization. International Workshop: Health as a Cross-Cutting Issue in Dialogues on Water for Food and the Environment. http://whqlibdoc.who.int/hq/2004/WHO_SDE_WSH_04.02.pdf. Accessed January 3, 2012.

28. Lindsay S, Kirby M, Baris E, Bos R. Environmental Management for Malaria Control in the East Asia and Pacific Region. http://www.who.int/water_sanitation_health/publications/whowbmalariacontrol.pdf. Accessed January 3, 2012.

29. Mergler D. Review of neurobehavioral deficits and river fish consumption from the Tapajos (Brazil) and St. Lawrence (Canada). *EnvironToxicol Pharmacol.* 2002;*12*:93–99.

30. U.S. Environmental Protection Agency. Pesticides: Reregistration. Atrazine. http://www.epa.gov/oppsrrd1/reregistration/atrazine/atrazine_update.htm. Accessed January 2, 2012.

31. Rusiecki J, De Roos A, Lee WJ, Dosemeci M, Lubin JH, Hoppin JA, Blair A, Alavanja MCR. Cancer incidence among pesticide applicators exposed to atrazine in the Agricultural Health Study. *J Nat Cancer Inst.* 2004;*96*(18):1375–1382.

32. World Health Organization. Chemical hazards in the water: Atrazine. http://www.who.int/water_sanitation_health/dwq/chemicals/atrazine/en/. Accessed January 3, 2012.

33. Hayes T, Haston K, Tsui M, Hoang A, Haeffele, Vonk A. Feminization of male frogs in the wild. *Nature.* 2002;*419*(3):895–896.

34. Hayes T. More feedback on whether atrazine is a potent endocrine disruptor chemical. *Environmental Science and Technology.* 2009;*43*(16):6115.

35. U.S. Environmental Protection Agency. Pesticides: Reregistration Atrazine update. 2011. http://www.epa.gov/oppsrrd1/reregistration/atrazine/atrazine_update.htm. Accessed January 3, 2012.

36. Worldmapper. Deaths from Drowning. http://www.worldmapper.org/display_extra.php?selected=479. Accessed January 25, 2012.

37. United Nations. Millennium Development Goals. Goal 1 Eradicate extreme poverty and hunger. http://www.un.org/millenniumgoals/poverty.shtml. Accessed January 25, 2012.

38. Heyman DJ (ed.). *Control of Communicable Diseases Manual.* 19th ed. Washington DC: An Official Report of the American Public Health Association; 2008.

39. Hunter D. *The Diseases of Occupations.* 3rd ed. London: English Universities Press; 1964.

40. U.S. Geological Survey. Fact Sheet. Mercury Contamination of Acquatic Ecosystems. 1997. http://water.usgs.gov/wid/FS_216-95/FS_216-95.html. Accessed June 19, 2012.

41. Vandenberg LN, Hauser R, Marcus M, Olea N, Welshons WV. Human exposure to bisphenol A (BPA). *Reproductive Toxicology.* 2007;*24*:139–177.

42. Government of Canada. Chemical Substances. http://www.chemicalsubstanceschimiques.gc.ca/challenge-defi/batch-lot-2/bisphenol-a/index-eng.php. Accessed January 25, 2012.

43. Baker N. Huffington Post Canada January 25, 2012. The goods on a bad plastic. http://www.huffingtonpost.com/nena-baker/bisphenol-a-the-goods-on_b_211105.html. Accessed January 25, 2012.

44. Springer M. NBC Connecticut. Connecticut Bans BPA. June 5, 2009. http://www.nbc-connecticut.com/news/local/Connecticut—Bans-BPA.html. Accessed January 25, 2012.

45. National Workgroup for Safe Markets. No Silver Lining. An investigation into Bisphenol A in canned foods. http://ej4all.org/contaminatedwithoutconsent/downloads/NoSilverLining-Report.pdf. May 2010. Accessed January 25, 2012.

46. Centers for Disease Control and Prevention. Food Safety and Raw Milk. http://www.cdc. gov/foodsafety/rawmilk/raw-milk-index.html. Accessed January 26, 2012.

47. Weisbecker A. A legal history of raw milk in the United States. *Journal of Environmental Health*. 2007;*69*(8):62–63.

48. Liu J, Ren A, Yang L, Gao J, Pe Li, Ye R, Qu Q, Zheng X . Urinary tract abnormalities in Chinese rural children who consumed melamine-contaminated dairy products: a population-based screening and follow-up study. *Can Med Assoc J.* 2010;*182*(5):439–443.

49. Belay ED, Schonberger LB . The public health impact of prion diseases. *Annu Revi Public Health*. 2005;*26*:191–212.

50. Food and Agriculture Organization of the United Nations. The State of Food Security in the World 2009. Economic Crises—impacts and lessons learned. Rome 2009. http://www. fao.org/docrep/012/i0876e/i0876e00.htm. Accessed June 20, 2012.

51. World Health Organization. Food Security. http://www.who.int/trade/glossary/story028/ en./. Accessed January 26, 2012.

52. Pelletier DL, Frongillo EA Jr, Schroeder DG, Habicht JP . The effects of malnutrition on child mortality in developing countries. *Bull World Health Organ*. 1995;*73*:443–448.

53. Rice AL, Sacco L, Hyder A, Black RE . Malnutrition as an underlying cause of childhood deaths associated with infectious diseases in developing countries. *Bull World Health Organ*. 2000;*78*:1207–1221.

54. Food and Agriculture Organization of the United Nations. The State of Food Insecurity in the World: 2011. How Does International Price Volatility Affect Domestic Economies and Food Security? http://www.fao.org/docrep/014/i2330e/i2381e00.pdf. Accessed June 20, 2012.

55. White F. Development assistance for health—donor commitment as a critical success factor. *Can J Public Health*. 2011;*102*(6):421–423.

56. Shah A. Global Food Crisis 2008. August 10, 2008. http://www.globalissues.org/article/758/global-food-crisis-2008. Accessed January 26, 2012.

57. Purcell R. The Current Food Situation and the UN Level Task Force on Food Security. http://archive.unctad.org/sections/wcmu/docs/CIMEM2_p19_Purcell_en.pdf. Accessed June 20, 2012.

58. Food and Agriculture Organization of the United Nations. (2011). Women in Agriculture: Closing the Gender Gap for Development. Rome, 2011. http://www.fao.org/docrep/013/ i2050e/i2050e.pdf. Accessed January 26, 2012.

59. Jones G, Steketee RW, Black RE, Bhutta ZA, Morris SS . How many child deaths can we prevent this year? *Lancet*. 2003;*362*(9377):65–71.

60. World Health Organization. Manual on the Management of Nutrition in Major Emergencies. Geneva, 2000. http://www.who.int/nutrition/publications/emergencies/ 9241545208/en/index.html. Accessed January 26, 2012.

61. Global Alliance of Improved Nutrition. About Gain. http://www.gainhealth.org/ about-gain. Accessed January 26, 2012.

62. Manan F. A comprehensive review: The role of vitamins in human diet 1. Vitamin A-nutrition. *J Islamic Acad of Sci*. 1994;*7*(4):221–223.

63. World Health Organization. Global Health Risks: Mortality and burden of disease attributable to selected major risks. 2009 . http://www.who.int/healthinfo/global_burden_ disease/GlobalHealthRisks_report_full.pdf. Accessed January 26, 2012.

64. World Health Organization. Iodine Status Worldwide. WHO Global Database on Iodine Deficiency. http://ceecis.org/iodine/01_global/01_pl/01_01_who_%20status_world-wide_04.pdf. Accessed January 3, 2012.

65. Thompson B. Food Based Approaches for Combating Iron Deficiency ftp://ftp.fao.org/ag/agn/nutrition/Kapitel_21_210207.pdf. Accessed January 3, 2012.

66. Water Related Diseases: Anemia. http://www.who.int/water_sanitation_health/diseases/anemia/en/. Accessed January 3, 2012.

67. Thompson B, Amoroso L . Combating micronutrient deficiencies: Food based approaches. http://www.fao.org/docrep/013/am027e/am027e00.pdf. Accessed January 3, 2012.

68. World Health Organization. Child and Adolescent Health and Development. http://www.emro.who.int/cah/imci-about.htm. Accessed January 24, 2012.

69. World Health Organization. Focusing on Anaemia: Towards an Integrated Approach for Effective Anaemia Control. http://www.who.int/nutrition/publications/micronutrients/WHOandUNICEF_statement_anaemia/en/index.html. Accessed June 20, 2012.

70. World Health Organization. Globalization, Diets, and Noncommunicable Diseases. http://whqlibdoc.who.int/publications/9241590416.pdf. Accessed June 20, 2012.

71. Dietary Guidelines for American: A Historical Overview. http://www.nal.usda.gov/fnic/pubs/bibs/gen/DGA.pdf. Accessed January 3, 2012.

72. Hite AH, Feinman RD, Guzman GE, Satin M., Schoenfield PA, Wood RJ . In the face of contradictory evidence: Report of the Dietary Guidelines for Americans Committee. *Nutrition*. 2010;*26*:915–924.

73. Iqbal R., Anand S, Ounpuu S, Islam S, Zhang X, Rangarajan S, et al. Dietary patterns and the risk of acute myocardial infarction in 52 countries. *Circulation*. 2008;*118*:1929–1937.

74. Jacobs DR, Steffen LM . Nutrients, foods, and dietary patterns as exposures in research: a framework for food synergy. *Am J Clinical Nutrition*. 2003;*78*(suppl):508S–513S.

75. Hu, FB . Globalization of food patterns and cardiovascular risk. *Circulation*. 2008;*118*:1913–1914.

76. Sobal J. Commentary: Globalization and the epidemiology of obesity. *Int J Epidemiol*. 2001;*30*(5):1136–1137.

77. Cutler DM, Glaeser EL, Shapiro JM . Why have Americans become more obese? *J Economic Perspect*. 2003;*17*(3):93–118.

78. Draper C, Freedman D . Review and analysis of the benefits, purposes, and motivations associated with community gardening in the United States. *J Community Practice*. 2010;*18*:458–492.

79. *MMWR*. Multistate outbreak of Salmonella infections associated with peanut butter and peanut butter-containing products. United States 2008–9. 2009;*58*(04):85–90.

80. U.S. Food and Drug Administration. FDAs investigation. http://www.fda.gov/Safety/Recalls/MajorProductRecalls/Peanut/FDA%E2%80%99sInvestigation/default.htm. Accessed January 26, 2012.

CHAPTER EIGHT

1. World Development Report 1993. Investing in Health. World Development Indicators. New York, NY: World Bank, Oxford University Press; 1993. http://files.dcp2.org/pdf/WorldDevelopmentReport1993.pdf. Accessed October 25, 2011.

2. World Health Organization. Health Topics. Health Systems. WHO. Geneva. 2012. http://www.who.int/topics/health_systems/en/. Accessed October 2, 2012.

3. Mills AJ, Ranson MK . The design of health systems. Chapter 10 In: Merson MH, Black RE, Mills AJ (eds.). *International Public Health—Diseases, Programs, Systems and Policies.* Gaithersberg, MD: Aspen Publishers; 2001.

4. Chan M. Address at WHO Congress on Traditional Medicine. Beijing, November 7, 2008. http://www.who.int/dg/speeches/2008/20081107/en/index.html. Accessed February 12, 2010.

5. Perlman A, Sabina A, Williams A, Njike V, Katz D . Massage therapy for osteoarthritis of the knee: a randomized controlled trial. *Arch Intern Med.* 2006;*166*(22):2533–2538.

6. Preyde M. Effectiveness of massage therapy for subacute low-back pain: a randomized controlled trial. *Can Med Assoc J.* 2000;*162*:1815–1820.

7. American College of Physicians. Position Paper: Achieving a high-performance health care system with universal access: what the United States can learn from other countries. *Ann Intern Med.* 2008;*148*:55–75. http://www.annals.org/content/148/1/55.full#T1. Accessed October 27, 2011.

8. The Commonwealth Fund. A Private Foundation working towards a high performance health system. http://www.commonwealthfund.org/About-Us.aspx. Accessed October 28, 2011.

9. Magnussen J, Vrangbaek K, Saltman RB (eds.). Nordic health care systems: Recent reforms and current policy challenges. World Health Organization 2009 on behalf of the European Observatory on Health Systems and Policies. Open University Press, McGraw-Hill Education. Maidenhead, England. http://www.euro.who.int/document/e93429.pdf. Accessed February 21, 2010.

10. White F, Nanan D . A Conversation on Health in Canada: revisiting universality and the centrality of primary health care. *J Ambul Care Manage.* 2009;*32*(2):141–149.

11. Guyatt GH, Devereaux PJ, Lexchin J, et al. A systematic review of studies comparing health outcomes in Canada and the United States. *Open Medicine.* 2007;*1*(1):E27–E36. http://www.pnhp.org/PDF_files/ReviewUSCanadaOpenMedicine.pdf. Accessed October 25, 2011.

12. Supreme Court of the United States. National Federation of Independent Business et al vs Sebelius, Secretary. Health and Human Services et al. Certiorari to the United States Court of Appeals to the Eleventh Circuit. No 11-393. Decided June 28, 2012. As cited in the Washington Post: Full text of the Supreme Court health-care decision. June 28, 2012. http://www.washingtonpost.com/wp-srv/politics/documents/supreme-court-health-care-decision-text.html. Accessed June 29, 2012.

13. Balabanova D, McKee M, Mills A . *Good health at low cost' 25 years on. What makes a successful health system?* London School of Hygiene and Tropical Medicine. 2011. http://nexus-clients.co.uk/ghlc/wp-content/uploads/2011/10/GHLC-book.pdf. Accessed October 27, 2011.

14. The World Health Report 2000—Health systems: improving performance. Geneva, 2000. http://www.who.int/whr/2000/en/whr00_en.pdf. Accessed October 25, 2011.

15. Nayani P, White F, Nanan D . Public-private partnership as a success factor for health systems. *Medicine Today.* 2006;*4*:135–142. http://www.phabc.org/files/Nayani_White_Nanan_Public-Private_Partnership-pg135–142.pdf. Accessed October 27, 2011.

16. Nutbeam, D . Health literacy as a public health goal: A challenge for contemporary health education and communication strategies into the 21st century. *Health Promotion International.* 2000;*15*(3):259–267.

17. World Health Organization. Ottawa Charter on Health Promotion. First International Conference on Health Promotion. Ottawa, 21 November 1986. WHO/HPR/HEP/95.1 http://www.who.int/hpr/NPH/docs/ottawa_charter_hp.pdf. Accessed October 26, 2011.

18. Universal Declaration of Human Rights, Article 25(1), 1948. http://www.un.org/en/documents/udhr/. Accessed February 22, 2010.

19. Bruntland GH. World Health Organization Message from the Director-General. In: *The World Health Report 1999—making a difference.* Geneva: WHO; 1999.

20. The Bangkok Charter for Health Promotion in a Globalized World (11 August 2005). WHO; 2011. http://www.who.int/healthpromotion/conferences/6gchp/bangkok_charter/en/. Accessed October 25, 2011.

21. Stuckler D, Basu S, McKee M . Global health philanthropy and institutional relationships: how should conflicts of interest be addressed? *PLoS Medicine.* 2011;*8*(4):e1001020. Doi: 10.1371/journal.pmed.1001020.

22. Boehm F. Regulatory Capture Revisited—Is There an Anticorruption Agenda in Regulation? IRC Symposium 2010. http://docs.watsan.net/Downloaded_Files/PDF/Boehm-2010-Regulatory.pdf. Accessed Nov 17, 2011.

23. Public Health in America. Essential Public Health Services. Adopted: Fall 1994, Source: Public Health Functions Steering Committee, Members (July 1995). http://www.health.gov/phfunctions/public.htm. Accessed October 25, 2011.

24. Hemmings J, Wilkinson J . What is a public health observatory? *J Epidemiol Community Health.* 2003;*57*:324–326.

25. Lewis S., Kouri D . Regionalization: Making sense of the Canadian experience. *Healthcare Papers.* 2004;*5*(1):12–33.

26. Touati N, Roberge D, Denis J-L, Pineault R, Cazale L, Tremblay D . Governance, health policy implementation and the added value of regionalization. *Health Policy.* 2007;*2*(3):97–114.

27. Frankish CJ, Kwan B, Ratner PA, Higgins JW, Larsen C . Challenges of citizen participation in regional health authorities. *Soc Sci Med.* 2002;*54*(10):1471–1480.

28. Neville D, Barrowman G, Fitzgerald B, Tomblin S . Regionalization of health services in Newfoundland and Labrador: perceptions of the planning, implementation and consequences of regional governance. *J Health Serv Res Policy.* 2005;*10*(suppl 2):S2:12–21.

29. Population Health and Wellness. Ministry of Health Services Province of British Columbia A Framework for Core Functions In Public Health—Resource Document. March 2005. http://www.phabc.org/pdfcore/core_functions.pdf. Accessed October 27, 2011.

30. Public Health Laboratory Service. NDPB Report 1997. London. http://www.archive.official-documents.co.uk/document/caboff/pubbod97/phls.htm. Accessed March 9, 2010.

31. European Agency for Safety and Health at Work (EU-OSHA). http://osha.europa.eu/en. Accessed March 9, 2010.

32. European Parliament. Common Policies. Health and Safety at Work. http://www.europarl.europa.eu/parliament/expert/displayFtu.do?language=en&id=74&ftuId=FTU_4.9.5.html. Accessed March 9, 2010.

33. Caribbean Epidemiology Centre (CAREC). http://new.paho.org/carec/index. php?option=com_content&task=view&id=24&Itemid=122. Accessed October 25, 2011.

34. CARPHA Caribbean Public Health Agency. Official Website. http://www.carpha.org/. Accessed September 30, 2012.

35. Public Health Institutes of the World (IANPHI). http://www.ianphi.org/. Accessed May 13, 2012.

36. White F, Nanan D. International & global health. Chapter 76 in: Wallace-Maxcy-Rosenau-Last, *Public Health & Preventive Medicine*. 15th ed. New York, NY: McGraw-Hill; 2008; 1251–1258.

37. Multilateral Organisation Performance Assessment Network (MOPAN) http://www. mopanonline.org/. Accessed October 25, 2011.

38. MOPAN Common Approach—WHO Report 2010 (Part I). http://static.mopanonline. org/brand/upload/documents/WHO_Final-Vol-I_January_17_Issued1_1.pdf. Accessed October 25, 2011.

39. World Health Organization—Bangladesh. http://www.whoban.org/current_programs. html. Accessed August 19, 2010.

40. Global Alliance of Improved Nutrition. About GAIN. http://www.gainhealth.org/ about-gain. Accessed January 26, 2012.

41. OECD. The Paris Declaration and Accra Agenda for Action. http://www.oecd.org/doc ument/18/0,3343,en_2649_3236398_35401554_1_1_1_1,00&&en-USS_01DBC.html. Accessed August 8, 2010.

42. White F. Development assistance for health—donor commitment as a critical success factor. *Can J Public Health*. 2011;*102*(6):421–423.

43. UN General Assembly Resolution No. 2626, October 24, 1970. http://daccess-dds-ny. un.org/doc/RESOLUTION/GEN/NR0/348/91/IMG/NR034891.pdf?OpenElement. Accessed July 5, 2012.

44. The Helen Keller Foundation for Research and Education. http://www.helenkellerfounda-tion.org/. Accessed October 25, 2011.

45. The Carter Center. Waging Peace. Fighting Disease. Building Health http://www.carter-center.org/index.html. Accessed October 25, 2011.

46. Health Alliance International. The NGO Code of Conduct for Health Systems Strengthening Initiative. http://ngocodeofconduct.org/. Accessed January 21, 2012.

47. White F, Nanan D . Community health case studies selected from developing and developed countries—common principles for moving from evidence to action. *Arch Med Sci*. 2008;*4*(4):358–363.

48. Ham C. Priority setting in health care: learning from international experience. *Health Policy*. 1997;*42*:49–66.

49. White F. De la evidencia al desempeno: como fijar prioridades y tomar buenas decisiones. *Current Topics. Pan American Journal of Public Health*. 1998;*4*:69–74.

50. Australian Agency for International Development (AusAID): AusGUIDElines. 1. The Logical Framework Approach. 2000. Last Updated 2th June, 2003. http://portals.wi.wur.nl/files/ docs/ppme/ausguidelines-logical%20framework%20approach.pdf. Accessed July 5, 2012.

51. Nanan D, White F, Azam I, Afsar H, Hozabri S . Evaluation of a water, sanitation and hygiene education intervention on diarrhoea in Northern Pakistan. *Bull World Health Organ*. 2003;*81*:160–165.

52. Department of Health and Human Services. Healthy People 2010. Mid-Course Review: summary and future directions. 2006. http://www.healthypeople.gov/data/midcourse/html/execsummary/future.htm.

53. National Center for Health Statistics. Health People 2000 Final Review. Library of Congress Catalog Card Number 76–641496. http://www.cdc.gov/nchs/data/hp2000/hp2k01.pdf.

54. Department of Health and Human Services. Healthy People 2010. All objectives, sub-objectives and indicators: http://www.healthypeople.gov/data/midcourse/html/focusareas/FA27Objectives.htm.

55. Institute of Medicine. The Future of the Public's Health in the 21st Century. November 2002. National Academy of Sciences. Washington DC. 2003. The full text of this report is available at http://www.nap.edu.

56. Senate Democrats. The Patient Protection and Affordable Care Act—Detailed Summary. http://dpc.senate.gov/healthreformbill/healthbill04.pdf. Accessed July 1, 2012.

57. Action Plan for the Western Pacific Declaration on Diabetes: From Evidence to Action. http://www.idf.org/webdata/docs/WPDD_PoA_2010.pdf. Accessed August 23, 2010.

58. Colagiuri R, Short R, Buckley A . The status of national diabetes programmes: A global survey of IDF member associations. *Diabetes Research and Clinical Practice.* 2010;*87*: 137–142. http://blogimages.bloggen.be/diabetescheck/attach/35639.pdf.

59. Pan American Forum for Action Against Disease. 22 December 2009 Update. http://new.paho.org/hq/index.php?option=com_content&task=view&id=1820&Itemid=1594. Accessed October 25, 2011.

60. Barcelo A, Vovides Y . Editorial. The Pan American Health Organization and World Diabetes Day. *Rev Panam Salud Publica.* 2001;*10*(5):297–299.

61. White F, Nanan D . Status of national diabetes programmes in the Americas. *Bull WHO.* 1999;*77*:981–987.

62. Giffin R, Robinson S (eds.). *Addressing the Threat of Drug-Resistant Tuberculosis.* Washington, DC: The National Academies Press; 2009. http://www.nap.edu/catalog.php?record_id=12570. Accessed June 6, 2012.

63. Internal Displacement Monitoring Council (Norway): Training Modules. http://www.internal-displacement.org/802570F8004CoA58/(httpPages)/27E7C556E3549FC880257 0A100471F33?OpenDocument. Accessed October 28, 2011.

64. *Health Services Organization in the Event of Disaster.* Washington, DC: Pan American Health Organization; 1983.

65. Guha-Sapir D, Vos F, Below R, Ponserre S . Annual Disaster Statistical Review 2010.The numbers and trends. Centre for Research on the Epidemiology of Disasters (CRED), Université catholique de Louvain—Brussels, Belgium. http://www.cred.be/sites/default/files/ADSR_2010.pdf. Accessed October 28, 2011.

66. World Conference on Disaster Risk Reduction. Hyogo, Japan. January 18–22, 2005. Hyogo Declaration. Extract from the final report of the World Conference on Disaster Reduction. http://www.unisdr.org/2005/wcdr/intergover/official-doc/L-docs/Hyogo-declaration-english.pdf. Accessed October 28, 2011.

67. 2011 United Nations Global Assessment Report on Disaster Risk Reduction (GAR11). http://www.preventionweb.net/english/hyogo/gar/2011/en/home/executive.html. Accessed October 28, 2011.

68. FEMA—Federal Emergency Response Agency. http://www.fema.gov/. Accessed August 31, 2010.

69. Grepen KA, Savedoff WD . 10 best resources on health workers in developing countries. *Health Policy Plan.* 2009;*24*(6):479–482. Doi: 10.1093/heapol/czp038. http://heapol. oxfordjournals.org/content/24/6/479.full. Accessed June 7, 2012.

70. International recruitment of health personnel: global code of practice. Resolution adopted by the Sixty-third World Health Assembly, Geneva, May 2010—available on http://apps. who.int/gb/e/e_wha63.html. Accessed June 7, 2012.

71. World Health Organization. The World Health Report 2006: working together for health. Geneva, 2006. http://www.who.int/whr/2006. Accessed June 7, 2012.

72. Figure 8-2 adapted from Figure 1 in: White F. Capacity building for health research in developing countries: a manager's approach. *Pan American Journal of Public Health.* 2002;*12*:165–171.

73. OECD Development Statistics Online. In: White F. Development Assistance for Health—Donor Commitment as a Critical Success Factor. *Can J Public Health.* 2011;*102*(6):421–423.

CHAPTER NINE

1. Baxter PJ, Baubron J-C, Coutinho R . Health hazards and disaster potential of ground gas emissions at Furnas volcano, São Miguel, Azores. *J Volcanology and Geothermal Research.* 1999;*92*(1–2):95–106.

2. Cronic SJ, Sharp DS . Environmental impacts on health from continuous volcanic activity at Yasur (Tanna) and Ambrym, Vanuatu. *Int J Environ Heath Res.* 2002;*12*(2):109–123.

3. Hong S, Candelone J-P, Turetta C, Boutropn C . Changes in natural lead, copper, zinc and cadmium concentrations in central Greenland ice from 8250 to 149,100 years ago: their association with climate changes and resultant variations of dominant source contributions. *Earth and Planetary Science Letters.* 1996;*143*:233–244.

4. Rosman KJR, Chisholm W, Hong S, Candelone J-P, Boutron CF . Lead from Carthaginian and Roman Spanish mines isotopically identified in Greenland ice dated from 600 B.C. to 300 A.D. *Environment, Science and Technology.* 1997;31:3413–3416.

5. Delmas RJ, Legrand M . Trends recorded in Greenland in relation with northern hemisphere anthropogenic pollution. International Global Atmospheric Chemistry (IGAC) Project, IGACtivities Newsletter No. 14, September 1998. http://igac.jisao.washington. edu/newsletter/highlights/1998/pascnl.php. Accessed January 13, 2012.

6. Awang MB, Jaafar AB, Abdullah AM, Ismail MB, Hassan MN, Abdullah R, Johan S, Noor H . Air quality in Malaysia: impacts, management issues and future challenges. *Respirology.* 2000;*5*(2):183–196.

7. Bates DV, Caton RB . A citizen's guide to air pollution. 2nd ed. Vancouver: David Suzuki Foundation; 2002.

8. Intergovernmental Panel on Climate Change. http://www.ipcc.ch/organization/ organization.shtml accessed December 13, 2011.

9. Union of Concerned Scientists. *Climate Hot Map. Global Warming Effects Around the World.* Cambridge, MA: Union of Concerned Scientists; 2011. http://www.climatehot-map.org/. Accessed December 8, 2011.

10. Hinzman L, Bettez N, Bolton WR, et al. Evidence and implications of recent climate change in Northern Alaska and other Arctic Regions. *Climatic Change*. 2005;*72*:251–298. Doi: 10.1007/s10584-005-5352-2.

11. Wilder-Smith A, Chen LH, Massad E, Wilson ME . Threat of dengue to blood safety in dengue-endemic countries. *Emerging Infectious Diseases*. 2009;*15*(1):8–11.

12. Patz JA, Martens WJ, Focks DA, Jetten TH . Dengue fever epidemic potential as projected by general circulation models of global climate change. *Environ Health Perspectives*. 1998;*106*(3):147–153.

13. White F. Editorial: Climate Change and the Expanding Global Reach of Dengue Fever—Warnings Unheeded? *International J Medicine Public Health*. 2011;*1*(3):1.

14. Greenwood M. Epidemics and crowd-diseases: an introduction to the study of epidemiology. London, UK: Williams and Norgate Ltd.; 1935.

15. Greenwood M. Medical statistics from Graunt to Farr. *Biometrika*. 1942;*32*:204.

16. IPCC Fourth Assessment Report (2007). Working Group II Report: Impact, adaptation and vulnerability. http://www.ipcc.ch/publications_and_data/ar4/wg2/en/contents.html. Accessed January 8, 2012.

17. Schumacher EF. *Small Is Beautiful: A Study of Economics as if People Mattered*. London, UK: Sphere Books Ltd.; 1974.

18. Khushk WA, Fatmi Z, White F, Kadir MM . Health and social impact of improved stoves on women: a pilot intervention in rural Sindh, Pakistan. *Indoor Air*. 2005;*15*(5): 311–316.

19. White F. Editorial: Rational energy choices in the wake of Fukushima. *International J Medicine Public Health*. 2011;*1*(4):1–2.

20. Organization for Economic Cooperation and Development (2010). Comparing Nuclear Accident Risks with Those from Other Energy Sources OECD Nuclear Energy Agency NEA No. 6861. ISBN 978-92-64-99122-4. http://www.oecd-nea.org/ndd/reports/2010/nea6862-comparing-risks.pdf. Accessed October 10, 2011.

21. The World Bank. Pilot Program to Conserve the Brazilian Rain Forest. Last updated: 2009-08-12 (PPG7) http://web.worldbank.org/WBSITE/EXTERNAL/COUNTRIES/LACEXT/BRAZILEXTN/0,,contentMDK:20757004~pagePK:141137~piPK:141127~theSitePK:322341,00.html. Accessed January 10, 2012.

22. Stanford Encyclopedia of Philosophy. Environmental Ethics. First published Mon Jun 3, 2002; substantive revision Thu Jan 3, 2008 http://plato.stanford.edu/entries/ethics-environmental/#EarDevEnvEth. Accessed January 10, 2012.

23. Air quality in British Columbia, a public health perspective. http://www.health.gov.bc.ca/pho/pdf/phoannual2003.pdf. Accessed January 2, 2012.

24. Cleveland C, Kubiszewski I, Miller M . United Nations Conference on Environment and Development (UNCED), Rio de Janeiro, Brazil. In: The Encyclopedia of Earth. 2007. http://www.eoearth.org/article/United_Nations_Conference_on_Environment_and_Development_(UNCED),_Rio_de_Janeiro,_Brazil. Accessed January 13, 2012.

25. World Population Day 2011: The World at 7 Billion. http://www.unfpa.org/public/home/sitemap/world-population-day. Accessed January 8, 2012.

26. Weiss BD, Hart G, Pust RE . The relationship between literacy and health. *Journal of Health Care for the Poor and Underserved*. 1991;*1*(4):351–363.

27. Kickbusch IS. Health literacy: addressing the health and education divide. *Health Promotion International*. 2001;*16*(3):289–297.

28. Wilkinson RG. Putting the Picture Together—Prosperity, redistribution, health and welfare. In: Marmot M, Wilkinson RG (eds.). *Social Determinants of Health*. Oxford: Oxford University Press; 1999; 258–274.

29. Health in the European Union—trends and analysis. In: Mladovsky P, Allin S, Masseria C, Hernández-Quevedo C, McDaid D, Mossialos E (eds.). *European Observatory on Health Systems and Policies*. Copenhagen, Denmark: World Health Organization; 2009.

30. Population Issues in the 21st Century: The Role of the World Bank. HNP Discussion Paper. April 2007. http://siteresources.worldbank.org/HEALTHNUTRITIONANDPOPULATION/Resources/281627-1095698140167/PopulationDiscussionPaperApril07Final.pdf. Accessed January 13, 2012.

31. Commission on Social Determinants of Health. Closing the gap in a generation World Health Organization. Geneva. 2008. http://www.who.int/social_determinants/thecommission/finalreport/en/index.html. Accessed June 26, 2012.

32. Migration: World on the Move. http://www.unfpa.org/pds/migration.html. Accessed January 4, 2012.

33. International Organization for Migration. http://www.iom.int/jahia/Jahia/about-iom/mission/lang/en. Accessed January 11, 2012 .

34. Climate change challenges Tuvalu. *German Watch*. 2004. http://www.germanwatch.org/download/klak/fb-tuv-e.pdf. Accessed December 8, 2011.

35. White F. Climate Change: Will there be any winners? *Global J Medicine Public Health*. 2012;*1*(3):1–2.

36. World Health Organization. The World Health Report 2006—working together for health. http://www.who.int/whr/2006/en/index.html. Accessed January 11, 2012.

37. Labonte R, Packer C, Klassen N, et al. The brain drain of health professionals from Sub-Saharan Africa to Canada. African Migration and Development Series No. 2 (Crush J ed.) Southern African Migration Project, IDASA South Africa; Queens University, Canada; University of Ottawa, Canada. http://www.queensu.ca/samp/sampresources/samppublications/mad/MAD_2.pdf. Accessed January 11, 2012.

38. Kinfu Y, Dal Poz MR, Mercer H, Evans DB . The health worker shortage in Africa: Are enough physicians and nurses being trained? *Bulletin of the World Health Organization*. 2009;*87*:225–230. Doi: 10.2471/BLT.08.051599. Accessed June 27, 2012.

39. UNCTAD Secretariat. The Least Developed Countries Report 2007—Knowledge, technological learning and innovation for development. United Nations Conference on Trade and Development. United Nations. New York and Geneva. http://www.unctad.org/en/docs/ldc2007_en.pdf. Accessed January 11, 2012.

40. Kumar P. Providing the providers-remedying Africa's shortage of health care workers. *N Engl J Med*. 2007;*356*(25):2564–2567. http://content.nejm.org/cgi/content/extract/356/25/2564 http://www.nejm.org/doi/full/10.1056/NEJMp078091. Accessed January 11, 2012.

41. Ethical Restrictions on International Recruitment of Health Professionals to the U.S. Resolution proposed for adoption (2006). http://www.apha.org/programs/globalhealth/section/advocacy/globalihtest2.htm. Accessed January 12, 2012.

42. Food and Agriculture Organization. The State of Food Insecurity in the World Economic crises—impacts and lessons learned, FAO Food and Agriculture Organization of the United Nations, Rome. Full report available as PDF via http://www.fao.org/publications/sofi/en/. Accessed January 13, 2012.

43. Dawe D, Drechsler D . Hunger on the Rise. International Monetary Fund. *Finance & Development*, 2010;*47*(1):40–41. http://www.imf.org/external/pubs/ft/fandd/2010/03/picture.htm. Accessed October 2, 2012.

44. United Nations Convention on Desertification (UNCCD) Homepage http://www.unccd.int/convention/menu.php. Accessed January 12, 2012.

45. Gnacadja L. As cited in: UN warns of 70 percent desertification by 2025 (AFP)—October 3, 2009. http://www.google.com/hostednews/afp/article/ALeqM5gpEL4aRMhxPRfbFmt V6ZY70IwmFQ. Accessed January 13, 2012.

46. Lal R. Potential of desertification control to sequester carbon and mitigate the greenhouse effect. *Climate Change*. 2001;51:35–72.

47. World Health Organization. Food Safety. http://www.who.int/foodsafety/en/. Accessed December 14, 2011.

48. World Health Organization. Food Production to Consumption. http://www.who.int/foodsafety/fs_management/en/. Accessed December 14, 2011.

49. WHO Collaborating Centre for Research on the Epidemiology of Disasters (CRED). The International Disaster Database (EM-DAT). http://www.emdat.be/. Accessed January 13, 2012.

50. International Strategy for Disaster Reduction (ISDR). http://www.unisdr.org/who-we-are/mandate. Accessed January 13, 2012.

51. United Nations Office for Disaster Risk Reduction. International Strategy for Disaster Reduction. Strengthening climate change adaptation through effective disaster reduction. Briefing Note 03. http://www.unisdr.org/files/16861_ccbriefingnote3.pdf. Accessed June 28, 2012.

52. Tibbets J. Louisiana's wetlands: a lesson in nature appreciation. *Environ Health Perspect*. 2006;*114*(1):A40–A43. http://www.ncbi.nlm.nih.gov/pmc/articles/PMC1332684/. Accessed June 28, 2012.

53. Riegelman RK, Albertine S . Undergraduate public health at 4-year institutions. *American Journal Preventive Medicine*. 2011;*40*(2):226–331.

54. The Educated Citizen and Public Health. Association of American Colleges and Universities. 2012. http://www.aacu.org/public_health/index.cfm. Accessed January 12, 2012.

55. OXFAM. Horn of Africa Transfer for Adaptation. Project Brief. http://portal.iri.columbia.edu/portal/server.pt/gateway/PTARGS_0_2_5494_0_0_18/HARITA%20Update%20 August%2011%202009%20short.pdf. Accessed January 5, 2012.

56. OXFAM Horn of Africa Risk Transfer for Adaptation—HARITA quarterly report: October 2010–December 2011 http://reliefweb.int/node/401787. Accessed January 5, 2012.

57. OXFAM. *Horn of Africa Risk Transfer for Adaptation (HARITA) Quarterly Report*: July 2011–September 2011.

EPILOGUE

1. Hardin G. Parenthood: Right or Privilege? [Editorial] *Science*. 1970;*169*:427.

2. Taylor R, Rieger A . Rudolf Virchow on the typhus epidemic in Upper Silesia. *Sociology of Health and Illness*. 2008;*6*(2):201–217. http://onlinelibrary.wiley.com/doi/10.1111/1467-9566.ep10778374/pdf. Accessed September 19, 2011.

Index

Index entries followed by *t* indicate a table; by *f* indicate a figure.

CPSIA information can be obtained at www.ICGtesting.com
Printed in the USA
BVOW06*2318020116

431448BV00008B/14/P